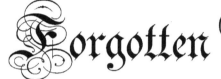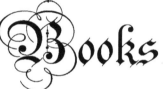

ISBN 978-1-330-31457-9
PIBN 10024022

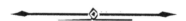

MEDICAL

NOTES AND REFLECTIONS.

———•———

BY

HENRY HOLLAND, M.D., F.R.S.,

FELLOW OF THE ROYAL COLLEGE OF PHYSICIANS, AND PHYSICIAN EXTRAORDINARY
TO THE QUEEN.

———•———

φαίνεται ουτε περας, ουτε τελευτην εχων· ότι προ τε της αρχης, αλλη αει φαίνεται
αρχη· μετα τε την τελευτην, έτερα ὑπολειπομενη τελευτη. — PLATO (*de Scientia*).

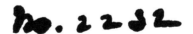

Philadelphia:
HASWELL, BARRINGTON, AND HASWELL,
293 MARKET STREET.
NEW ORLEANS: JOHN J. HASWELL & CO.
1839.

PREFACE.

THE title of this volume is chosen as being that which most nearly expresses its contents. Though appearing now as detached papers, they are founded chiefly upon notes made in the course of twenty years of medical practice in London. During nearly the whole of this time, I have been accustomed to preserve notices, not merely of particular cases, but also of such general reflections as were suggested to me by actual observation. At the expiration of the period named, I have thought it well to look back upon these various memoranda; to give something of more definite form to those which seemed worth preserving; and to compare the whole, as well with my own present impressions, as with the actual state of knowledge on the several subjects in question. This volume is the result of a revision and selection so made. But as its form, though sanctioned by precedents of high value, is not altogether common, it may be right to add a few words more, in explanation of the motive and manner of publication.

It seemed to me, looking at them as impartially as I was able to do, that there were, among these papers so revised, a certain number which might be likely to contribute in some degree to medical knowledge, or to the exactness of our views in practice. I have had regard to these objects only, as justifying publication; and as a principle of selection out of the materials before me. In making this selection, I have put aside a great deal as relating to subjects of inferior importance; still more, from finding that many of my notes related to facts or opinions no longer new. What I have retained includes much that will be familiar to all who have carried observation and study into their medical life. But this was inevitable, without wholly omitting many subjects of great interest; and it would have been presumptuous to offer a work composed, as this has been, from materials acquired in the course of active practice, as one of original research.

Every physician has, in his progress, some particular occasions or facilities capable of being converted to good. The opportunities of private practice, from which almost exclusively my own observations are drawn, do not furnish the same striking conclusions as those of hospitals; nor the large classes of facts, which form the statistics of medicine, and are so fruitful of results. Yet such is the scope of the subject, that a prolonged experience, with due regard to the nature and sufficiency of the evidence, may from this more limited source derive much to aid other methods of research, and to enlarge the general amount of medical knowledge.

What I would fain hope may be found in this volume is, a just view of some of the relations of diseases, as well to each other as to the healthy functions of the body;—the correction of some doubtful or erroneous views in practice;—suggestions which may be useful as regard particular classes of remedies;—and reflections on certain

points of physiology, in which, without any pretension to experimental inquiry, it appeared to me that something might be gained
by arranging the facts and inferences in a new form.   On topics
of the latter class I have sought especially to associate pathology
with physiology, the morbid with the natural and healthy states of
the body ; believing this principle of modern inquiry to be above all
others fertile in sound conclusions, and far from being yet worked
out to its full extent.   If I might venture on giving any distinctive
character to the volume, it would be that of aiming throughout at
this object.

In one instance only have I indulged in any mere speculation ;
and this only interrogatively, as to an old hypothesis, regarded in
its relation to modern science, and to the history of a remarkable
disease.   Many other points I have put as questions ; finding them
as such in my notes ; and thinking it well, whenever it could be
done, thus to mark the objects most open to inquiry.   I have further
taken the privilege, (which more than twenty years' experience
may perhaps be allowed to sanction,) of commenting on certain
usage and details of practice, in which the character and usefulness of the profession, and, through them, the welfare of the public,
are materially concerned.

On each subject treated of, I have brought together my notes
in the manner best suited for perspicuity ; adding whatever seemed
necessary to give greater completeness to the reasoning, or to
connect it with the inquiries of others on the same topics.*   In
effect of this, much of the volume has been wholly written anew.
I had at one time proposed the insertion of a greater number of
the cases upon which its materials were founded ; but I abandoned
the intention, from a wish not to increase the size of the work,
which this must largely have done.   And for the same reason I
have abridged into the form of notes many topics on which I had
originally written at greater length.

As respects the arrangement of the subjects, it will be found a
very desultory one; such as naturally arose out of the miscellaneous
materials employed.   In a few instances only have I thought it
worth while to bring topics expressly together for their mutual
elucidation.   To have attempted this further would imply a more
complete and consecutive work than that now offered to the public.

These, I think, are all the circumstances which need be stated
in explanation of the form and matter of the volume.   It will deeply
gratify me, if hereafter I find cause to believe that it has contributed
to science by any right views in the philosophy of medicine, or to
practical good by any suggestions of value regarding the treatment
of disease.

---

* On the latter point great deficiencies are inevitable.   In these days of various
research, actively pursued in so many countries, it would require more reading
than is compatible with actual practice to collect together all that has been done
on these subjects ; nor would a single volume suffice for the mere references
needful to such a work.

CONTENTS.

MEDICAL NOTES, ETC.

CHAPTER I.

ON MEDICAL EVIDENCE.

THERE can be few better tests of a sound understanding, than the right estimation of medical evidence ; so various are the complexities it presents, so numerous the sources of error. The subjects of observation are those in which Matter and Mind are concurrently concerned ;—Matter, under the complex and subtle · organization, whence vitality and all its functions are derived,— Mind, in its equally mysterious relations to the organs thus formed ; —both subject to numerous agencies from without,—both undergoing great changes from disease within. Individualities of each have their influence in creating difficulties, and these amongst the most arduous which beset the path of the physician.* Few cases occur strictly alike, even when the source of disorder is manifestly the same. Primary causes of disease are often wholly obscured by those of secondary kind. Organs remote from each other by place and function are simultaneously disturbed. Translations of morbid action take place from one part to another. Nervous affections and sympathies often assume every character of real disease. While remedial agents are rendered uncertain in effect by the various forms of each disorder, by the idiosyncrasies of the patient, by the difficulty of securing their equal application or transmission into the system, and finally, by the unequal quality of the remedies themselves.

These difficulties, the solution of which gives medicine its highest character as a science, can be adequately conceived by the medical man alone. It is the want of this right understanding which makes the mass of mankind so prone to be deceived by imposture of every

---

* Idiosyncrasy, as arising in most cases from inappreciable causes, is the most absolute and inevitable difficulty in medical evidence ; since no accumulation of instances, such as might suffice for the removal of all other doubts, can secure us wholly against this source of error.

kind; whether it be the idle fashion as to a particular remedy; or the worse, because wider, deception of some system, professing to have attained at once what the most learned and acute observers have laboured after for ages in vain.

It must be admitted, indeed, that this matter of medical testimony is too lightly weighed by physicians themselves. Else whence the so frequent description of effects and cures by agents put only once or twice upon trial; and the ready or eager belief given by those, who on other subjects, and even on the closely related questions of physiology, would instantly feel the insufficient nature of the proof.[*] Conclusions requiring for their authority a long average of cases, carefully selected, and freed from the many chances of error or ambiguity, are often promulgated and received upon grounds barely sufficient to warrant a repetition of the trials which first suggested them. No science, unhappily, has abounded more in false statements and partial inferences; each usurping a place for the time in popular esteem; and each sanctioned by credulity; even where most dangerous in application to practice. During the last twenty years, omitting all lesser instances, I have known the rise and decline of five or six fashions in medical doctrine or treatment; some of them affecting the name of systems, and all deriving too much support from credulity or other causes, even among medical men themselves.

Look at what is necessary, in strict reason, to attest the action and value of a new remedy or method of treatment. The identity or exact relation of the cases in which it is employed,—a right estimate of the habits and temperament, moral as well as physical, of the subjects of experiment,—allowance for the many modifications depending on dose, combination, quality of the medicine, and time of use,—due observation of the indirect or secondary, as well as direct, effects,—and such observation applied, not to one organ or function alone, but to the many which constitute the material of life. All these things, and yet more, are essential to the completeness of the testimony. All can rarely, if ever, be reached; and hence the inevitable imperfections of medicine as a science. But more, doubtless, of truth and beneficial result might be attained, were these difficulties rightly appreciated, and the means of obviating them kept more constantly in view.[†]

In no class of human events is the reasoning of "*post hoc, propter hoc*," so commonly applied by the world at large, as in what relates to the symptoms and treatment of disease. In none is this judgment so frequently both erroneous and prejudicial. It would seem as if the very complexity of the conditions necessary to sound evidence tended to beget acquiescence in that which is lightest and most in-

---

[*] Id credunt esse experientiam, quando semel vel bis faustam, vel infelicem, in certo morbo a sumpto medicamento annotarunt efficaciam.—*Hoffman.*

[†] Amongst the other difficulties of evidence in such cases must be noticed the ambiguity of all language as applied to denote and distinguish sensations; an evil familiar to every medical man, and only to be obviated by watchful experience.

sufficient for truth. The difficulties occurring in practice from this source are great, and require a right temper as well as understanding to obviate them.

Nor is there any subject upon which words and phrases, whether applied to diseases or remedies, exercise a larger influence. Terms have descended to us, which we can hardly put aside,—maxims which fetter the understanding,—and methods of classification, which prevent the better suggestions of a sound experience. And these are among the evils most aggravated by public opinion, ever prone to be governed by names, and particularly in all that concerns the symptoms and treatment of disease. The deeper the interest belonging to the subject, the greater the liability to error.

But in medical doctrine and theory also, there is scarcely less of difficulty from the nature of the evidence concerned. If example were needed to illustrate this, it might be drawn from what relates to the history of fever, whether idiopathic or symptomatic in kind. Here centuries of research, amidst facts of daily occurrence, have yet left some of the most important questions wholly unresolved; such is the difficulty of obtaining unequivocal proofs, of nature essential to a just theory. The same with respect to the doctrine of inflammation; a question which spreads itself, directly, or indirectly, over every part of pathology. Here the most various and refined inquiry, aided by the highest powers of the microscope, has not yet made it certain whether there be an increased or diminished action of the capillaries of the inflamed part; or in what mere turgescence differs from inflammation.*

The history of contagious diseases furnishes another instance scarcely less remarkable. It is the common belief, and one plausible enough in its first aspect, that the laws of contagion are simple and readily learnt. No mistake can be greater than this. All parts of the subject, even the circumstances most essential to practice, are wrapt up in doubt; and the evidence is of so intricate a kind, and so much disturbed by seeming exceptions, that the best judgments are perpetually at fault upon it. The same remark may be extended to other classes of diseases, where time and the most acute observation have hitherto failed to extricate truth from the multitude of conditions present. And it is no less true in relation to the various remedies we employ, even those most familiar, and seemingly simplest in use. The difficulties already noticed as belonging to the evidence of their effects, extend yet further, and more remarkably, to theory of their action; and our knowledge has scarcely yet passed the threshold of this inquiry.

It must be admitted, however, that the methods of research in medicine at the present time have gained greatly in exactness, and the just appreciation of facts, upon those of any previous period:— a natural effect of increasing exactness in all other branches of

---

* The active renewal of controversy on these points among modern writers shows at once their importance, and the insufficiency of the knowledge yet obtained on the subject.

science. A very especial advantage here has been the application of numerical methods and averages to the history of disease; thereby giving it the same progress and certainty which belongs to statistical inquiry on other subjects. Averages may in some sort be termed the mathematics of medical science. The principle is one singularly effectual in obviating the difficulties of evidence already noticed; and the success with which it has been employed of late by many eminent observers, affords assurance of the results that may hereafter be expected from this source. Through medical statistics lies the most secure path into the philosophy of medicine.*

In looking further to the chance of overcoming these difficulties in the future, regard must be had to the principle, now verified in so many cases, that in proportion to the complexity of phenomena, is augmented also the number of relations in which they may be surveyed and made the subjects of experiment.† The application of this principle to medical science is every day becoming more apparent. Each new path of physical knowledge opened, each single fact discovered, has given guidance more or less direct towards the objects still unattained in physiology and the treatment of disease. The unexpectedness of some of the relations, thus determined and converted to use, is the best augury for further advances in this direction of pursuit.

A due estimate among medical men themselves of the nature of the proofs with which they have to deal is now more especially needful, when the older doctrines of physic and physiology are all undergoing the revision required by modern science, and when new medicinal agents are every day produced upon trial; many of them dangerously active in their effects, many suggested by analogies which need to be verified by the most cautious experience. Hasty and imprudent belief may here become a cause of serious mischief; the wider in its spread, as the minds most prone to this credulity are those most ready also to publish to the world their premature conclusions; and thus to mislead the many who found their own practice upon faith in others; or who seek after novelty, as if this were in itself an incontestable good.

It must, however, be added, that on questions of medical evidence there may be an excess of scepticism as well as of credulity. Sometimes this occurs in effect of a temperament of mind (not uncommon among thinking men) which is disposed to see all things under doubt and distrust. There are other cases, where the same feeling, not originally present, grows upon the mind of physicians who have been too deeply immersed in the details of practice. The

---

* The inquiries which so greatly distinguish M. Louis as a pathologist, may be noted as eminent examples of this method, which is now pursued with great success by many physicians in our own country.

† M. Comte, in his "Cours de Philosophie positive," has defined this as a general law, through which compensation is made for the difficulty or impossibility of giving a mathematical form to certain branches of physics; such particularly as relate to the phenomena of organic bodies.

hurried passage from one patient to another precludes that close observation, which alone can justify, except under especial circumstances, the use of new remedies or active methods of treatment. From conscience, as well as convenience, they come to confine themselves to what is safe, or absolutely necessary; and thus is engendered by degrees a distrust of all that lies beyond this limit.

Though such scepticism be less dangerous than a rash and hasty belief, it is manifestly hurtful in practice, and an unjust estimate of medicine as a science; both as it now exists, and as it is capable of being extended and improved. No one can reasonably doubt that we have means in our hands admitting of being turned to large account of good or ill. Nor is it more reasonable to distrust the knowledge gained from a faithful experience as to the manner of using these, and others which may hereafter become known to us, safely and beneficially for the relief of disease. It is clear that between the two extremes just noticed, there is a middle course, which men of sense will perceive; and to which they alone can steadily adhere, amidst the many difficulties besetting at once the judgment and the conduct of the practitioner.

I am the rather led to these remarks on the nature of medical evidence, and the causes, moral as well as physical, affecting it, looking at the wonderful advances which have been made in all branches of science; not by the addition of new facts only, but even yet more by new methods and instruments of research, and increasing exactness in every point of inquiry. The dissimilarity of the proofs, and the greater difficulty of their certain attainment, must ever keep practical medicine in the rear of other sciences. But its still wider scope of usefulness requires that the distance should be abridged as far as possible; and that no occasion should be lost, by improved methods as well as new facts, by more cautious observation, and greater exactness of testimony, of maintaining its fit place among the other great objects of human knowledge.

CHAPTER II.

ON HEREDITARY DISEASE.

THE subject of hereditary temperament and tendency to disease is still largely open to inquiry. Future research will probably lead to an increased estimate of the influence of this cause on all the conditions of individual life, and not least on those of disease. Looking to analogy in plants and lower animals, we see in every direction the wide and various transmission of incidental varieties in each species; generally depending on combinations of natural

causes; sometimes effected by human care and design. The general law, as respects man, seems to be that so ably developed by
Dr. Prichard; viz., that all original or connate bodily peculiarities
tend to become hereditary; while changes in the organic structure
of the individual from external causes during life, end with him, and
have no obvious influence on his progeny.*

I know not that this principle could have been in any way anticipated, or otherwise derived than from actual observation of facts.
Nor is it certain that many exceptions do not exist to it; especially
in the wide circle of structural changes from the effect of disease,
as well as more notably in those instances where necessities of
situation alter certain parts of the organization of animals, and
where the continuance of such change is needful to their preservation under these new circumstances.† Nevertheless, as a general
law, it may be deemed highly probable, if not wholly proved; and
it is one fruitful of important inferences, both in physiology and
pathology. It comes in direct relation to the subject of hereditary
diseases: and though the manner of their transmission be still a
mystery, hidden in the same obscurity as the more general fact of
the reproduction of the species, yet are we able to reason upon the
effects, and to class them in certain relation to each other, and to
the healthy and natural condition of the human frame.

· It would be needless, and beyond my purpose, to cite the numerous examples of hereditary peculiarities of conformation, function,
and tendency to disease. Such instances are familiar to us in
common life,—in history and books,—and yet more especially and
frequently in the practice of medicine. I have, indeed, been led to
put together these remarks on the subject, from the numerous examples I find among my notes and recollections, to which I have
desired to give a more definite form, illustrative of their relations
to each other, and to the general laws of animal life. As I have
already remarked, we are still only partially acquainted with the
number and singular variety of such cases. The greater exactness
of modern observation is ever placing before us new and wonderful instances, in which the most minute peculiarities or defects, in
structure and function, are transmitted from one generation to another. Scarcely is there an organ or texture in the body, which
does not give its particular proof of these variations, so transmissible; and we might almost doubt the permanence of the type of our
species, thus largely and unceasingly infringed upon, were we not
permitted to see something of those more general laws, by which
the Creator has set limits to the change, and made even the deviations subservient to the welfare of the whole.

* Researches into the Physical History of Mankind.
† The effects of domestication come under the latter view, where changes
originally individual to the animal are propagated to its posterity; reaching
gradually, as it would seem, a certain range of duration for each, beyond which
definite causes interfere to prevent a further change. If other animals than those
now possessed were needed for the uses or luxury of man, there is little doubt
that human care alone might greatly extend the number of these varieties.

For in considering this hereditary tendency to disease, whether arising from structure or less obvious cause, it is needful to regard it in connexion with, or rather as part and effect of, that great general principle, through which varieties of species have been spread over the globe, with obvious marks of wise and beneficent design. The laws upon which these diversities depend, and by which they are limited, allow wide scope to their existence without injury or disorder of the general system. In the instances where such effects do occur, we discern some part of the modifying causes, even amidst the profound obscurity which conceals from us their original source.*

This subject, indeed, cannot be rightly pursued, without referring to those recent inquiries into the original types and development of animal life, from the simplest to the most complex forms, which form a new field within the great domain of human science. Such researches into what has been termed Embryology, though Hervey and Hunter prepared the way for them, have latterly engaged much less attention in England than among the naturalists of France and Germany.† The boldness, or even rashness, of some of the generalizations which have been attempted, particularly in the doctrine of fundamental unity of structure and design, must not prevent us from looking to a large increase of sound knowledge from these inquiries, based as they are upon a close and minute observation of facts. Their bearing upon the question of hereditary conformation and peculiarities, whether in families, tribes, or races of men, will be obvious to all who have studied this curious subject, and the controversies which have grown out of it. Dismissing the notion of a single primitive germ, or absolute unity of animal type, as a thing not proved, and probably incapable of proof; and putting aside further some fanciful analogies which have defaced the inquiry, we yet must admit that comparative anatomy is ever carrying us

* That there are fixed laws of design by which the permanence of species is secured, must be admitted as a general fact,—the result of all observations hitherto made on animal organic forms both living and extinct. The very circumstance of the frequent repetition of analogous and parallel series of forms, under different physical conditions, and at different geological epochs, though admitting some doubt as to its interpretation, is nevertheless most favourable to this opinion. Still we are not entitled to deny to the followers of Geoffroy St. Hilaire the *possibility* that it may be otherwise; and that research may hereafter disclose to us some evidence that species are not immutable. If this were eventually proved, it would in no wise affect the great argument of Natural Theology. A law presumed at one time to be universal, would be found collateral or subordinate to a still higher law; further removed, it may be, from our comprehension of its details, but involving the same proofs of design as the basis of the whole.

† In France, Geoffroy St. Hilaire, Lamarck, Blainville, Dumas, and Serres; in Germany, Meckel, Tiedemann, Baer, Spix, Valentin, &c., have been the most conspicuous of those lately engaged in the inquiry. In the former country, Cuvier sought to stay the extremes into which these doctrines have occasionally been carried. The sound and perspicuous understanding of this admirable man, while ever pursuing the highest generalizations to which facts would conduct him, had the power, no less important, to resist all inordinate speculation, and to recognise the bounds as well as the capacity of human research.

back, by successive steps, to simpler and more fundamental types
of animal life;—to conditions of structure, common to large and
seemingly remote classes of created beings.* If descending again
in the series, we make the progress of development the basis of our
views, and follow this downwards from more general forms to those
which are successively subordinate, even as far as to families and
individuals of the same species, we connect the subject of hereditary aberrations with this more general law; finding reason from
analogy to expect that such should occur, and that they should be
carried into extreme variety and minuteness. The different parts
of structure and function become more special, or individual, at
each step of descent; never losing, however, their relation to the
original common type; and in the instances at least of individuals
of the same species, tending ever to recur to it, when the causes of
change are modified or withdrawn.

This manner of pursuing the inquiry, through the unity or analogy of structure in corresponding organs, is probably the most
conformable to nature, and the most likely to lead to correct conclusions from the facts observed. Among other results already
obtained from it, is a more just view as to the nature of what
have been termed monsters; which, though still regarded as deviations, more or less, from the natural type, are so for the most part

* It is still a subject of dispute where this progress upwards to simpler and
more general forms is stopped by essential differences of type, or whether such
do at any point in the series really exist? whether there are separate circles of
analogies, as defined by the four great classes of Cuvier, or whether these are
but artificial limits, subordinate to a type pervading all the forms of animal life?
Professor Whewell, in his History of the Inductive Sciences, and Dr. Roget, in
his Bridgewater Treatise, have discussed these questions, as to general types
and unity of design, in a happy spirit of philosophical inquiry. Some valuable
papers on the same subject, by Dr. Martin Barry, will be found in the Edinburgh
Philosophical Journal. Other eminent naturalists in our own country have now
entered upon the investigation.

I have never, as already stated, seen cause to think the argument of Natural
Theology at all affected by these inquiries; even when pushed to the speculations
of a primitive germ, or original unity of type. Its truth indeed is far above the
reach of what, after all, are but subordinate researches, even if they could by
possibility attain the proofs of what these terms express. The chain is lengthened, and its parts are connected together by new and unexpected links. But
still it is a chain of designed organization throughout; and if we simplify the
first of these links, it is but to render more wonderful the number and perfection of the varieties which are evolved in definite forms from this elementary structure. If the parts in man have all their analogies or models in lower
animals; or if, according to one view proposed, we regard the several organs of
the human embryo as passing through all the gradations of lower types, before
reaching their perfect development in man, still the great argument remains the
same. The progressive elaboration throughout all its stages is definite and
designed,—the points are fixed at which each deviation has its beginning from
the more common antecedent forms,—the limit of change is fixed in each particular case. If there be an argument for the unity of creation, more complete and
comprehensive than another, it is that which is furnished by the recent progress
of comparative anatomy; enabling the observer, by the uniformity of general
laws, to predicate from a single minute part of structure all the more important
generic characters of the animal to which it belongs.

in the sense of an interference or arrest at particular periods of development; displacing organs only partially evolved, or suspending the progress of structure in parts yet imperfect. The advance here from the old notion of a *lusus naturæ* is obvious, and the details into which the doctrine has been carried form a remarkable feature in physiological science. Though exceptions exist to the law propounded by some naturalists, that every particular monstrosity in man has its analogy in the natural state of the same parts in some inferior animal, the fact is nevertheless so general as to justify its being regarded as a principle in the development of animal life.

It can scarcely be needful to say, that these views are simply illustrative of relation in a series of effects. While augmenting our knowledge in this way, and leading us up to the threshold of the mystery, they give us no power to pass beyond it. The insuperable nature of the limit is even rendered more obvious, when thus approached, than as it is seen from more distant points of view. While we find cause of wonder at the extraordinary transmission of resemblances from parent to offspring, we must admit the equal wonder that there should ever be deviations from this likeness. The one case is in reality as great a miracle to our understandings as the other.

The hereditary tendency to disease, regarding the subject in its most general light, shows itself either in the anormal conformation of particular organs or textures, or in the presence and transmission from parent to offspring of certain morbid products, either altogether new, or vitiated in kind, or faulty by excess.* Pursuing the subject more closely, it may be inquired, whether these morbid products are in reality all referrible, as effects, to variations in some part of organic structure, producing or evolving them; so that the solids of the body alone, by their conformation and texture, carry on such peculiarities through successive generations? or, whether the animal fluids also, and particularly the blood, may not be concerned in the transmission thus taking place?

This is a question involving much curious but doubtful speculation, nor does the actual state of our knowledge afford any certain answer to it. We can go little further than to say, that the evidence as to the agency of the solids, and the changes they severally undergo, is more distinct and complete; but we are not justified in denying that the blood may also take on morbid conditions, directly transmissible to offspring. The question, in truth, here involves the origin of the blood itself, in relation to the solids of the body; and merging in this, its import to the subject before us is less than might at first be supposed. So close is the mutual connexion of the animal solids and the blood, in growth, function, and change, that it is scarcely possible, even were it practically needful, to separate them in this inquiry. The faulty organization of certain parts of

* I have not used the term *monstrosity* here, as this in common language expresses only extreme cases of mal-conformation; depending on the same principles, but from obvious causes more generally prevented from becoming hereditary.

the former may produce morbid changes in the latter; or the fluids of the body, already vitiated from other cause, may alter and deprave the texture of the solid parts.

If there were reason for going further into this question, it might fairly be argued, that, however difficult to conceive a fluid like the blood, ever in motion and change, being capable of hereditary taint, yet is not this really more difficult to understand than a character or peculiarity conveyed by descent to any part of the solids of the body. The blood has vitality in every sense in which we can assign it to the latter. Under some views it is the portion of the animal frame which is especially so endowed. Its first appearance, in the *area vasculosa* of the germinal membrane of the embryo, is prior to the existence of those very organs which, after birth, chiefly minister fresh materials to it :—and though undergoing constant change, it has this in common with the animal solids; and with those equally, which are most frequently the subjects of hereditary affection. The morbid changes, moreover, which it undergoes, are often the effect of inconceivably minute portions of foreign matter brought into the circulation; as denoted in the effect of various poisons, in the exanthematous disorders, and other instances familiar in the history of disease.

Examples of the anormal conformation of particular organs, transmitted by descent, are alike numerous and familiar. If peculiarities of external form and feature, whencesoever originally derived, tend so speedily to become hereditary,—affecting, as we see on every side, not families alone, but, by intermixture and descent, whole races of mankind,—we can have no doubt that deviations of internal structure, (whether they be of deficiency or excess, or of any other nature,) are similarly transmitted ; and with them propensities to, or conditions of, morbid action in the parts thus organized. Though the direct proof is not equal for the two cases, and though the effects resulting are of such different importance, yet is it certain that the peculiarities, so carried on from one generation to another, have reference for both to one common law. And it is to the same principle that we must look for explanation of the difference in the average duration of life in different families ;—a fact well attested in itself, notwithstanding the many exceptions which the laws or social usages of mankind are ever inducing upon it. Those deviations from the primitive or common type of the species, which occur chiefly in the bony structure, integuments, or muscular fabric ; producing varieties in the outward form and feature, in the texture or colour of the skin, hair, &c., may exist to great extent, without affecting in any important way the health or natural functions of the individual. On the other hand, much smaller deviations from this type, in the internal organs of circulation, respiration, digestion, absorption, or secretion,—or in the brain and nervous system,—may produce morbid actions, painful in progress and fatal in result: each class of deviations alike transmissible to progeny, under the same general law.

This distinction is obviously one of summary importance in the history of disease, and capable of very wide application. It throws light upon the connexion of various morbid states, by giving the relation to a common physical principle in their cause ; and this principle one which is associated with other of the more general laws of life. There is no reason to doubt that hereditary peculiarities of structure are as frequent and varied, perhaps as extensive, in the internal organs, as in the external parts of the body. Analogy would suggest this as probable ; and it is confirmed in great measure by observation ; more extensively as the examination is rendered more minute. On the same grounds it may be presumed that there is a general ratio between the resemblance of external features, and that of internal parts of structure. The child most like its parent in traits of countenance and figure has probably closest kindred with him in other and more minute points of conformation. The evidence here is chiefly that of similarity of morbid affections in such cases,—a fact almost indisputably ascertained, and which, if the views contained in this chapter be correct, affords the best proof we can reasonably seek for. In the instance of gout it has been observed, that the children most resembling the gouty parent have greatest liability to the disorder. This can only be explained by supposing a corresponding likeness in those parts of internal structure which are chiefly concerned as causes or seats of the disease.

It must be admitted indeed that this inquiry is still incomplete in many of its parts ; and, on first view, it might appear that such internal deviations were much less extensive than those of outward conformation. But we can scarcely name any organ of importance which dose not afford evidence of diseased actions, derived from structure and transmissible by descent. And looking to the textures more widely diffused through the body,—as the different vascular systems, the nerves, &c., we have every reason to suppose, though the proof be less direct, that they are subject to hereditary variations of structure, not merely in detached parts of each system, but throughout those minute branches and terminations where the most important functions of the body, both animal and vital, may be presumed to take place.

On a subject of this nature, however, it is not sufficient to refer merely to the vague division of external and internal parts. The distinction between the animal and vital organs is at the foundation of every such inquiry, and each particular question must be brought into connexion with it. The fact may be considered as ascertained, that the vital organs are subject to more frequent and extensive deviations from the natural type than those of animal life ; the principle of symmetry (essential it may perhaps be deemed) in the latter, requiring, for the integrity of the functions, that all such deviations should be limited in extent.* A presumption might hence

* It is a remarkable attestation of this fact, that where anormal varieties of the muscles occur (a much rarer event than in the vascular system), there seems a strong tendency in these varieties to become symmetrical for the two sides.

arise, that the tendency to transmission by descent would follow the same law, and the parts belonging to organic life offer more frequent cases of hereditary malconformation than the animal organs. I know not that this question of relative frequency has ever been explicitly answered.   There is, however, enough of proof to make it probable that no disproportion exists of the kind, just indicated ; and that anormal structure in the parts of animal life is quite as liable to be transmitted as in the organic.   Taking the obvious instances indeed, these may appear more numerous ; but as the difficulty of observation is much greater in the latter case, it is enough to rest in the fact that both the great divisions of life are liable to this general law, and probably not in any different degree.

Though it becomes needless, from their frequency, to enumerate many special instances of hereditary malconformation and tendency to disease, yet some general facts may be noticed from their singularity, or in illustration of other parts of the subject.   One of these is the wonderful extent to which such congenital deviations are carried, not only as respects the variety of the parts affected, but also their individuality and minuteness.   I will notice here a few of the examples as to the latter point which have come under my own notice ; without looking to the many, more or less authenticated, which might be taken from medical works, or other sources of information.

An instance is known to me of hydrocele occurring in three out of four successive generations, in one family,—the omission adding to the singularity of the fact, from its depending on a female being the third in the series, in whose son the complaint reappeared.   I am acquainted with a family, in which there are three examples, the father and two children, of inability to distinguish red as a colour. Another example, resembling the last, is known to me, where three brothers, and two or three children of their families, have the inability to distinguish between blue and pink.   Instances of this kind as an hereditary defect are far from infrequent.*.   I have known squinting to occur in every one of five children, where both parents had this defect.   The repetition of cases of deaf and dumb children in the same family is well known to those who are concerned in institutions for the relief of this congenital defect.   An example has recently occurred to me of that remarkable affection, the *suffusio dimidians*, existing in a father and his daughter ; and brought on in each by circumstances singularly alike.   In another family I have seen several instances of the peculiar tremor tendinum of the hands and arms, which is sometimes called the shaking palsy ; and which here occurred in young persons of sixteen or eighteen, as well as in those more advanced in life.   In this case, too, I had proof of the peculiarity having gone through at least three generations.   Similarity in the form and setting of the teeth, as well as in the colour

---

* An interesting case of this congenital defect, where it was also hereditary, is given in the Med. Chirurg. Transactions, vol. ix., p. 363.

of the hair, is often observed between parents and children; and lefthandedness, from whatever this proceeds, sometimes takes the character of a family peculiarity. In a family where the father had a singular elongation of the upper eyelid, seven or eight children were born with the same deformity, two or three other children having it not. In like manner I have seen enlarged tonsils occurring in almost every individual of a numerous family, without other cause by which to explain it.

Eneuresis in children, from whatever source arising, occurs sometimes in so many individuals of the same family, as to make it almost certain that it has a common congenital origin. What is not less remarkable, as an instance of similar specialty, emphysema of the lungs has been ascertained to depend in the majority of cases on hereditary influence, independently of any disposition to tubercular pulmonary disease.* Another instance which may be termed special, though belonging to a part of structure diffused over the whole body, is the hemorrhagic diathesis. Though I do not find in my notes any well marked examples of its hereditary nature, except where confined to the lungs and connected with phthisical constitution, yet some are recorded so explicit as scarcely to leave the fact in doubt ; and remarkable further, for the seeming limitation of these instances to the male sex. Nor is there indeed greater difficulty of comprehension here, than where a more limited portion of structure is concerned. The points of question are the same in each case ; and the solution, if ever obtained, must be common to both. I might add to these many similar instances; but they are too familiar to require further recital. It will be remarked, that all are perfectly congruous with, and in no respect more wonderful than the common transmission from parent to offspring of external features, in the peculiarities of which no diseased action is involved.

There are some examples of anormal structure or disease, which, though frequently occurring in detached instances, yet are so especially numerous in certain localities, as to give suspicion, in the absence of other sufficient causes, that hereditary tendency is much concerned. Such is the goitre of particular districts, no consistent explanation of which has yet been given, founded on local circumstances of climate or mode of life. The *plica polonica* is another instance to the same effect. I might apply the same remark, though with greater doubt, to that curious affection, the *trismus nascentium*, prevalent in particular localities, and these widely different in all physical circumstances.† The great frequency of stone in the

---

* This fact we owe to the late Dr. Jackson, of Boston, in America, a physician whose life was too early terminated.

† When in Iceland, in 1810, I had the opportunity of collecting some facts as to the singular frequency of this disease in the Vestmann Isles, on the southern coast of this island. On these desolate rocks, the population of which does not exceed 160 souls, I found that, in a period of 25 years, 186 infants perished of this disorder, under the age of 21 days ; of which 161 died between the fourth and tenth days after birth ; 75 on the eighth day. Though the condition of life

bladder, in certain districts where there is no obvious peculiarity of air, food, or water, as a probable cause ; and the common tendency to lithic acid deposits in the same family, may admit of like explanation. And this is further sanctioned by the certain connexion of the calculous with the gouty diathesis.

Seeking then for the most general expression of facts, we may affirm that no organ or texture of the body is exempt from the chance of being the subject of hereditary disease. Or, in other words, every part is susceptible of deviations from the normal type or natural structure, capable of being conveyed to offspring ; and of producing morbid actions, which are thus, under the name of disease, often propagated through successive generations.

A singular variety in this general law is that which Duchesne and others have termed Atavism ; where a bodily peculiarity, deformity or disease, existing in a family, is lost in one generation ; reappearing in that which follows. One curious instance of this is mentioned above, where the omission depended on change of sex in the series. There may be many analogous cases, in which the part of structure affected by hereditary disease is such as to be disguised or superseded by other casualties in the bodily conformation of the individual. Or, if the animal fluids be directly concerned in the transmission, we may conceive these liable to be more readily affected by causes of variation, so that the same morbid influence is directed to one part rather than another. But these explanations, if such they be, do in no way apply to the numerous cases where, the sex and all obvious circumstances being the same, a disease or deviation from common structure is missing in one or more individuals of a family series, recurring in their children. Here we pass at once into the obscurity which wraps over all that belongs to this great function of life, the reproduction of the species. But the same analogy, or rather unity of plan, is still present to us. If one generation escapes in the transmission of an hereditary disease, so do we often find some strongly marked feature of face or figure lost in one of a family, but reappearing in his children. The proof is hereby strengthened of that general relation which pervades all these phenomena, and which makes the simple resemblance of an external feature the exponent of other cases, in which the most severe diseases are conveyed from parent to offspring.

Connected with the foregoing is another curious variety in the transmission of disease, if so it may be termed, which has been little noticed by medical authors; the case, namely, of several children of a family being affected in common with some given malady, of which there has been no token on the side of either parent. An example has lately occurred to me in one family, of three sons and a daughter, every one of whom underwent an attack of hemiplegia

of these poor people is singularly destitute, fish and the eggs of sea-fowl being their sole aliment, yet is it not so different from that of the Icelanders of the main land as to explain the frequency of this fatal disorder among them ; and it would seem as if some constitutional and hereditary causes were concerned.

before the age of forty-five, though neither father nor mother had been similarly affected. I find another instance in my notes, where three brothers severally suffered hemiplegia, and about the same period of life, without any record of the like event in the family. I have recently seen a fatal case of cerebral disease, with epileptic fits, in a young lady of twenty-four; two sisters of whom had died about the same age with similar symptoms, though neither parent had been subject to such disorder. I am acquainted with a family in which four children have died during infancy from affections of the brain, without any like instances in the family on either side. In another family, without any similar disease in the parents, three or four children had epileptic fits.

I have notes of several similar instances; chiefly, as I think, but not exclusively, disorders of the brain and nervous system. I have known three cases of *diabetes mellitus* in brothers, under ten years of age, in the same family; one of them fatal in result.* In another instance, four cases of ascertained disease of the heart, all fatal about the same period of life, occurred to my notice in the brothers and sisters of one family; without any suspicion, as far as I could learn, of the parents having been the subjects of this disease. By a singular coincidence, another instance is known to me, where four brothers died, between sixty and sixty-five, of ossification and other disease of the heart; but here there appear to have been prior cases of the same kind in the family. In the instance of the deaf and dumb, already referred to, the examples are frequent and curious of several children being thus affected (five out of a family of eight, four from a family of seven), without similar defect existing in the parents. At the School for the Deaf and Dumb in Manchester, in 1837, there were forty-eight children taken from seventeen families, the total number of children in these families being 106; and giving therefore an average of nearly three such cases in each family. Out of these instances, there appears but one in which the defect was known to exist in either parent; and we may rightly therefore consider this as one of the most striking examples of the fact under consideration.†

Some of these examples may perhaps be referred to the condition last mentioned, of the revival of an hereditary disorder, absent in one or more generations. But proof to this effect is wanting in other cases: and the remarkable fact remains, of several children of the same parents being affected in common with a given malady, of which there are no certain prior examples in either family. All physiology is at fault as to the solution of this phenomenon.

A yet further variety in the hereditary transmission of disease is

* Several instances are related by Dr. Prout, in which this disease showed an hereditary character.

† As a curious variation of the same general conditions, a case is known to me, where the children of parents, each deaf and dumb, are themselves free from that defect. In another large family I have known almost every child short-sighted, without either parent being so.

its limitation, more or less complete, to the males or females of the family affected.   This fact is illustrated by two or three of the instances already given, and seems well attested in the case of the hemorrhagic diathesis.*   In the more familiar example of gout, the same condition may be admitted to a greater extent.   The circumstance most remarkable here is the frequent evidence of transmission through the female of a morbid tendency or action, not observable in herself during any part of life.   This indeed is only the case of the singular phenomenon of atavism, already noticed; but still more interesting to physiology, as being more special, and including the relation of the sexual peculiarities to the other functions and changes of the system.   Considering the subject in its most general light, it appears certain that the cause of action in such cases cannot be altogether dormant, though not attested by the usual signs of its presence.   We may better find explanation in differences of the seat and manner of action, whether depending on sexual structure, or on other less obvious conditions.   It cannot be doubted that such differences exist, modifying the influence of every one material agent upon the body; and thereby giving, it may be presumed, a totally different aspect to the effects of the same physical cause.   I shall have other occasions to remark on the wide application of this principle to the phenomena of disease.

Looking at what may hereafter be learnt on these curious subjects, the most obvious source of knowledge is the observation of corresponding facts in other animals.   Here our means of inquiry are greatly increased by adding direct experiment to the mere observation of facts.   The results obtained from breeding, especially in the domestic animals, are infinitely valuable in this respect; and replete with curious inferences, all more or less applicable to the case of man.   The whole subject of specialties of structure and function, whether natural or obtained by artificial means, is full of the same interest; and forms the most direct line along which to carry research into the types and development of animal life.   The physiology of plants affords similar illustrations; though more remote, from the wider difference in their organs and mode of existence.†   Much has been attained on these subjects; but more yet remains behind.   Though the principle of life and reproduction be still a mystery at the root of the inquiry, all the effects resulting from this principle may become better known, their connexions de-

* Examples to this effect will be found in the Archives Générales, Oct. 1833, and July 1835; one or two of them made more remarkable by the transmission of the diathesis through females, themselves unaffected in this way; and further by the very frequent concurrence of the hemorrhagic with the rheumatic constitution.

† I may cite, as an excellent example of the mode of pursuing this research, the work of Gallesio, little known in this country, " Storia della Riproduzione Vegetale." Pisa, 1816. Gallesio takes the genus Citrus as his subject, and, from his experiments upon these plants, draws conclusions which apply largely to the production of varieties, monsters, and hybrids, in vegetable life.

termined, and the relations explained by which they take the forms of hereditary disease.

Many interesting but difficult inquiries arise out of those diseases, where the hereditary evil is not of one organ or texture, but seeming to pervade every part of the body,—showing itself at intervals, and especially at certain periods of life,—and frequently shifting its action suddenly from one part to another. Gout and scrofula in their various forms, and perhaps also the cancerous diathesis, will here occur as the most familiar examples. The very difficulty of the research gives proof of the extent to which it may be applied, in extending and correcting our pathological views. In gout, for instance, admitting, what can scarcely be denied, a morbid ingredient in the blood as the cause of the disease, it may be asked whether hereditary gout depends on the transmission of some part of structure, favouring the formation of this matter, or on some faulty texture of the kidneys or other excreting organs, whose office it may be to remove it from the body? Or further, if it be that gouty matter is merely an excess of some ingredient natural to the blood, whether the determination to the joints, forming the fit of active gout, is the effect of hereditary conformation of these parts; the absence of which peculiarity in others allows this excess to show itself in very different appearances of disease?

I have noticed these questions more in detail, when treating elsewhere of this disorder. They apply equally perhaps, though this relation has been less followed, to those forms of acute rheumatism (a name unfortunately vague in its use), where there is every proof, from the nature of the symptomatic fever, from the peculiarity of the secretions and deposits, and from the metastasis to internal parts, that the disorder is one of the whole habit, and probably depending on some peculiar state of the blood. There is sufficient evidence to show that this disease is of hereditary kind; though perhaps more dependant than gout on occasional exciting causes from without.* Many similar inquiries will apply to the scrofulous or tubercular constitution; admitting it, indeed, as a single form of cachexia. It may be asked whether this congenital temperament consists in a certain texture of solid parts, vascular or otherwise, giving liability to peculiar deposits at certain periods of life? or whether, in a specific morbid state of the circulating fluids, producing such deposits in the parts of the body most prone to receive them? The latter view, as in gout, may be admitted as the more probable one, and for the same reasons. Indeed, however different the diseases in many respects, yet certain general relations subsist between gout and scrofula;—in their hereditary nature; in their respective connexion with particular periods of life; in the proofs of a morbid matter peculiar to each; in the variety of forms in which this morbid cause shows itself in different persons; and in

* The most ample proof is that furnished by the large experience of Chomel, who rates as high as one-half the proportion of rheumatic cases where the parents had suffered under the same disease.

the frequency and facility of translation from one part to another. These analogies lead us to no common cause; but they show causes operating by certain common laws; and, in a case where there is still so much to be learnt, all such relations are of value. Hereafter we may be able, by these and similar means, to associate together diseases now widely apart in our nosologies,—gaining thereby a classification more just, and of greater practical usefulness, than any we now possess.

In the scrofulous temperament, even more than that of gout, we have a remarkable diversity in the forms the disease takes, and the organs it attacks. But it is worthy of note, that there appears a general tendency to the same form in the same branch of a family thus affected; still more in children of the same parents. I may mention, as a striking example, the number of cases of blindness, partial or complete, in some families where this temperament exists. In others, the disposition is as strongly marked to affections of the joints;—in others, again, to pulmonary consumption in its more common form. These are instances of the tendency to specialties before noticed, extending to morbid structure or functions, as well as to those of healthy kind.

What has been just said of the scrofulous diathesis applies by parity of all essential characters to the carcinomatous habit. Though the proofs are more limited by the comparative infrequency of the disorder, it is certain that this also is often an hereditary disposition of body, tending to the production of morbid growths, more especially at certain periods of life. If, as alleged, the lymphatic temperament is that particularly disposed to carcinoma, the question again arises, (but without any further facility for solving it,) whether this connate tendency consists in a state of the solid tissues, or of the fluids circulating through them? In using the term of lymphatic habit, we are not indeed entitled to carry our meaning beyond some of the more obvious effects of a constitutional cause, the nature of which, whether affecting the solids or fluids, is still unknown to us.

Those disorders of the skin which depend on the general habit, however such temperament be termed, may be regarded in the same light, and are evidently prone to become hereditary. I have recently seen three cases of psoriasis in the children of one family, where there was strong predisposition to gout. The coincidence of this complaint with gouty habit I have observed in many other instances. Certain impetiginous eruptions belong also to a family constitution, such as is often termed scorbutic, and are obviously transmitted from parents to children.

I may notice here another singular disease, the *pellagra* of Lombardy, in which, together with the peculiarity of a local limitation, there occurs a very singular succession of symptoms, beginning with a cutaneous affection of leprous character, passing through various stages of cachectic disorder, and ending generally, after the lapse of a few years, in fatuity or death. I have had much opportunity of observing this curious disease in all its forms.* There can be no doubt from circumstances of its hereditary nature, though there is difficulty in tracing it back in Lombardy for more than eighty or a hundred years, and equal difficulty in assigning the causes which give it existence in this district alone.

Other diseases might be mentioned, offering questions no less difficult than those stated above. Spasmodic asthma, for example, sometimes shows an hereditary character. I have known the complaint to occur in four successive generations; and often so numerously in the same family as to make it certain that a common cause was concerned. This cause is presumably one of structure:—yet it would be difficult to affirm it to be so, or to state in what part the peculiarity is likely to exist. Here perhaps the nervous system may be chiefly looked to: and there is certainly nothing to disprove the possibility that irregular structure of certain parts of this system may be transmitted by descent, so as to become a source of the disordered actions of asthma.

I have already, indeed, noticed the strong tendency to hereditary character in disorders of the brain and nervous system. This is a very remarkable part of the subject; involving, as it does, every variety and degree of morbid affection, from simple head-ache to the worst forms of epilepsy and palsy. It is further a topic of deep interest, as including the various conditions of hereditary insanity, —instanced not merely in particular families, but even in districts and communities, where from local circumstances there has been little intermixture with the rest of the world. From the latter disease thus occurring, we gather the important conclusion, that some deviation in physical structure, whether obvious or not, is the cause of the aberrations it presents. In no other way can we conceive the transmission of the tendency from one generation to another. It may be that part of the fabric of the brain is concerned, far too minute for the most subtle research to follow; and this indeed might be presumed, looking at the nature of the functions affected. But still, whenever the transmission occurs, we are bound by all analogy to infer the presence of a morbid material cause, upon which the phenomena primarily depend.†

* A paper I wrote on the Pellagra, was published in vol. viii. of the Medico-Chirurgical Transactions. There are many points of great interest in the history and pathology of this disorder. Its first appearance seems to have been in the Alto-Milanese; but in the early part of this century, it had spread increasingly over the greater part of Lombardy, and to the shores of the Adriatic Sea. I have seen the disease as far eastwards as Friuli, at the foot of the Carinthian Alps. There are some districts in the Alto-Milanese where the pellagrosi form one-fifth or sixth of the whole population. And at the time I visited the Lunatic Hospital at Milan, out of nearly 500 patients of both sexes, about one-third had been brought thither in effect of this disorder.

† Here again, as so often before, we are called upon to note the close relation of particular morbid phenomena to more general laws; and, in the present case, to those laws which determine the varieties of character in nations and communities of men. Hereditary deviations in excess, such as come under the character of insanity, are corrected or limited by the usages of society. Those variations

There is much that is curious in the tendency to head-aches thus transmitted by descent, and often going through whole families with similar character. The cause here presumably varies in different instances. Sometimes, and especially perhaps where they are periodical, the affection may belong to the gouty habit, and to the matter of gout in the circulation. In other cases, anormal structure of the vessels of the head may be concerned : in others, again, some peculiarity in the nervous substance itself.

In hereditary affections of the nerves, as in those of other parts, it is extraordinary in what minute peculiarities the tendency often shows itself. It is difficult indeed in some of these cases to distinguish what is due to imitation alone: but in other instances, where this is excluded by circumstances, we find nevertheless nervous habits and disorders of the parents reappearing in the offspring to a singular extent. These entailed disorders are certainly more numerous than is generally supposed; and probably the source of many morbid states, apparently remote in kind. As respects their origin, they may all be referred to the general principles we have been considering.

Connected with this part of the subject is the remarkable fact of an hereditary temperament, in which are blended together the elements of various disease, both of body and mind, with some of the highest mental qualities and endowments. Instances are frequent, where in the same family we find almost every individual possessing some strongly marked peculiarity; such peculiarities often very different in aspect, yet all having reference to some single point in constitution from which the several effects diverge. Or the life of one individual, so circumstanced, may itself afford example of the most singular extremes of state, equally to be referred to some common cause.

Another fact still to be noticed regarding hereditary constitution, in its relation to disease, is, the disposition of individuals of the same family and generation to be similarly affected under any given maladies; even such as have no apparent connexion with the peculiarity of family habit. There are indeed various chances of error in observations of this kind; and many exceptions will occur. Nevertheless, examples free from ambiguity must be familiar to every medical man, where disorders assume a certain marked character in the same family, as regards the severity of the symptoms, the organs especially attacked, and the effects they leave behind. Such is the case with hooping-cough and various infantile complaints —with exanthematous and epidemic diseases—and with others less

from the common type (if we may apply this term to mind as well as body) which are not so controlled, may, in the infancy of any community, and in combination with other causes, become the basis of those more permanent traits which we designate as the character of a people. Such diversities existing, as they actually do, and being in many cases perpetuated within human record, must be derived in some part from this source. Or if we could suppose it otherwise as to origin, it must at least be admitted that this cause is concerned in their perpetuation among races of men.

definite in their course of symptoms. In the instance of twins, these coincidences show themselves in still more remarkable degree. And it is likely, in general, that they should be most distinct in early life, when extraneous causes have yet done little to alter congenital likeness in structure and habit.

I find in my notes some curious instances, where two children of a family, with strongest likeness to each other in feature, figure, and habits, have shown similar resemblance in the symptoms of the disorders affecting them, and in their idiosyncrasy as to particular remedies.

No new difficulties occur in the explanation of these facts. Every morbid cause must have definite effect on certain parts of structure; and, if these are alike in two or more individuals from family descent, the presumption is, that any diseased actions ensuing will exhibit corresponding likeness in kind and degree. What here we might expect on theory, we find to be realized in the facts. And connected with these is the result, well attested by experience, that there is a general tendency towards the same duration of life in those of the same family,—often obviated by individual constitution or the incidents of life, but never perhaps wholly absent. In some instances this may be referred to the likeness in particular structures; but we must probably look still further and deeper for the causes concerned in this remarkable effect. The research indeed brings us immediately to the great mystery of the transmission of life itself—under the conditions of a fixed average duration to each species, and with subordinate variations belonging to particular series in the same species.

It is another fact in the history of hereditary diseases, meriting attention on various accounts, that many of these have a well-marked tendency to evolve themselves at particular periods of life, differing for each. This is true, not only as to those which are termed constitutional, such as gout and scrofula, where it might more easily perhaps be anticipated, but applies also to some cases where the hereditary disposition seems limited to a particular organ, as the heart, or the brain. These circumstances find their explanation in the general views already stated. When the disease depends upon anormal conformation of some organ, it may be brought into active shape, either by the accumulated effect of exciting causes long continued, or by the operation of new causes, coming into operation at certain periods of life. If there be cases in which we may suppose the blood concerned in transmitting hereditary taint, a point already considered, still it is conceivable (especially as we know that this fluid undergoes actual alteration at different ages) that some changes in its quality or distribution may bring the morbid principle into activity at one time rather than another. Or, without referring to such direct alteration in the blood itself, the changes successively taking place in the solid tissues of the body, particularly those of secretion, may so operate upon this fluid as to cause the commencement at a certain period of morbid changes, whether of deposit or other kind of action, which had not before occurred. To seek to carry explanation beyond these very general views would be merely to substitute vague phrases for actual knowledge.

I have not hitherto alluded to the question, which has been discussed and differently answered by different authors, from which parent the predisposition to disease is more frequently derived? The difference of opinion here probably results from the actual approach to equality in the occurrence of the respective cases. The question, in fact, merges in the more general one as to the transmission of physical resemblances from parent to offspring; these being, as we have seen, the chief source of similarity in morbid affections. And as such resemblances, both of lineament and structure, proceed from each parent, according to laws of which we are ignorant, but seemingly in proportion nearly alike, the diseases therewith connected must be considered under the same relation, and as being probably derived equally through the two sexes.*

Viewing the subject of hereditary disease in all its parts, one question yet arises:—whether, and to what extent, there may be continued progress of change in the organization or other material cause of the disease through successive generations?—or, where are the limitations to such changes, and whence derived? The general answer to this question may be drawn from the views already stated; and particular facts in illustration of it are best deduced from the growth of varieties in animals and plants, whether casual or designed. The conclusion presumably is, that the repetition of circumstances producing variation tends in itself to augment or confirm this, whether disease be the effect or not,—but that the original type of the species is ever present in opposition to the changes thereby induced; defining their extent, differently perhaps for different parts of the structure, but still with an eventual and certain limit to all.

It is unnecessary to point out the important relation to practice of all that concerns hereditary tendency to disease. The subject is one which meets us at every step, and to which our attention is perpetually required, as an exponent of symptoms, as affording some of the most certain means of prognosis, and as directing us in many particulars to the right course of treatment. No judicious practitioner will neglect the resources hence derived; which it is probable may be largely augmented in future, both by increased attention to them in practice, and by the actual extension of our knowledge in this branch of physiology.

There is yet wanting to our medical literature a work which may embrace this subject in its whole extent, and with the aids derived from other departments of science. What I have given here is but

* Dr. Nasse, of Bonn, treating of the tubercular diathesis, considers that the disposition to disease is more commonly derived from the mother than the father. The general opinion seems to have been the reverse of this; but neither view, as far as I know, is supported by such amount of averages as to warrant its adoption.

an outline of this; and the examples are drawn chiefly from my own observations in practice. These of course may be greatly extended in number and variety, and I must add further that they will require much more specification and exactness than I have been able to give in this general view. It is not enough, for instance, to speak of diseases of the heart collectively, at a time when the morbid anatomy of this organ ·is minutely investigated, and averages of weight and admeasurement obtained for its different states. And it will be readily perceived that the more precise and minute the definition of parts subject to hereditary affection, the greater is the hope of further insight into this remarkable phenomenon,—the more certain the aids afforded to the treatment as well as theory of disease.

———————

CHAPTER III.

BLEEDING IN AFFECTIONS OF THE BRAIN.

Is not depletion by bleeding a practice still too general and indiscriminate in affections of the brain, and especially in the different forms of paralysis? I believe that the soundest medical experience will warrant this opinion. The vague conception that all these disorders depend upon some inflammation or pressure, which it is needful to remove, too much pervades and directs the practice in them: and, if the seizure be one of sudden kind, this method of treatment is often pursued with an urgent and dangerous activity. Little heed is taken of the many cases where the symptoms depend upon irritation alone,—or on loss of nervous power,—or on deficient circulation of the blood within the brain,—or on altered qualities of this blood,—or, it may be, on morbid changes in the nervous substance itself. Theory might suggest that, in some of these various cases, the loss of blood would lead to mischief.—Experience undoubtedly proves it; and there is cause to believe that this mischief, though abated of late years, is still neither infrequent nor small in amount.

It is certain indeed that there is a state of brain, best perhaps represented to us in its general effect of diminished nervous power, which tends to produce sometimes spasmodic seizures, sometimes delirious or maniacal affections, sometimes palsy of different parts of the body—these effects being in nowise obviated by depletion, but rather increased by all such means; while they are relieved by remedies which tend to excite the energy of the sensorium, and to augment the general power. I have known cases of this kind where bleeding has immediately been followed by convulsions of epileptic character; occasionally by amaurosis or deafness; more frequently still by rambling delirium; and where wine or other cordials have as speedily abated these tendencies. The fevers of typhoid type, or those which are called nervous, in default of a better name, afford constant examples of delirium depending on this peculiar state of the sensorium. In cases of large and sudden hemorrhage, as in that of the uterus after childbirth, the whole system is often put into a state of seeming excitement; and the head in particular affected with acute pain, throbbing, and vertigo; which symptoms often continue for a considerable period, and are best removed by such means as gradually and equably restore the circulation and nervous power. Delirium, preceded generally by vertigo, is known as an effect of extreme starvation, without other obvious disease, as frequently recorded in the narrative of shipwrecks, &c. The condition of the patient in delirium tremens, on whatever proximate cause this may depend, is one of the most marked instances of that state of brain which any large depletion might hurry on to fatal result. Here indeed the treatment is not often mistaken; but in many cases essentially the same, though less distinct in symptoms, and less obvious in their origin, the mischief done by large bleeding is long continued, and sometimes of irreparable kind.

In the valuable experiments of Sir Astley Cooper, (Guy's Hospital Reports, No. III.,) the tying of the two vertebral arteries, which have seemingly a more important relation than the carotids to the cerebral circulation, brought on various forms of paralytic as well as spasmodic affection. Here we have direct proof that the brain, suddenly and largely deprived of blood, becomes liable to conditions apparently the same as those which we so often employ bleeding to obviate or relieve. They may be really different in many cases, and the facts show them to be so; but, where we have this source of ambiguity, it behoves that our practice be carefully guided by a reference to the constitution, habits, and age of the patient, as well as to the first obvious effects of the treatment pursued. I have known many instances where bleeding has been repeated to remove the very symptoms which it was next to certain it had been the means of bringing on.

In the experiments just referred to, sudden privation of blood produced a state of the brain which doubtless exists in effect of other causes of slower operation, manifesting itself in every grade of deviation from the healthy state. It would be difficult to define it by name; but presumably it has close relation to that already mentioned, where there is a deficient or altered nervous energy—testified in slighter cases chiefly by its influence on the mind and animal spirits; in those more severe, by the tendency produced to convulsive and paralytic affections. This temperament, doubtless depending on a physical cause in the organ, will be familiar to all who have attended to this class of disease. It appears to have much connexion in its nature with some of the changes which occur in the brain in old age; and possibly from similar causes as respects the supply of blood to this part. Anxiety and distress of mind long continued, or even the habit of overstrained intellectual labour, produce a similar state; and furnish much reason to the physician why he should exercise singular caution in all such cases. Certain it is that bleeding unduly practised in habits of this kind, and especially when the time of youth is past, depresses the nervous system, and through it, more or less, all the functions of the body, producing for a time a sort of premature approach to old age throughout the whole being. I have notes of some remarkable cases to this effect, in which the influence of the cause was unequivocally continued for a long period, passing even into years after the original occurrence.

In infancy also, when the brain and nervous system are more easily and critically affected by causes of excessive or deficient excitement, effects of the same kind follow great depletion, however produced. These, by a fatal error, are sometimes mistaken for proofs of inordinate action or of pressure; and a practice adopted of which it is difficult to recall the consequences, when once incurred.*

Even in those cases of cerebral disorder where the tendency to coma might give stronger presumption of pressure, I have sometimes had the most direct cause to believe that large bleeding induced paralytic attacks, which might otherwise have been spared.† These are instances in which absolute proof can scarcely be attained; but where the presumptive evidence may be such as nearly to approach to it. Two or three examples have occurred to me, in which, looking to the circumstances before and after, as well as to the immediate concurrence in time of the bleeding and paralytic seizure, it could hardly be doubted that they stood to each other in the relation of cause and effect. The existence of such instances, or even the suspicion of them, may well warrant a singular caution in this part of practice.

The state of coma is indeed a very ambiguous one, as respects our knowledge of its proximate cause. In the ordinary use of the term, the notion of pressure is associated with it by most practitioners, and this even in the cases where it seems but as an excess of the condition of sleep. But it is familiar to us also as a concomitant and token of the last stage of debility; and is often expressly induced by depletion and other depressing causes, as well as by those which are known to produce direct pressure on the brain.

* This important point in practice has been explicitly noted by some of our best medical writers; but experience shows that it is still not sufficiently enforced.

† In using the term cerebral here, as throughout this chapter, I have not thought it needful to advert to the distinction now established between the brain proper, and the system of the medulla oblongata. The relation of these respective parts in their morbid states is so complex and close, as far as our present means of diagnosis go, that, even in reasoning upon points of medical practice, it is necessary, if not expedient, to consider them together. Even if we had more certain methods of distinguishing them, we have yet no well-determined rule of practice to adapt to this distinction.

Even in children we have express instances of a state having all the characters of coma; but which is proved by the precursory causes, as well as by the effects of medical treatment, to depend on general feebleness of circulation and deficiency of nervous power. There is reason indeed to presume that the two states just alluded to are really distinct; and that the former is much more nearly akin to the condition of syncope than that of pressure. Or however related, as respects the nervous substance itself, so different in the operation of the causes producing it, as to require a method of treatment altogether opposite. Here then the governance of names must be put aside; and the more carefully, from that close resemblance of symptoms which makes the utmost discretion of the physician necessary, rightly to direct his practice for their relief. Nor can any rules be given, at once general and exact enough, to supersede the particular judgment in each case.

Vertigo, in all its degrees, is another symptom which often conveys alarm, from the idea of pressure on the brain, and leads to immediate depletion under this view. In some cases the inference and practice are just and beneficial. But there are others, and these, as I think, of frequent occurrence, where vertigo is the effect of causes wholly remote from fulness or over-action; being in fact a step toward syncope, and a proof of exhaustion of the nervous power. Here we require, not bleeding, but cordials, to restore the brain; and a wrong practice may lead into serious danger. As in the instance of coma, just mentioned, we must presume a wide distinction between states requiring a treatment so different, though the seeming resemblance of symptoms has led to the same name for both. The frequent occurrence of vertigo, in apparent good health, as well as under actual or threatened disease, is a reason for sedulously noting this distinction; which may generally be done by observation of other symptoms, or of the causes especially acting on the body at the time.

The difficulty of getting a correct nomenclature for morbid sensations applies peculiarly indeed to the head, of which the ambiguous use of the terms *light* and *heavy* may be taken as a familiar example. It must be owned, however, that the names here are not much more vague than the knowledge they represent. That state in which the head feels as if without weight or substance, common though it be, has not yet received any physical explanation. Many of the varieties of headache are as little defined by our knowledge of their cause as by the terms used in describing them,—though probably the greater number depend on different conditions of the circulation through the brain, of which conditions that of congestion or retarded circulation, varying in degree and in the vessels in which it may occur, is presumably the most frequent.

Among other symptoms which are still to be considered doubtful, as representing states of the brain, I may mention the dilatation of the pupil, and susceptibility of the retina. Direct observations show that these conditions depend for their degree upon different causes;

and accordingly we find, as a pathological fact, that, in cases of compression, concussion, or other disorder of the brain, we may have either contraction of the pupil, and a very sensitive state of the retina, or the reverse of this, without our being able securely to predict either of these states. Sometimes, too, they pass into each other; and each may occur in high degree, yet disappear without fatal or even mischievous consequence. Inequality in the pupils of the two eyes is perhaps to be taken as a more certain proof of some organic injury. But here also we can rarely affirm whether the dilated pupil concurs with the side affected or not; and other evidence is required to determine our practice as regards this distinction.

I mention these various sources of ambiguity, not to inculcate distrust of all practice in such cases, but merely to hold out caution against that indiscriminate principle of treatment which finds pressure in every altered condition of the brain ; and motive for bleeding in every transient irritation of parts, still but imperfectly known to us in their functions and diseases.

Even were the tendency to paralytic seizures as generally lessened by bleeding as common practice could imply, it does not thence follow that abstraction of blood from the brain should be needful or desirable in immediate sequel to such attack. In many cases it is undoubtedly otherwise. The paralysis, when depending on apoplexy, with extravasation of blood or serum, or on other cause of continued pressure, may come on by degrees, and admit of relief in its progress by emptying the vessels of the head. But often it occurs as an instant shock to a portion of the brain or spinal marrow, without any proof of extravasation or obvious cause of pressure ;—the shock itself being of momentary duration, though it leaves lasting effects on parts of the nervous system thereon depending. In these cases, and they are frequent, the physical causes of the change are little known to us. There are reasons for supposing that the nervous substance itself is often primarily effected. We have certainly no sufficient proof of mere pressure from fulness of vessels being concerned, to warrant large bleeding, especially after the stroke of palsy has actually occurred. The degree of coma attending and following these seizures is not alone sufficient cause for the practice; and will usually subside without it, where the original attack is not such as to endanger life.*

Looking indeed to the magnitude of the event between, common

* The question as to what constitutes the cure of paralysis is not less difficult than that as to the causes of original seizure ; our ignorance of the structure involved forming the difficulty in each case. The medullary fibres are presumably the parts immediately affected,—but whether by effusion between them, which is removed by absorption ; or by any breach of continuity which is repaired ; or by conditions yet more remote and subtle, we are unable to affirm. From the operation of causes affecting the brain alone, it may be inferred that in hemiplegia the morbid change takes place at or near the origin of the motor fibres ; but the evidence of other kinds of paralysis would show that this is not a necessary part of the phenomenon.

reason would suggest a doubt whether the same treatment can be desirable immediately before, and after a stroke of palsy. I do not mean to give this the weight of an argument. From the nature of the circumstances, it is extremely difficult to bring unequivocal proof on the subject; but there is much cause to believe that the practice of bleeding in the latter case is often injuriously pursued. The risk, I believe, will generally be less from waiting a certain time,—to observe the effect of what has occurred upon the circulation, the breathing, and the sensibility,—than from hastily taking away blood, at the moment of a great shock to the brain, and before we can rightly appreciate its consequences. This effect upon the greater functions of life gives us in fact the best information we can have in guidance of further practice. But this we forfeit in great part, by the disturbance any large depletion makes in the system, and particularly in the organs upon which these functions depend. The practical importance of this consideration may readily be understood.

Even where evidence is obtained of the fitness of bleeding soon after one paralytic attack, for the prevention of another, the question still remains as to the manner of this,—whether by copious depletion at once, or by smaller bleedings, repeated as observation may suggest. And this question the practitioner, while prepared for boldness in all fit and urgent cases, is bound always to keep before him; seeing especially that any great excess in the remedy may hurry on the very mischief it is sought to prevent. I believe that in most cases the latter method is to be preferred. It accords better with the state of our knowledge of those disorders; involves no irretrievable step; and in its progress affords the information most requisite to decide how far it should be carried into effect. Paralytic cases there presumably are of such nature, that a few ounces of blood taken away at regular intervals will ward off a recurrence of the attack, which any large and sudden depletion would probably hurry on. The proof here can seldom be explicit; but the presumption is one I have often been led to entertain.

These remarks, and the cautions they suggest, are familiar to many, and to such needless. But I feel assured, from what I have seen, that they ought to be carried further into general practice. The use of the lancet is easy, and gives a show of activity in the practitioner at moments when there appears peculiar need of this promptitude. Current opinions and prejudices are wholly on the side of bleeding; and the complexity and danger of the cases tend to obscure the results of the treatment pursued. The physician needs all his firmness to decline a practice thus called for; where the event is so doubtful, and where death may be charged upon his presumed feebleness or neglect.

While making these remarks, however, I must be understood as recognising, in the fullest sense, the value and need of this remedy, promptly and vigorously used, in various cerebral diseases, or in prevention of such, where well-marked symptoms lead to their anticipation. And I dwell upon this the more earnestly, lest, while merely inculcating a cautious discrimination as to the cases for its use, I may seem to be seeking reasons against the practice altogether. In active inflammation of the brain or its membranes—in many states of pressure from congestion in the head, topical or general, without inflammation—in cases where extravasation may be presumed to be going on—and even in other conditions of cerebral irritation less definite than these, we have no method of treatment equally effectual; and safety often depends solely on the speed and sufficiency of its employment. But almost in the same ratio with the necessity of the remedy in the above cases is the importance of refraining from depletion in other instances, often with difficulty to be distinguished from the former. And, in the right direction of diagnosis and treatment here, we have the best proof that the mind of a practitioner is equal to the most difficult exigencies of his profession.*

There are one or two lesser points in the treatment of affections of the brain deserving more discrimination than they usually obtain. One of them is the general use of ice, or other cold applications, to the head. Any influence of cold, through its effect on the capillary vessels of the scalp, is at least ambiguous in these cases; and though its direct sedative effects on the nervous system may afford more certain warranty for the practice, yet these require to be distinguished and watched over in their progress. For even where relief is distinctly obtained from cold suddenly applied to the head, as after intoxication, it by no means follows that this application, long continued, will produce or maintain a like benefit. It is well known in various parts of practice how far it is otherwise; and that the effect of cold upon the circulation and nervous system is sometimes even reversed, according to the manner and amount in which it is applied. Or allowing, as I readily do, that there may be a distinct sedative effect from cold, beneficial in cases of inflammation of the brain or its membranes, will this equally apply to apoplectic cases, where pressure occurs from fulness of vessels or extravasation? If the relief to some kinds of headache be alleged, it must be remembered that other headaches are increased by this means. The same disparity doubtless exists as to the more serious affections of this organ, requiring discrimination wherever we can exercise it. Unfortunately these are cases in which generally patients can render least aid. Sometimes they are manifestly uneasy under the application of cold. Their feeling, whenever it can be ascertained, is better than any other test.

I believe that patients labouring under affections of the brain are too indiscriminately forced to a raised position of the head, with a view of lessening the flow of blood or congestion there. Such effect it undoubtedly has; and in many, perhaps most, of these cases

* There is great practical value in the writings of Dr. Marshall Hall on the principle and methods of bleeding in cerebral disorders.

it is a prudent precaution. Sometimes, however, it is employed
without any good to compensate for the discomfort thereby produced. And, further, there are many cases, like those already alluded
to, where the diminished energy of the brain seems to require a full
and equable circulation through it; and where the symptoms are
aggravated by the compulsion of a raised posture. The effect of
sudden recumbency in relieving faintness is a familiar illustration of
this; and conversely, the vertigo which frequently occurs, especially
in a weakened state of body, upon suddenly rising from a couch.
Headache moreover in some instances is brought on, or much augmented, by the upright posture, and subsides when this is changed.
In general we may gather from observation which position of the
head is best—by the colour of the face, by the state of breathing,
and by the action of the heart or other functions, if the patient be
unable to express his own sensations. Perhaps altogether the respiration is the most certain test we can employ in the absence of the
latter.

Bleeding by leeches from the hemorrhoidal vessels might be much
more frequently employed than it is in affections of the brain, as
well as in those of the spinal cord. I know no mode in which a
given quantity of blood can be removed with equal effect in the
cases where this is required. It may be difficult to give strict
anatomical reasons why this should be so; but what we know on
the curious subject of the changes of balance in circulation will
furnish at least illustration of it. And we have especial argument
for the practice, in the frequent alternation of bleeding hemorrhoids
with headaches, and other graver affections of the head; and also
in the serious effects which sometimes ensue upon the suspension of
such discharge, after it has long been habitual to the system.*

In the foregoing remarks, particularly those which relate to bleeding in affections of the brain, I have spoken of these disorders in a
way which may seem too general and vague for practical purposes.
In explanation of this, I would make one or two remarks. In the
first place, I think the object likely to be best fulfilled, of deterring
from indiscriminate bleeding, by broadly pointing out the great
practical disparity of certain conditions of the brain, which have
some appearances in common; and which even produce (though
doubtless in different way) some similar effects upon other parts of
the body. The attention of the practitioner, if well awake to this
distinction, will rescue him from a blind adherence to the one
method of instant treatment, so generally in use. It will further
direct him to those special indications,—whether derived from the
general habit of the patient, from the action of the heart and arteries,
from the respiration, or from change in the functions of the brain
itself,—which may give better and safer guidance to his practice.

* Dr. Prichard's proposal for the application of pea-issues along the whole
course of the sagittal suture, is deserving much attention, in cases where we
seek to obtain the closest and most effective access for counter-irritation to
the brain.

Secondly, while fully admitting the value of what has been written on diseases of the brain, and the great advances recently made to their better classification, I can scarcely think the latter object to be yet duly attained.* This remark applies alike to the diseases depending on inflammation of the brain and its membranes; on altered circulation in the organ from other causes; or on extravasation or effusion within the cavity of the cranium. Still more expressly does it apply to lesions, general or partial, of the nervous substance itself. Here the difficulties of exact observation, and ignorance of the functions of particular parts, have hitherto precluded any such intimate knowledge as might furnish a basis for classification and treatment; and we are compelled rather to look to changes in vital condition, than to actual pathological states, in reasoning on the subject.† That there are diseased conditions of the nervous substance, more numerous and varied than those hitherto described, may well be admitted both from analogy and from notice of effects not easily referrible to any other cause. Nor can it be doubted that many of these will hereafter become known to us; the path for research being widely open, and the methods and instruments of inquiry much better fitted for success than heretofore.

Meanwhile, in this yet imperfect arrangement of cerebral disorders, there is cause for treating of bleeding as a general question of practice, even without express reference to the forms of particular disease. And, from the difficulty as well as importance of this question, it is better perhaps that the medical man should have it constantly before him in this light, than that his judgment should be submitted to rules and nosological distinctions, the application of which to actual disease involves almost as great risk of error as he can incur in proceeding without these technical aids.

* It is impossible not to advert here to the valuable work of Dr. Abercrombie, which has done so much towards a right arrangement of these difficult and important diseases. Also to Dr. Bright's Treatise on Diseases of the Brain and Nervous System, (vol. ii. of his Medical Reports,) in which a very good basis of classification is proposed and followed. And, further, to the Memoir on Injuries of the Brain and its Membranes, by Sir B. Brodie, in vol. xiv. of the Med. Chirurg. Transactions.

† I may instance the question, still undecided, whether the state of *ramollissement* of the brain can ever occur without preceding inflammation. Dr. Abercrombie's opinion, that there are two distinct causes of this state, is probably that nearest the truth. The difficulty of obtaining unequivocal proof in these cases is hardly to be understood by those who do not know them on experience. The diagnosis in lesions of the brain is not aided by those external physical signs which have lately obtained such invaluable application to diseases of the chest.

CHAPTER IV.

ON SUDORIFIC MEDICINES.

It must have occurred to the observation of most practitioners, that, of the direct evacuant remedies, sudorifics are amongst those which can least be depended upon; and this even in cases where natural perspiration is one of the symptoms statedly present. It will, I think, be further admitted, that perspiration produced by artificial means rarely corresponds, in the degree of benefit obtained, with that occurring from natural causes:—and, further, that it is a class of remedies where discrimination of effect is singularly vague as regards the several medicines so denominated. These indeed are points which different observers will differently estimate; yet I believe the facts will be so far allowed, as to give some interest to a consideration of their cause.

Does not this uncertainty chiefly depend on mistaken views of perspiration, as a part and symptom of disease? In general opinion, it seems to be regarded as an active cause of change, and usually of amendment, in the existing disorder; and practice is founded for the most part upon this impression. May it not more justly be considered as effect and proof of such change taking place; frequently beneficial in kind, but by no means invariably so? The distinction is obviously important; inasmuch as it involves the question, how far, and by what means, this action is to be sought for as a direct object in the treatment of disease.

In their employment of sudorific remedies, physicians at all times have manifestly dwelt much on the fact, that many disordered actions, and especially those of the simple febrile paroxysm, and certain of the phlegmasiæ, are suspended in immediate sequel to natural sweating. Proofs as to this mode of inference might be largely drawn from medical writers, were it necessary; nor is the reasoning devoid of plausibility. Setting aside all question of peccant humours, and obvious and general evacuation from the body, followed by mitigation of disorder, is a fact in pathology which could never escape notice, and might readily suggest the idea of like advantage from perspiration artificially obtained. Nevertheless, there is great cause to doubt the justness or extent of this inference, and the propriety of much of the practice founded upon it.

In this inquiry, it is needful first to be considered, how far the natural action, which it has been sought to imitate, is really remedial in kind. It would advance us very little here to enter into the various theories as to the functions of the capillaries and exhalant vessels. The probable statement seems to be, that what is termed perspiration in the widest sense involves two separate processes—one a mere physical act of simple evaporation of moisture from the sur-face,—the other an act of specific secretion by vital power, and affected therefore expressly by the various states of the circulation and nervous system. The latter is that with which we are here concerned: and, looking to the character of this function, it must be admitted as not impossible that what are called critical sweats. may be really the cause of the relief which ensues upon them. But this admission by no means proves the fact to be so; and there are various presumptions, more or less strong, which may be brought against it.

First, the occurrence, often observed, of similar and equal relief under the same course of previous symptoms, without intervening perspiration. This will be familiar to all who are accustomed to note the phenomena of fever. Here remissions or intermissions take place; always, no doubt, with an altered state of the vessels of the skin, but often with little or no actual perspiration succeeding to the hot stage. Even in the simple paroxysm of ague, which affords the best case for the inference now in question, this absence of a distinct sweating stage is occasionally observed ; in other forms of fever, idiopathic or symptomatic, much more frequently. It may be difficult to say, why this resolution of fever or inflammation should occur in some cases with copious perspiration, in others with little or none. But, the fact being so, it is safer and probably more correct to regard the sweating stage or critical sweat, when it hap-pens, as one in the series of changes constituting fever, rather than as the cause of the relief to symptoms that ensues.

The second point I would advert to is, the frequent occurrence of natural perspiration in morbid states of the body, without any such relief, and sometimes with aggravation of disorder. Proofs of this may be drawn from common experience in continued fevers, pneumonia, acute rheumatism, and various other diseases attended with fever, where profuse or long-continued sweating often occurs, with doubtful benefit or even manifest disadvantage to the patient.* The perspirations in hectic fever, though marking the several pe-riods of remission, yet augment the distress of the patient, and in-crease his weakness. In the fever attending the epidemic influenzas, the more general state of the skin is that of a clammy perspiration, manifestly not producing any remission of the symptoms. Even in the exanthematous fevers, where it might be inferred from the eruptive symptoms that diaphoresis would be more uniformly bene-ficial, and a legitimate object of treatment, cases constantly happen where natural sweating is attended with no obvious good; and where the attempt to force it out by medicines or other means is dis-tinctly injurious to the patient.

* The remark of Hippocrates is warranted by fact, ιδρως πολυς αμα πυρετοισιν οξεσι γιγνομενος φλαυρον. And elsewhere, καν πυρετοισιν ιδρως επιγενηται, μη εκλειποντος του πυρετου, κακον. These are among the numerous prognostics which he derives from perspiration, as a symptom in the course of disease, and an ex-ponent of changes taking place in the body.

Many other instances will occur, more or less directly, in illustration of the same point. In those complaints usually termed bilious, and where there is accumulation, or disordered change of secretion, in the digestive organs, perspirations break out often and copiously, without any relief to the system. The same happens in various disorders of the alimentary canal; an effect of the intimate sympathy between this great internal membrane and the surface of the body. A tendency to perspiration is the consequence of purging in an excess; as indeed of all causes which, even without fever, tend to debilitate the body. These instances, though less determinate than those of simple and symptomatic fever, yet illustrate the same general view. If perspiration be regarded as an index of the change of symptoms, rather than as the cause of such change, it may be expected to occur in many cases, where it does not indicate any favourable alteration, and where in fact none such takes place.

Looking indeed to the various circumstances under which this symptom appears, we have reason to infer that the state of the exhalant vessels producing it is not a single and uniform one; but that at least two, possibly more, conditions are necessary to explain the different manner in which perspirable matter is thrown off. I doubt whether sufficient inquiry has been directed to this point. It seems probable that one of these states may be simple relaxation of the vessels; the reverse of that which exists during the hot stage of fever, and indicating therefore a more entire removal of the febrile state,—another, a forced and active state of the same vessels, by which fluid is thrown out, but with little diminution of heat or febrile symptoms. Other causes of variation might be conjectured, to explain these differences of effect, as well as the phenomena of partial sweats, indicating some unequal pressure on the vessels in different parts of the body.* Without attaching much weight to these explanations, it is certain that perspiration differs as respects the state of the vessels, and also as to the nature of the matter perspired,—the latter variation probably depending on the former in most cases; though there may be others where the reverse is true, and where the condition of the blood in the extreme vessels may determine the state of the orifices through which exhalation takes place. On this subject I have made some observations, but they need to be extended and confirmed before I can state them in distinct shape.

Recurring, however, to the question of sudorifics as a remedy, it may be alleged that something is due both to the quantity of perspirable matter thrown off by the skin, and to the quality of this, as ridding the blood of superfluous or noxious ingredients. It cannot be denied that there may be influence from these causes. But the little proportion in many cases between the amount of perspiration

---

* The ancient physicians attached more importance than we do to the "sudores non per totum corpus æquales," as a bad symptom in disease. They are connected, doubtless, with the same general causes which produce local determinations of blood, and variations of vascular action, in different parts of the body.

and the degree of relief attending the remission of fever, and the frequency of copious perspiration without any relief at all, proves that this at least is only partial and accessory. As respects the latter circumstance, viz., the nature of the matter thrown off, it offers undoubtedly a question of greater difficulty. We have not yet sufficient knowledge of the varieties of this, especially under morbid conditions of the body, to be entitled to deny the influence of such changes; and the researches which show that a function analogous to that of respiration is exercised by the skin, and varied by disease, make it probable that, in perspiration, the excretion of carbon through this channel may be considerably increased in amount.* Still it is very doubtful whether these presumed changes of quality in the matter perspired can have much effect on the course and character of disease; seeing that perspiration is one of the least constant symptoms, even where usually present, and that the relation is very uncertain between its amount and the relief that ensues.

The presumed influence of perspiration in reducing animal heat admits of the same general remarks. Even admitting that there is no doubt as to priority in the order of occurrence, the frequent continuance of morbid heat under excessive perspiration shows that there is no certain ratio between the two symptoms, and lessens the value of this relation to the purposes of practice.

Looking cursorily to medical history on the subject before us, it would appear that the use of internal sudorific medicines was comparatively infrequent among the Greek and Roman physicians. Collecting the passages in Hippocrates which relate to this point, I doubt not that Dr. Freind was justified in believing, that by this great physician sweating was regarded much more as a prognostic sign than as an instrument of cure.† The practice, even if originating earlier, gained ground chiefly in the middle ages; was extended by the larger introduction of chemical medicines into the Pharmacopoeias; and naturally allied itself with the humoral pathology, and the notion of expelling peccant matters from the body. It is well known how far the custom was carried, at a period not distant from our own, of forcing perspiration by external heat, confined air, and stimulating sudorifics; and this more especially in fevers and exanthematous disorders. No more beneficial change has occurred in modern practice than the abandonment of these methods; nor any more conspicuous in its effects on the rate of

---

* The experiments of Dr. Edwards on the Batrachians with soft skins show to what extent this function, resembling respiration, may take place through the cutaneous vessels; and confirm the observations which had before been made on the human body. From the researches of the same eminent physiologist, as well as the anatomical observations of Breschet on the skin, we are entitled to infer a distinction in quality of ingredients between perspiration by secretion and the simple moisture which is evaporated from the surface of the skin.

† Etenim sudor perpetuò apud Hippocratem non ut curandi instrumentum, sed tantum ut præsagii nota præponitur.—*Comment. Novem de Febribus, Londin.* 1717.

mortality in disease. Yet we have cause to ask whether there be not still too much influence from this source! supported as it is by popular prejudices, and by maxims transmitted from one generation to another. The excitement of perspiration is still often made a direct object of treatment in cases where, even when not injurious, it has little value except as an exponent of the state of other symptoms.

Nor indeed can we draw this inference equally from perspiration artificially obtained as from that of natural occurrence. In many diseases, perhaps more than our medical philosophy has hitherto dreamt of, there is much mischief done by forcibly disturbing and altering the train of symptoms which forms the wonted course of the disease. No point is more difficult in the theory of medicine, none which puts to closer test the practical judgment of the physician, than the knowledge where boldly to break into, or cut short, the course of a malady,—where to confine the treatment to such means as may simply mitigate the symptoms, obviate any irregularity in their course, or prevent injury to particular organs. The question is one which has had influence, more or less direct, upon medicine and medical schools in every age. In some diseases there can be no reasonable doubt which of the respective plans should be pursued. But even in these more marked cases there is need of greater discrimination than is usually employed; and to the young practitioner, more especially, it is often matter of much difficulty, not only to form his judgment, but to carry this judgment into action. A firmness is required from him, which may show itself in boldness and vigour, when these are needed; and no less in forbearance (whatever the solicitations to the contrary), when a disease is pursuing its course mildly, and without any unwonted symptoms.

This forbearance, often the most difficult virtue, may fairly be inculcated as to the use of sudorific means, at those periods of diseases of definite course where sweating does not generally or naturally occur. The attempt to force it at such times, even if successful, is a very dubious benefit; and under many methods of treatment for this purpose becomes a very positive injury. The effect in question, however, is by no means so easily obtained as we commonly suppose. The perspiration attributed to medicines employed is very often a symptom in the natural progress of the malady, or depending on other causes in the animal economy. We have, for instance, every reason from direct observation to conclude that the state of sleep, as such, tends to increase perspiration, separately from all influence of other agents. I doubt not that the diaphoretic medicine often obtains for itself the credit of an effect due chiefly to this cause. Even where more obviously the result of internal remedies, it would seem that these are effectual in the greater number of cases, rather by abating fever, and changing the course of actions in the system, than by direct influence on the exhalant vessels.

The employment of sudorifics may indeed be regarded, on the

whole, as less determined by method or reasonable experience than that of other evacuant remedies; and every candid physician will admit his frequent disappointment in this part of the treatment of disease. The doubtful views on which their general use is founded, will best explain the uncertain effects of the particular medicines brought under this class. The antimonial preparations, though so largely employed from their presumed action on the skin, may nevertheless be noted in proof of this. There is reason to suppose that their beneficial effect in fevers and inflammations is mainly owing to the influence they have in diminishing the force of circulation, and thereby lessening the febrile action, which prevents secretion from the surfaces as well as from the glandular textures of the body. And their employment is generally more successful in proportion as this principle is kept in view, and the act of perspiration regarded as an effect of secondary kind.

The reputation of James's Powder as a diaphoretic may have depended in part on this sedative action upon the circulation; but still more, as I believe, upon the sweating regimen employed together with it. The comparative neglect of this regimen, as well as the smaller and less frequent doses of the medicine now used, will explain its lesser efficacy in modern practice, of which we often hear complaint. There is much reason, further, to presume that its value was always rated too high.

The latter remark will apply to the general use of antimonials in cutaneous disorders, where a direct effect on the skin is sought for. A fair estimate of the evidence here will lead to reasonable doubt whether this practice is ever of much avail. The proofs indeed are usually so far obscured by the conjunction of other means that little can be securely gathered from them.

With respect to the stimulating sudorifics, as they have been termed, it may fairly be presumed that most of them act as such only by exciting a certain degree of febrile action, followed by relaxation of the exhalants—a doubtful benefit in any case, and often a certain source of mischief. Sydenham strongly reprehends this practice as it existed in his time; and other physicians have, at succeeding periods, repeated his censure. Yet even now it cannot be said to be wholly discarded.

Of the various internal means for obtaining diaphoresis, I believe that opium, in one or other of its forms, is the most uniformly certain and beneficial. Its action, in conformity with the views just stated, may be considered to depend on its power of allaying inordinate circulation, or other excitement of the system. This opinion is justified, as well by the other effects of opium as by the similar influence of various narcotics on the state of the skin.

I allude more especially to opium as a diaphoretic, because I believe that in our modern practice we too much neglect the various and beneficial resources afforded by this medicine. Its action in this way probably depends chiefly on its power of allaying excitement of the vascular system. Whatever be thought of Lind's re-

commendation of opium in the hot stage of ague, it is certain that
in various states of fever and inflammatory disorder, where preceded by sufficient evacuations, no medicine can be more safely
used as a sudorific, or with greater collateral advantages.   This is
strongly urged by Dr. Freind, in the third of his Commentaries on
Hippocrates ; to which I further refer, as containing some excellent
observations on the sudorific plan of treatment in fevers — one of
the earliest efforts to change the opinions before held on this part
of practice.

I have spoken elsewhere of the use of simple diluents as a means
of · exciting perspiration, too much neglected in modern English
practice.   The influence of blood-letting in producing the same
effect doubtless arises from its diminishing what may be called, in
default of a better term, the tension of the general circulation, and
thereby relaxing the vessels of the skin and other surfaces.   Here
then, also, while admitting that some benefit may be derived from
the perspirable matter thrown off, we must regard the act of perspiration principally as an index of the favourable change taking
place in the vascular system at large.

Limiting these remarks, however, chiefly to sudorifics of internal
use, I say nothing of the various external means employed to the
same end; even though they might illustrate in many points the
views already stated.   Nor do I propose here to apply these views
to particular cases of disease.   My object is merely to offer suggestions which may tend to render our notions on the subject more
simple and precise: and I venture to lay down the following posi-
tions as founded on sufficient evidence : —

First, that it is more reasonable, as well as beneficial in practice,
to have regard to the changes in the circulation producing diaphoresis than to the action of sweating itself.   And, secondly, that
the amount of perspiration is rarely a just measure of the good obtained ; and that to make this a primary object is likely to give a
wrong and injurious bias to the treatment of disease.

It may be alleged that these are needless refinements of principle,
not required by the present state of medicine among us: and I
willingly admit that there has been in this instance a greater
change in actual practice than in the general views upon which it
is professedly founded.   It was impossible, with increasing exactness of observation, to escape the conviction that in febrile and inflammatory disorders the direct cooling methods of treatment are
the safest and most beneficial ; and these accordingly have been
gaining ground to the exclusion of such as were previously in
common use.   Still there remains something to be done to render
this change more general and complete.   And yet further, it is of
importance to give stability to all such practical results, by fixing
them upon principles which cannot be changed with the fashions
that affect particular medicines or methods of treatment.

commonly recognised as produced by disorder of the sensorium upon the animal and vital organs.

If immediately after an attack of cramp, the attention be kept fixed on the limb so affected, a tendency will be felt to renewal of the spasm; and sometimes it will actually recur from this continued excitement to the part.

I have known asthmatic patients in whom a certain degree of this affection was generally brought on by seeing others suffering under the same disorder—a fact analogous to the act of yawning, already mentioned. And another more singular case is that of an expected impression on some part of the body, producing, before actually made, sympathetic sensations or movements in other parts which are wont to be thus affected by the impressions in question.* These instances, while involving other curious points in physiology, illustrate the dependence of such morbid sympathies, and acts of imitation, on the more general principle which forms the subject before us.

If now, dispensing with other examples, we come to the examination of this principle in our constitution, many perplexities occur at the outset; nor is it paradoxical to say that some of these depend on the familiarity of the subject. It may appear little better than a truism to affirm, that the attention of the mind directed to any particular part makes us conscious of sensations derived from it, more distinct in kind or augmented in degree. While the close connexion between this act or faculty of attention, and the whole class of mental emotions, offers a ready analogy for the many cases where parts of functions are manifestly disturbed by the mind thus directed to them.

Analogy, however, is here not explanation. And the seeming familiarity of the subject depends on this agency being so entirely incorporated with our existence—so integral a part of the mind in its relation to the bodily organs—that all proof or reasoning upon it appears superfluous. Yet looking to this very fact, how much is there to be inquired regarding a faculty thus remarkable,—by which, under the action of will, the mental consciousness is directed to separate portions of the body; individualizing itself, as it were, with the part; and not merely augmenting the sensations thence derived, but affecting more or less for the time its actual state and functions. The latter is obviously the point of greatest moment in the question: because if showing, as I have sought in many instances to do, that the physical state or action of a part is altered from this cause, the ambiguity is removed which belongs to the supposition of altered sensation alone. As far as I am aware, the subject has not been sufficiently examined under this view; though in the various forms

* An example occurs to me at this moment where the expectation of any strong pressure of the hand instantly creates uneasiness, approaching to pain, in the perinæum; this effect in greater degree invariably following actual pressure.

which the theory of a vital principle has taken, we have proof of the influence of these facts upon the course of speculation.*

The difficulties of language, which surround all topics of this nature, beset us here in many points; and even the term of *consciousness*, though more precise than most others, has its ambiguity, as applied respectively to the operations of thought and emotion, where it is the index of personal identity; and to the relations of mind and body, where it is difficult to separate it from the very acts themselves in which these relations consist. All writings on the subject give proof how hard it is to define that, which, though real in itself, blends its reality in one way or other with every part of our existence. The term *sensation* has yet more especially been exposed to ambiguous and widely different uses, and with still greater injury to all sound reasoning and results. This indeed is one of the points where we tread on the very confines of the knowledge possible to man; light and darkness mingling so strangely, that we seem ever to be obtaining glimpses along avenues, which are speedily closed by impenetrable obscurity.

The most explicit manner of pursuing the inquiry seems to be through the question, whether any physical explanation can be found for the phenomena? whether that transference of consciousness by volition to particular parts, which we have called attention of mind, takes place through some branch of the nervous system, as volitions are conveyed to the muscular organs? or whether, in default of proof to this effect, our inquiries must end as they begun, by simply recognising that essential relation of the sensorium to every part of the body, which forms the individuality of the whole being?

There is one consideration, principally, which makes it almost certain that a function of the nerves is concerned in the results before us. This is the fact (a very important one in physiology) that the peculiar relation of the mind to the bodily organs, of which we are treating, is not alike or equal in degree to all parts; but that it seems to exist for each in some proportion to its nervous sensibility, or perhaps also to its vascularity in the healthy state:—and, still further, that the attention, strongly concentrated on one part,

---

* The *Archæus* of Van Helmont, and the *Anima* of Stahl, (as well as the πνευματα of Galen and earlier writers,) have reference to the agency which is the subject of this chapter. It is obvious that each author sought by such phrases to express an active immaterial principle, producing and controlling the actions of the system, by an operation neither chemical nor mechanical, but in fact identical with life itself. It was the need and effort to find something intervening between mind and body,—some middle agency that might give a show of explanation of the actions of the former upon the latter,—which suggested these terms, and gave a sort of reality to them. In sound reasoning, it is plain that we acquire only new names by their adoption, and no increase of real knowledge.

" There is a connexion of the living principle in the powers of one part with those of another, which may be called a species of intelligence." This is a happy expression of John Hunter, applicable here and to many other questions in this part of physiology.—*Croonian Lecture on Muscular Motion.*

precludes for the moment any similar effort being exercised towards another. Admitting these circumstances as founded on observation, they lead directly to the inference that the nerves are in some manner excited by the act of attention, and that all particular and local effects on the body are produced through their agency.

Upon this conclusion, however, rises another question equally difficult, viz., with what other function of the nerves this action is most closely allied, and through what class of nerves it is carried on ? Those of voluntary motion can scarcely be admitted, seeing that motion in this sense is no part of the effect, and that the influence extends to parts over which we have little or no voluntary power. The only employment of will here is in giving this partial direction to the consciousness. If, on the other hand, we suppose the nerves of sensation concerned, we must admit two several actions in opposite direction along the same tract of nerve; a condition of which we have no well-assured proof. In neither of these functions therefore, nor in the nerves ministering to them, can we find any sure explanation of the phenomenon before us, though it has various and close relation to both, as they mutually have to each other.

In considering this intricate subject, it is impossible not to advert again to the connexion between attention, as a state of mind, and the whole class of mental emotions; a relation the more important to be noticed, because it is testified to us by many similar effects of both on the bodily organs, and may afford therefore some presumption that the same nervous agency is concerned in each case. An examination of individual consciousness will afford the best proof as to this relation. The difficulty in following it out, and that which makes it obviously needful to discriminate between the two cases, is the explicit power of the will in directing the attention of mind to particular parts. A faculty exists here distinct from mental emotion, though variously complicated with it, and especially in those instances where the attention is strongly excited by sensations derived from any organ. As a power it is equally definite as that by which we change or give direction to the trains of thought, and indeed closely allied to it in many respects.

Reverting to the question, whether there be any especial nervous action by which we thus direct the attention of mind to different organs ?—and if any, what are the nerves engaged in it?—the admission must be made that we are not furnished with any means to solve the difficulty. I have tried to obtain proof in cases where there was palsy either of the nerves of sensation or of voluntary motion. But though some of the results seemed to show loss or enfeeblement of the power, particularly in the first class of cases, there was too much ambiguity from other sources to admit of certain inference. The effects upon the circulation of a part, from the consciousness thus directed to it, appear so immediate, that we might perhaps suppose the nerves belonging appropriately to the vascular system to be engaged in producing them. But, in truth, the difficulty here is one which extends largely over all that relates to the functions of the nervous system. Scarcely yet have all its parts been defined in reference to the two great functions of sensation and volition; while the ganglionic system, and the various nerves of organic life, are still only partially known to us in their proper actions, and yet more obscurely in their intricate connexions with the nervous powers of animal life.

The physiological fact treated of in this chapter has close relation to the faculty the mind possesses, of withdrawing itself wholly or partially from objects of sense, which yet physically impress the external organs in the same way as when fully perceived:—shifting itself to other sensations, sometimes by direct effort of the will, sometimes in effect of other causes. Every moment of life affords instances in illustration of this. We live indeed, it may be said, in a series of acts or states, each involving the exercise of some particular faculty or sense, to the exclusion more or less of others: but all so blended, and in such subordination to the identity of the being, that we are speedily at fault in seeking to divide or analyse the succession. I doubt, however, whether sufficient notice has been taken of the voluntary power the mind possesses, of separating and arranging anew objects equally and simultaneously present to the organs of sense. The phenomena both of vision and hearing offer perpetual examples of this sort of analysis of compound sensations. It is one of the bases of our intellectual existence, and well deserves all the research that can be made into its modifications.*

Every instance of this nature, and all the topics indeed of this chapter, are subordinate to the great inquiry regarding the relation of consciousness in the sentient being, to those functions of the different organs of sense, which connect this being with its own bodily organization and with the world without. This in truth is the fundamental mystery of animal life. The difficulty, as well as importance of the questions it involves, increase, as we rise from the simpler forms of existence to those where the intellectual and moral faculties are more fully developed. In man these phenomena take their most complex character; and the ever changing relation of individual consciousness in the sentient unity, to the different bodily and mental actions which form the totality of life, illustrates best, though it may not explain, the endless varieties and seeming anomalies of human existence. Instincts, habits, insanity, dreaming, somnambulism, and trance, all come within the scope of this principle; which points out, moreover, connexions among them, not equally to be understood in any other mode of viewing the subject.

* In such inquiry simple examples are the best. I am looking at this moment upon a paper of somewhat intricate pattern, covering the walls of the room. Though the pattern is one and the same, as received on the retina, yet, by special and separate acts of attention to the particular relations of its parts, I can divide it successively into three or more distinct patterns, each producing for the time a separate impression on the mind. A certain or even difficult effort, and some time also, are required for making the translation from one apparent pattern to another; and there is difficulty in retaining any one impression before the mind, so that it does not blend with, or pass into the others. Experiments of this kind may be variously combined and multiplied.

CHAPTER VI.

ON POINTS WHERE A PATIENT MAY JUDGE FOR HIMSELF.

WHAT are the circumstances in which the suggestions of the patient himself may safely or expediently be admitted in the treatment of disease? Every prudent physician will make himself aware of these, in as far as they can be reduced to anything like rule; and guide his practice more or less closely by them.

First,—the patient may almost always safely choose a temperature for himself; and inconvenience in most cases, positive harm in many, will be the effect of opposing that which he desires. His feeling here is rarely, if ever, that of theory; though too often contradicted by what is merely such. It represents in him a definite state of the body, in which the alteration of temperature desired is that best adapted for relief, and the test of its fitness usually found in the advantage resulting from the change. This rule may be taken as applicable to all fevers, even to those of the exanthematous kind; where, with an eruption on the skin, the balance between the outer and inner surfaces of the body, and the risk of repression, might seem, and actually are, of greatest importance. In whatever stage the eruption be, if the patient expressly seeks for a cooler atmosphere or cooling applications, they may be fully conceded to him, without fear of ill result; and,under the guidance chiefly of his feelings as to the time during which their use may be continued. Except in some cases of vitiated sensation from nervous disease, I have scarcely ever known the judgment of a patient practically wrong on these points; and in this case of exception the error itself is of very little consequence.

Secondly,—in the majority of instances of actual illness, provided the real feelings of the patient can be ascertained, his desires as to food and drink may safely be complied with. Whatever be the physical causes of the relation (and·they are yet beyond our research), the stomach itself is the best expounder of the general and more urgent wants of the system in this particular. But undoubtedly much care is needful that we be not deceived as to the state of the appetites, by what is merely habit or wrong impression on the part of the patient, or the effect of the solicitation of others. This class of sensations is much more nurtured out of the course of nature than are those which relate to the temperature of the body. The mind too becomes much more deeply engaged·with them: and though in acute illness they are generally submitted again to the natural law, there are many lesser cases where enough remains of the leaven of habit to render every precaution needful. With such precautions, however, which every physician who can take schooling from experience will employ, the stomach of the patient becomes a valuable guide,—whether it dictate abstinence from or recurrence to food,—whether much or little in quantity,—whether what is solid or liquid—whether much drink or little,—whether things warm or cold,—whether sweet, acid, or saline,—whether bland or stimulating to the taste.*

As respects limitation of food, indeed, the "tempestiva abstinentia" is often with the patient himself an urgent suggestion of nature, especially in cases where fever is present. It is a part of the provision for cure which we hold in our hands ; and if not sufficiently regarded, all other remedies lose greatly of their value. Here, then, we are called upon to maintain the cause of the patient, for such it truly is, against the mistaken importunities which surround him, and which it sometimes requires much firmness to put aside.

It is not wholly paradoxical to say that we are authorized to give greatest heed to the stomach, when it suggests some seeming extravagance of diet. It may be that this is a mere depravation of the sense of taste; but frequently it expresses an actual need of the stomach, either in aid of its own functions, or, indirectly, under the mysterious law just referred to, for the effecting of changes in the whole mass of blood. It is a good practical rule in such cases to withhold assent, till we find, after a certain lapse of time, that the same desire continues or strongly recurs; in which case it may generally be taken as an index of the fitness of the thing desired for the actual state of the organs. In the early stage of recovery from long gastric fevers, I recollect many curious instances of such contrariety to all rule being acquiesced in, with manifest good to the patient. Dietetics must become a much more exact branch of knowledge, before we can be justified in opposing its maxims to the natural and repeated suggestions of the stomach, in state either of health or disease.†

These remarks, I am aware, may be liable to cavil in various ways. But restricting them, as I do at present, to the case of actual illness, and even then rather as a guidance than as a positive rule, I believe they will be found not merely admissible but useful in general practice.

Thirdly,—as regards exertion of body, posture, continuance in bed or otherwise, the sick may generally be allowed their own judgment, provided it is seen to be one dependent on bodily feelings alone. And so equally with respect to fresh air, methods of exercise, and times of repose. In these things, as on points of diet,

---

* There may seem some exception to be made for those cases, where urgent thirst gives the wish for liquids of a kind hurtful to the stomach. But it is the fluid alone which is the object of desire; and when the choice is before the patient at the moment, he will usually take that which most simply satisfies this natural want.

† Aretæus says judiciously, in a passage which applies to all parts of this subject, Εστω τοισι καμνουσι χαριτες, και το καθαρως απαν δραν, και τοισι επιθυμιησι επεσθαι τ ιατρον μη μεγαλα βλαπτοντα· αριστον γαρ τοδε, ην μη καρτα ωφελουντων οριξις ηκη.

suggestions, founded on careful notice of the feelings of the patient, and watchfulness as to the effect of the first trials, are all that is required from the physician; and more than this often does mischief. I have often witnessed the ill effects of minute interference in such matters; whether arising from excess of caution, or from the mischievous spirit of governing everything by medical rule and authority; without appeal to the feelings of the patient, even where these may securely be taken in evidence.

The most important exception to this rule is in certain nervous and dyspeptic disorders of chronic kind, where it is needful to urge bodily exertion upon the patient, in contradiction to his own sensations, and sometimes even where the first trials are seemingly unsuccessful. With moderate care in observation, the tests of fitness here are so simple that there can be little chance of any error leading to injurious consequences.

As respects mental exertion during illness or convalescence, much more caution is needful. Here the patient is usually less able to estimate his own power, and is more entirely at the discretion of those around him. The present condition of life among the higher classes produces as much of evil from excesses of moral and intellectual excitement, as from those of the stomach: and it is equally difficult to place watch and reasonable restraint upon them. In these instances, and they are of constant occurrence, the judgment of the physician, as well as firmness in his manner of interference, are urgently required. But in ordinary cases, and under more tranquil methods of life, he may leave much to the discretion and feeling of power in the patient himself; with simple injunction that this feeling should be duly consulted before any change is made.

Fourthly, The prudent physician, without sacrificing his science or authority, may often draw knowledge from his patient as to the fitness of particular medicines, or the fitness of employing medicines at all. Frequently it happens that the latter, at some period or other of his disorder, usually when convalescence has begun, expresses strongly his feeling that medicine will do no further good, and that his future progress is best left to nature alone. Provided it be clearly seen that this does not arise from any whim or perverseness of mind (and the feeling may exist wholly without such), the medical man is bound to give attention to it, as suggestion at least for his further treatment. And if continued and repeated, at a time when the urgent symptoms of disorder are past, it may for the most part be rightly acquiesced in,—certainly so far as to make trial of the effects of the change which, being of negative kind, can rarely produce much evil, even if it fail of good.

Looking fairly, indeed, at the common course of practice in this country, I believe more mischief to be done by needless protraction of the use of medicines, than by any premature abandonment of them;—a point, if true, requiring attention to all such means as may best contribute to its reform. And the case just stated is one

7*

of those where the practitioner may often effect this, in the way most conducive to the general welfare of his patient.

There are other instances, as mentioned above, where the persevering distaste to a particular medicine, or method of treatment, will not only sanction, but call for its disuse, though the authority of all ordinary experience be in its favour. On points of this kind a discreet forbearance is as needful to the physician as firmness. And the best rule is, not to be implicitly subservient to rule:—a maxim essential in all cases to the right practice of medicine, seeing the many contingencies which are ever arising in contradiction to its soundest methods and precepts.

CHAPTER VII.

ON THE CONNEXION OF CERTAIN DISEASES.

It will probably be one of the most certain results of future inquiry to associate together, by the connexion of causes of common kind, diseases now regarded as wholly distinct in their nature, and arranged as such in our systems of nosology. This remark applies very widely throughout all the genera of disease; but in no instance so singularly as to some of the disorders of contagious or epidemic kind; scarlatina, measles, booping-cough, erysipelas, the infantile fever, dysentery, epidemic catarrh or influenza, &c. Without affirming the *materies morbi* to be the same in any two of these disorders, —presuming it to be different in most of them,—and admitting the diversity of the symptoms,—yet relations there probably are, closer and more peculiar than any which have yet been ascertained, or made the basis of classification. And these are, without doubt, some of the most interesting objects of pathological research.

On the most general view of the subject, numerous conditions will be found capable of giving different aspect even to the effects of a common cause of disease. Season of the year; peculiar states of the atmosphere as to heat, moisture, weight, or electricity; circumstances of locality; the age of individuals exposed; their different temperaments; the influence of foregoing disease; the incidental direction of the morbid cause to some particular organ or texture of the body;* and still more the quantity or intensity of the virus

* An illustration of this occurs in the *glanders* and *button farcy* of horses; the virus being proved by inoculation to be nearly, if not wholly, identical; but affecting under the former name the lymphatics of the internal surface, under the latter those of the skin.

There is reason for the same inference as to the virus of hydrophobia; the variation in the effect of which on different animals may be presumed to depend, not merely on their diversity of habits, but also on the difference of parts more directly or more severely affected by this remarkable poison. The most exact observations we have on the subject are those by Dr. Wagner, in vol. i. of *Hecker's Annals*, 1836.

itself:—all these and other circumstances may be conceived as producing such modifications, and thereby concealing the common origin of many disorders. From this complication of conditions the difficulties of inquiry are considerable, but still of a nature to be overcome by future observation.

Referring more especially to the disorders mentioned above, does it not happen that measles, scarlatina, hooping-cough, and infantile fever, are often singular concurrent in particular districts, and about the same periods of time? And, as a variation of this fact equally illustrative, is it not common to find one of these disorders exceedingly prevalent in certain localities; while at the same time, in contiguous places, another of them equally prevails? Many instances to this effect come within my recollection; too strongly marked, as it seems to me, to be attributable to chance alone. Similar examples, more or less distinctly noted, are not uncommon in medical authors. If it be alleged that they prove only the influence of certain seasons and particular localities in evolving the virus of two or more of these diseases, or in creating a state of body favourable to their reception, still here are connexions which it is important to denote, and to follow into their several consequences.

Morton, as is well known, considered scarlatina and measles to be varieties of the same disorder. It would be difficult to establish this opinion by any proof; and the actual points of diversity are indeed insurmountable;—especially the negative fact, that one disease has never been known by infection to produce the other; and the certainty that the infectious matter of each, though equally unknown to all observation of the senses, has different properties in relation not only to the human body, but also to other media, which are concerned in communicating the disease. Even the uniformity with which each disease manifests itself on different portions of the same texture,—as the inflammation of measles on the mucous membrane of the air passages, that of scarlatina on the membranes of the pharynx,—furnishes proof of different origin; and not less the difference in the character of the attendant fever, and of the sequelæ of the two disorders. Yet still there are some relations which cannot escape notice; and which in fact lead to the occasional difficulty of discrimination, in the early stages, and in certain forms, of each disease. The case related in the subjoined note involves only a succession of the one malady to the other; yet this so singular, in having twice occurred under circumstances similar as to interval, as strongly to warrant the suspicion, that there was some state of constitution liable in common to both.*

* The remarkable case alluded to was that of Lord ——, who at the age of fifteen had the measles in the ordinary way, caught at a public school, when prevalent there. This was followed about two months afterwards by scarlet fever, with ulcerated throat; which went on in the usual course, leaving behind the most extensive anasarca over the body which I have ever seen in sequel to this disease—cured by bark and steel, with blue pill and diuretics. Two or three years afterwards, Lord ——, when at Berlin, had the measles a second time. The physician who attended him in that city, entertained no doubt as to the nature of the disorder. And what forms the extraordinary part of the case, this

I have observed repeatedly that, during the seasons in which influenza has occurred as a general and severe epidemic, these two diseases of scarlatina and measles have been more than usually frequent; though in no instance, perhaps, reaching the extent to which they occasionally occur at other times:—and further, that during the actual prevalence of influenza, a class of cases has appeared of very singular and ambiguous kind, having many appearances analogous to each of these disorders, but particularly, as I think, to scarlatina. I noticed frequent cases of this nature during the influenza of the spring of 1833, when the scarlet fever was also very prevalent, and produced much mortality in London. A peculiar spotted efflorescence on the skin, generally attended with some angina, and occasionally with slight ulceration of the throat, were the symptoms chiefly marking this apparent relation; which was sufficient in degree to suggest the question, whether it arose from the concurrent action of two morbid causes? or from one virus capable of producing different forms of disease, according to the texture on which it fell, or other less obvious circumstances?* If hazarding an opinion on this obscure subject, it would be in favour of the former view. Though we have many instances of such seeming incongruity of two diseases, that one present in the system precludes the ingress of the other, still there is no foundation for a general law to this effect. On the contrary, we have various proof that morbid actions, derived from sources wholly different, may coëxist in the body; severally modifying each other, though under conditions scarcely even surmised in our present knowledge.

Not less worthy of notice are those curiously anomalous cases, which occur in conjunction with scarlatina, when this disease is

attack of measles was followed again, after the interval of a few weeks, by scarlet fever, unequivocal in its symptoms, according to the information I received—with desquamation, but no anasarca following it. It seems impossible to suppose mere casual coincidence here; and I do not see any equivocal circumstance in the case, unless it be thought possible that what was deemed measles in each instance was merely an imperfect manifestation of scarlatina, followed by the more regular form of the disease.

* I have observed also many of these ambiguous cases during the yet more remarkable influenza prevailing while I write this note (Feb. 1837). In one singular instance, I traced something like a separate course of the two diseases in one family; two children having well marked scarlatina, with ulcerated throat, eruption, and desquamation, in a house filled with cases of influenza. It is worthy of note, that the symptoms of influenza in these children preceded those of scarlet fever by several days; and appeared distinctly to recur in succession to the latter, as a fresh seizure, after an interval of two or three days almost free from disorder. At the same time, two other children of the same family showed the ambiguous symptoms described above, and another child passed from the influenza into a fever, having the typhoid or adynamic type.

I add a further note here regarding the latest of these epidemics, that of the early part of 1838. Scarlatina was again very prevalent in London at the same time; and I noted several of the anomalous cases cited above, though less remarkable than those of former years; possibly because the influenza itself was less severe in degree. Sir G. Baker notices the tendency to angina and erratic efflorescence of the skin in the remarkable influenza of 1762.

prevailing alone. In close contact with distinct and violent instances of the disorder, we find others where the influence of the same virus is manifestly present, but where the symptoms are incompletely evolved; often so partially, as to wear every appearance of other and different disorders, and frequently to obtain wholly different names; yet, amidst all these anomalies, capable by diligent observation of being referred to a common cause. I shall have occasion to speak again on this curious subject of the incomplete development of disease from a virus of given kind, insufficiently received for complete effect, or acting on peculiar temperaments of body.

Erysipelas and erythematous inflammations are frequently found to prevail during particular seasons, and in certain localities; and with many common characters. Such are, the affection of internal membranes, the translation of the inflammation to the skin, the frequent presence of fever of low or typhoid type, and the influence of this state of habit upon all casual injuries or disorders of the body occurring at the time.* An example may be given in the sort of epidemic character which puerperal fever often takes, in seasons when erysipelas is very prevalent; rendering it probable that there are some causes in common to the local and constitutional disease; if not indeed the same morbid cause to both, modified in its action by the texture affected, and by the individual peculiarities of each case. The presumption, now rendered almost certain, that both puerperal fever, and erysipelas in its ordinary character, become contagious under certain circumstances of type, season, or locality (and these seemingly alike in different instances), may be admitted in further proof of such a relation.† And further, we have reason to believe that there is increased tendency to both disorders during the prevalence of epidemic influenza; as was well attested with regard to the puerperal fever in the spring of 1838.

The hooping-cough among children has also been singularly concurrent with some of the epidemics already mentioned; particularly, as I find in my notes, with the influenza, which spread so universally over England in the summer of 1831, immediately before the first appearance of the Asiatic cholera in this country: and again

* In a very valuable manuscript narrative, by Dr. Hillyar, of the cholera which prevailed on board the Caledonia, when cruising between Sicily and Malta in the autumn of 1837, I find a curious notice as to the peculiar tendency to erysipelas in this ship for several successive years: a fact agreeing with what is known to occur in particular hospitals and locations on shore, but more striking here from the still closer limitation of the circumstances. The Caledonia during this time always bore the repute of being a sickly ship; a larger proportion than usual of the crew suffering under any existing epidemic, and with erysipelas generally as a concomitant malady.

For some curious facts bearing on this subject, see Dr. Budd's paper on the cholera, as it appeared on board the Dreadnought Hospital Ship, in October, 1837:—Med. Chirurg. Trans. vol. xxi.

† This statement has very little to do with the disputes that have existed as to the nature and treatment of puerperal fever or peritonitis; further than in confirming the opinion that at certain times, and under particular circumstances, the inflammation present has a different character from that which exists at another.

very remarkably with the similar, though less severe epidemic, which prevailed in London during the spring of the present year (1838).—The cases were numerous at both these periods, in which, in children especially, it was scarcely possible to draw distinction between the two disorders; and difficult to avoid the persuasion that some cause was concerned, common to both.

The infantile remittent fever, in its various forms, has equally prevailed during the period of some of these influenzas; and in such close concurrence as to give strong suspicion of a relation more intimate than that of mere coincidence of time. It may be urged again that there is nothing more in these various cases than a state of season favouring the evolution of distinct disorders, which can coëxist, and perhaps blend with each other. But the connexion of symptoms between hooping-cough and the infantile fever goes beyond this; and points at some common or similar cause, modified in its effects by acting on different temperaments or different parts of texture. The hooping-cough rarely prevails as an epidemic without being conjoined with great frequency of those bowel disorders among children, attended with remittent fever, to which, in their more marked form, this name of infantile fever has been applied.—And, if objection be made that the one disorder is infectious, the other not, it may reasonably be asked whether the latter assumption is certain? whether the occasional infection in this fever is not proved as clearly as in erysipelas or dysentery? and whether the mode of proof is not the same as for hooping-cough itself? My own belief is, that no such ground of distinction can fairly be taken between the cases in question.

I have often had occasion to notice a fact further illustrative of the subject before us. This is, the singular frequency, especially · among children, of ulcerations or eruptions of the mouth, fauces, nose, lips, and face, at those periods when bowel disorders, whatever their cause, are peculiarly prevalent and severe. The uniformity of the connexion, as well as the frequent translation from one form of complaint to the other, leaves no doubt of the relation here; and we must necessarily look to a common cause of irritation or disorder, affecting different portions of a continuous texture; as determined either by idiosyncracy of the patient, or different application of the cause itself. That the one form does occasionally, under such circumstances of variation, become a complete substitute for the other, I can as little doubt as I do the frequent interchange of these morbid actions, even between the most remote parts of the alimentary canal.

Facts of this nature, it should be observed, do not subserve to medical theory only, but are capable of much more useful application to practice than is generally given to them. What we can see externally in some cases, may be taken, with certain allowance, as an index to the state of parts concealed from sight. If in a given epidemic we find many children having the throat and mouth beset with irritable sores, it becomes a reasonable suggestion that drastic or frequent purgatives are unfit for the more numerous cases, where the same disorder is shown by irritation, depraved secretions, or even by torpor of the intestinal canal. Mercurial alteratives may be admissible, or even expressly indicated ; but other objects of treatment are for the most part best attained by mild remedies and a proper regulation of food ; the latter, moreover, being regarded rather as a medicinal agent, than a means of nutrition to the system. I find this conclusion so generally justified in my own experience, that I cannot hesitate in recommending it as a valuable rule in practice.

It is probable as a general fact, (and, if true, a very important one,) that the disorders already mentioned, incidental chiefly to childhood, have virtual identity with certain fevers or other diseases of adult age; the operation of the causes varying according to circumstances, of which difference of age may readily be admitted as the chief.—Dysentery will here suggest itself as one of these kindred disorders. It has various relations to the infantile fever, in the course of the symptoms, in the textures affected, and in the morbid lesions consequent upon it ; and perhaps no differences beyond what are compatible with a common cause, acting under different conditions. It is further worthy of remark, in pursuing this series or circle of relations, that dysenteric symptoms are generally frequent at the same period as the diseases just mentioned, as well as during the seasons when the influenza has appeared in its most severe epidemic form. I find it remarked in the notes I made on these epidemics, that the dysenteric tendency, as well as other forms of bowel disorder, became much more frequent when the influenza, in its first and more obvious symptoms, might be said to have subsided.* It may admit of doubt whether this should be regarded as a translation of morbid action from the same original cause, or merely as an indirect and casual effect, to which the system became more liable from the previous disorder. Either supposition may be true ; but I think the former, on the whole, the more probable one.

This connexion between epidemic dysenteries and pestilential disorders has been noticed by many writers; and numerous instances have been recorded in proof it. The occurrence of dysentery in sequel to the latter has led to an opinion that may be produced in such cases. by morbid exhalations from dead bodies. Even were this view admissible in some instances, it certainly is not so in that of the epidemic influenzas, as we have known them in our own country: and here the dysentery following may more reasonably be attributed to one of the causes stated above.

In referring thus frequently to these epidemic influenzas, which have so frequently and widely prevailed of late years, I may add

* It is worthy of remark, that dysentery occurred in London as a severe and fatal epidemic, in 1762, during the three autumnal months, beginning only a few weeks after the cessation of the fatal influenza of the same year. Sir G. Baker, who has well described both, designates them as " duo morbi memorabiles, qui in eundem annum, hic veris, ille autumni soboles, inciderint."

that no class of diseases lays open to us a larger field of practical inquiry; as relates not only to their own nature, but also to the connexion of other diseases, with which they are closely associated. In a succeeding chapter I have spoken more at length on this subject. The simultaneous or rapidly successive influence of a common morbid cause over large communities and countries, discloses relations which in no other way are equally accessible to research. In showing the various forms which a single disease is capable of assuming, it illustrates the nature and action of the circumstances which thus modify it, and especially the effect of particular textures in altering the aspect of the symptoms. We have not yet sufficiently drawn from this source of knowledge. It is probable that we may hereafter learn from it the virtual identity of many diseases; hitherto placed asunder by distinctions, which have foundation only in subordinate symptoms, thereby disguising from us what is most important both in pathology and practice. Or, if no such identity be proved, we may find evidence, scarcely less curious, of an endemic state of constitution, (be it called adynamic, or by any other name,) which, originating with the same causes that produce the symptoms of influenza, renders the body for a period more prone than usual to certain other disorders, the material causes of which are ever more or less present. Each mode of viewing the subject is probably correct in part, and they are perfectly compatible with one another.

In further illustration of this topic, I may briefly notice the singular analogy to the milder forms of typhus, and of intermittent fever, which these epidemics have occasionally presented. It would seem, as I infer from my own observation, that the former, a typhoid type, prevailed most at the time when the virus of the disorder was in its greatest activity. There is cause also to believe, from the history of the disease in its whole course and spread, that this type was more common in some localities than others. It is further certain that some constitutions were peculiarly liable to be thus affected. The tendency to intermittent symptoms, both tertian and quotidian in type, and often very regular in period, seemed to me more common when the disorder was abating: and here too it was manifest that individual habit had much to do in determining the nature of the symptoms taking this character.[*]

The typhus fever itself, in the graver form which we now rarely see in English practice, as well as in those milder shapes to which such various names are applied, has its probable connexion with other diseases; and especially, as some recent authors have supposed, with the contagious exanthemata or eruptive fevers.[†] That

---

[*] Sir G. Baker describes the same intermittent type in the fevers attending the influenza of 1762.

[†] Dr. Roupell has described a form of fever which prevailed in the Grampus Hospital Ship, in 1831, under the name of the *febris typhodes rubeoloida*, from its being accompanied in almost every case by a rash like that of measles. A similar fever, though somewhat less marked in character, was very frequent in

the relation here is beyond that of mere casualty can scarcely be doubted. Whether inquiry begin with the exanthematous disorder, or with pure typhus, equally are we carried into certain common symptoms, sufficiently close in character, and frequent in occurrence, to justify the belief of some community of origin. From the true petechial eruptions, which have at all times marked more or less the severe forms of epidemic typhus, to the slight and fading exanthematous spots of common epidemic fevers, we have every grade by which to connect the eruptive tendency with the other symptoms most essential to the character of these diseases. We can scarcely indeed touch upon this subject of fever (particularly that which our present knowledge obliges us to consider of idiopathic kind), without finding in it a bond by which to associate together numerous forms of disease; but withal a knot so intricate, that no research has hitherto succeeded in unravelling it.

Looking to the great influence of the several conditions of idiosyncracy, season, and locality, in producing varieties of disorder from a common cause, as in the instances I have stated, it is impossible to doubt that the same principle of inquiry might be carried much further into the history of disease. Other conditions may be added, to which I have already shortly alluded; such especially as the varying intensity of any given virus, and its action upon different textures in different persons, or upon the same texture in different parts of the body. That all these modifying causes exists is certain on the most superficial view of the history of disease. Their influence in determining its course and aspects is no less distinct than important. In the influenza, as it prevailed successively in 1831, 1833, 1836, and 1837, the action of the virus was chiefly upon the mucous membranes of the respiratory passages and alimentary canal; the symptoms varying according to the various local direction of this morbid cause. It appeared to me certain in evidence, not merely that the virus affected primarily a different portion of these membranes in different persons; but also that many of the phenomena of the disease, in its progress and sequelæ, depended on the removal of this action from one part to another.

In variations such as these, we have the probable index to relations of disease of a simpler and more elementary kind, than those upon which our present systems of nosology are founded. For while admitting, as must be done, that the causes just cited do greatly modify the aspects of a disease in individual cases, (still leaving assurance of its identity with some epidemic prevailing at

London a few weeks after the greatest violence of the influenza in 1837; attended in numerous cases with the same anomalous eruption. Again, during the early months of 1838, and concurrently with, as well as subsequently to, the influenza then prevailing in London, the same character of low or adynamic fever existed to considerable extent and fatality; attended with eruption, sometimes of scarlet, more frequently of dusky red spots. Instances of this nature are very frequent in medical history, though not always related in their proper connexion.

the time,) is it not possible, or even probable, that a given material cause of disease may occasionally be so far modified in action by causes more largely operative, whether atmospheric or otherwise, as to assume the aspect of another epidemic, and to obtain separate name as such? This is the furthest point to which the speculation can be carried;—not sanctioned indeed to this extent by any direct evidence (for in our ignorance of the material causes it is very difficult to procure proof), yet plausible enough to warrant its being entertained as one of the questions open to research.

One step towards future success in these inquiries will be the relinquishment of the two exclusive attention hitherto given, even by physicians themselves, to the eruptive part of certain maladies; an error which has naturally arisen from the obvious nature of the symptom, and the more ready diagnosis it affords. I allude here especially to the contagious exanthemata: in which diseases, the common facts of a virus received,—of its maturation for a certain time within the system,—of symptomatic fever,—and of the translation of morbid action from internal to external parts,—though far from proving identity of cause, yet indicate a series of similar morbid changes, and actions analogous in their nature and progress, amongst the most important in the whole history of disease. The eruption here is not itself the disorder; but one only, and that not always the most critical, of the series of changes composing it. Every one who has noted the variety of anomalous symptoms which arise from scarlet fever imperfectly developed, or the disorders which often precede by a considerable time the appearance of erysipelas on the surface, will at once recognise the truth of this statement. It may seem needless to draw attention to these circumstances; and yet it is not wholly so. The influence of names and of early opinions is not easily overcome; and here, as elsewhere, they have effect in withdrawing us from that method of pursuit which is best fitted to lead to further knowledge.

In writing on this subject, I might refer to many eminent authors who have touched upon it in parts; and more especially in what regards the relation of fevers and pestilential or epidemic diseases. The foregoing remarks form, indeed, a mere outline of one portion of the inquiry, and must be considered as such. But it is that portion which is the most remarkable in itself; and through its connexion with idiopathic fevers, and with the general principle of contagion, having the largest and most intimate association with every other class of disease.

CHAPTER VIII.

ON THE ABUSE OF PURGATIVE MEDICINES.

In a preceding chapter I have spoken of the excess or indiscriminate use of bleeding in affections of the brain. I allude here to another instance, in which the use of a most important class of remedies is converted into a frequent abuse, by wrong and indiscriminate employment,—without due regard to the natural powers of the body in health, or to the peculiar course of morbid actions in disease. If asked whether the use of purgative medicines, beneficial beyond all others under certain conditions, is not carried too far in modern English practice, I must affirm my belief that it is so; and each successive year of experience strengthens this conviction. It may be noticed as one of those instances of fashion in medicine, so largely sanctioned by reason and experience as to last beyond the ordinary term of mere novelties, yet so far carried into excess, that the same reason requires much abatement of the abuse. Two or three works of merited reputation on this subject,—the success of antiphlogistic treatment in many diseases which had formerly been dealt with otherwise,—and especially the great benefit of purgatives, ascertained in certain cases where such treatment had before been deemed injurious,—all these circumstances concurred, about the same time, to give new reputation to this mode of practice. It may be added, that the simplicity of the treatment favoured its adoption by medical practitioners; while it had further countenance from the prejudices of the world, always prone to accredit a method from which there are obvious and speedy results, however doubtful the benefit thence derived.

We cannot wonder that fraudulent advantage should be taken by empirics of a feeling thus general, and so far sanctioned by the habits of more regular practice. And the mischiefs hence arising are, in fact, notoriously great. One form of purgative drugs succeeds another in noxious fashion; a fictitious need is created; and the functions of nature are injuriously supplanted, even under reputed health, by the compounds of quackery and fraud. This evil can be lessened only by reasonable employment of these medicines among the profession at large: and hence a further motive for weighing well what is really their use, and what their abuse, in our present practice.

One of the greatest abuses undoubtedly is the system of giving daily purgatives, and insisting upon daily evacuation; making this the habitual management in health, and treatment in disease. Under both conditions, it is a notion fertile in mischief. Looking first to that of health;—it is certain that the natural constitution of different persons is very various as to this point; and that to seek by medical means for anything like a common rule, is in most cases an absurd and injurious interference with the natural functions. The practice of habitual purgatives unhappily prevails most in the cases where default of natural action arises from torpor of the intestinal canal. Yet these cases, so frequent among the higher classes of society, ought especially to be exempt from the irritation of strong or frequent medicine. Dyspeptic symptoms, with increased torpor, are the more immediate effects; and disease frequently comes on as the sequel and consequence of a long continued habit.

The colon, perchance, cannot readily or quickly propel its contents, though the earlier stages of digestion are well and easily performed. To remedy this defect, it is goaded by the constant use of cathartics, which injuriously fret the stomach and long tract of bowels through which they have to pass before reaching this part. The habitual irritation of the mucous membrane alters and depraves its secretions throughout the whole course of the alimentary canal, becoming thereby a further source of mischief and suffering to the patient. These disordered secretions are too often urged in proof of the need of further evacuation (an error sometimes arising from inexperience, sometimes from a graver source); and thus the practice proceeds, in a vicious circle of habit, from which the patient is rarely extricated without more or less of injury to his future health.

It is not enough considered, either by physicians or patients, that a certain distension of part of this canal by solid contents is even necessary to its healthy state. It is probable that this is more especially true as respects the colon and rectum. I cannot doubt, from observation, that these bowels, even if not actually assuming diseased state from constant irritation of the mucous membrane, are often much injured in their functions by the want of equable and sufficient distension, which the habit of purging implies. Distension by air, which is the alternative, produces various irritation, and impedes the proper peristaltic motions.*

In effect of the causes of disorder cited above, the nutrition of the body generally suffers; the processes of digestion are imperfectly performed; the ingesta are hurried forward without the due amount of change and separation taking place; and there is usually decay of flesh and strength. The expressions of Celsus, quoted below, are common to all the ancient medical authorities, and founded on the observation of facts.†

The effect of sudden and violent diarrhœa in depressing the vital powers is well known. Syncope is a frequent consequence;—death, when there is already great exhaustion, an occasional one. I have seen instances where a strong purgative, given directly after a

---

* Το υποχωριον εστω σκληρον· πληθος δε κατα τα εισιοντα.—*Hippocrat. Prædic.*

† Purgationes, ut interdum necessariæ sunt, sic, ubi frequentes sunt, periculum afferunt. Assuescit enim non ali corpus; et ob hoc infirmum erit; cum omnibus morbis obnoxia maximè infirmitas erit.

severe and protracted operation, or after a shock to the nervous system from accident, has produced very urgent danger by aggravating the tendency to collapse. In cases where there is the habit of constant irritation by purgative medicines, the tendency of result is the same, though the immediate effects are less rapid and obvious. The extent of highly sensitive surface, forming the canal of the bowels, gives great scope to this influence; and few consequences can be stated more certain than the gradual undermining of the vital powers by the abuse in question.

Disordered action of the heart, whether depending on disease, or on mere irritability of the organ, is often much aggravated by the habitual use of purgatives. Not unfrequently I have known it produced by this cause in nervous or dyspeptic constitutions, where the relinquishment of the habit becomes the most effectual cure. Such effects are readily explained, not only from the flatulence and acrid secretions thereby produced in the stomach and bowels; but also from the unequal balance and sudden changes in the venous circulation of these viscera, which always attend purging, and which affect directly the regular transmission of blood to the right side of the heart;—and further, it may be, by an impression upon the nervous centres, producing that sudden sinking which I have already noticed as frequent under any inordinate action of the bowels. A discreet judgment is the more needful here, because there are other cases where disturbance of the heart is the effect of congestion about the liver and other chylopoietic viscera, requiring large evacuation for its relief.

Every physician must be familiar with the frequent confession of patients, even of those most wedded to the habit, that they feel better on those days when there is no action of the bowels. Of such avowal we are bound to take advantage, unless there are circumstances especially to prevent us. It is difficult, in truth, to find a footing for relief in cases of this kind. The notion of instant remedy clings pertinaciously to such patients, and the mind becomes morbidly engaged to the habit. I have sometimes been successful in checking it, by expressly enjoining an action only on alternate days, as needful to health: thereby giving a new course to the sensations and to the imaginations which attend them. In regarding the extent to which this abuse exists, I am well persuaded that the judicious physician may do almost as much good by withdrawing medicines of this nature, as by their employment in cases of real need. And this, if it be a just opinion, is saying a great deal.

For while thus speaking as to the excessive use of purgatives in ordinary health, or in dyspeptic cases, where their abuse is the greatest, I would in nowise depreciate their value, as the most powerful means we possess in the treatment of disease;—nor deny that modern practice has carried them into successful use (both by themselves and in aid of the action of other remedies) where opposite principles of treatment had long unavailingly been employed.

In truth, there are cases where the bold and steady persistance
8*

in this method produces effects attainable in no other way. Such is especially the fact where the head is the part affected,—or the organs connected with the system of the vena porta,—or in certain cases of dropsical effusion, depending on disease of these organs, and where the kidneys refuse their office,—or again, where the body is disordered by certain morbid matters collected and circulating in the blood, the removal of which can thus only be speedily and sufficiently obtained. The latter case, of which I shall speak more at large elsewhere, is one of much importance in pathology. 1 may describe it briefly here as that attested in practice by the very large and long continued discharge of dark grimous matters, usually termed bile, and understood to come from accumulation in the liver ; but which I doubt not to be secreted from the membrane or glands of the intestines; and to be in fact a gradual separation from the blood of matters noxious to the system; such as produce, by reten- tion, various forms of active disease. The free and adequate use of purgatives gives proof here no less of the judgment than the boldness of the practitioner.

In the foregoing cases, and others might be added to them, this vigour is sanctioned to an extent even beyond that to which it is carried in ordinary practice. For it is not paradoxical to affirm that the practitioner who deals too familiarly with these medicines in all cases, is less likely to use them boldly and sufficiently where the need is greatest. The accustomed habit is carried on to the particular instance, and due discrimination is wanting in both.

And again, with respect to the amount of dose, in those cases where there is express demand for purgatives for the relief of disease, it is a frequent error, and often arising from the very cause just cited, to reduce this too much, and to substitute small repeated quan- tities for those capable of more instant and powerful effect. With . the exception of cases of very feeble vital power, where sudden changes of any kind involve risk, there is commonly less disturbance to the constitution from this decided practice, with fitting pauses between, than from the seemingly milder plan of small doses and daily repetition. And further it is to be noticed, that the large dose often produces action different in kind, as well as degree, from that of smaller amount; and is in this respect more beneficial in those instances where free evacuation is wanted from the system at large.

Yet, even in many forms of 'actual disease, it must be admitted that there is excess in our employment of these medicines, and some justification of the reproach which English practice has incurred on this score. In cases of actual obstruction of the bowels, where the name seems to lend a full sanction to the treatment, it may be affirmed that it is often-carried on too grossly and indiscriminately. If vomiting does not prevent it, and frequently indeed at the risk of bringing this on, purgative is hurried after purgative, with increase of dose, or adoption of more drastic medicines, at each successive step ;—often with little thought as to the causes of obstruction,—

with much danger of producing inflammation in the obstructed part or elsewhere,—and with no due allowance for the tendency which all parts have to resume a healthy action, if left in quiet.

I do not mean that purgatives should not be given in cases of obstructed bowels. But I wish to convey the caution, required, as I think, by the too uniform direction of practice in these instances; viz., that if there be distinct local pain, threatening inflammation in any part of the canal,—or much active irritation, with nausea and vomiting,—and if the first cathartic medicines, freely given, fail of success,—it behoves the physician well to consider whether he shall urge this treatment farther. There are doubtless cases where it is expedient to do so; but many others where the irritation of drastic purgatives hurries on the patient to danger or fatal result:—and this not unfrequently, where quiet; abstinence equally from food and medicine; leeches and fomentations over tender parts of the abdomen; or still better, in some cases, leeches to the hæmorrhoidal vessels; would have removed obstructions, and relieved the complaint.*

In these important cases of apprehended obstruction of the bowels, it is obvious, on the grounds just stated, that the first use of cathartic means should be the most vigorous, instead of the reverse. If the effect be obtained, it signifies little that the dose has somewhat exceeded the necessity. If otherwise, the chances of mischief by repeated and augmented irritation are spared, and we obtain the indications most to be desired for further treatment.

There can be no doubt of the fitness of using purgatives in the early stage of most fevers; though I believe it might be well in almost every case to let emetics have the precedence. But even in fevers there ought not to be daily purging, as is often practised; and the remark applies still more explicitly to many diseases of local inflammation, where this treatment persevered in becomes a certain source of mischief to the patient.† In inflammations of the chest, for example, as well as in other disorders of this part, cathartic medicines are often employed to a very injurious extent. The retention for a while of disordered secretions is generally much less hurtful, than the irritation created in thus incessantly forcing them away. And without recurring to ancient theories of fever, it may

* The latter point of practice has not been sufficiently attended to; though more on the Continent than in England. I doubt not that in various cases of visceral inflammation, obstruction, or disease, much more might be attained by drawing away blood from the hæmorrhoidal vessels than by the methods of treatment generally in use. Looking to the connexion of these vessels with the circulation through the liver and bowels, it is a strong presumption (and my experience justifies me in so stating it) that no given quantity of blood can be abstracted elsewhere, in cases of this nature, with equally good effect. The remedy particularly deserves trial in topical inflammation, with obstruction; and the influence of the state of the liver upon hæmorrhoids gives some proof of what may be obtained, in disorders of this organ, by bleeding from the vessels of the rectum.

† Εν τοισιν οξεσι παθεσιν ολιγακις και εν αρχησι τησι φαρμακιησι χρεισθαι, is the expression of Hippocrates, in his aphorism on this subject.

further be affirmed, that there is frequent injury arising from inter-ference with the ordinary course of a disease, when this is so far definite as to mark a series of changes connectedly taking place in the system.   In the exanthematous fevers more particularly, the use of strong and repeated purgatives, prior to or during the eruptive part of the disease, is often a well-marked cause of evil,—retarding or repelling the eruption, and transferring morbid actions to parts out of the ordinary course of the disorder.   This consideration includes some of the most important questions in pathology and practice; nor has it, as I think, been duly recognised in the treatment of diseases at the present day.*   The knowledge where to abstain is as valuable as that where to act.   To preserve the character of medicine as a science, each path must be kept open; and the practice be decided by a regard both to what is the natural and necessary course of symptoms, and to those new actions which it is in the power of medicine to produce.

Without embarrassing the question by endless nomenclature of fevers, I would remark that the disorder, often epidemic, to which the term of gastric fever is fairly applied, (where there is manifestly great disturbance, congestion, and depraved secretion of the chy-lopoietic organs without any symptoms of true inflammatory kind, but with tendency rather to a typhoid character,) is, on my experience, the form of fever most benefited by the full use of purgatives; not merely in clearing away disordered secretions already in the bow-els, but further, perhaps, by aiding their more speedy and effectual separation from the blood.

It will, I think, be found, that most physicians who have begun their practice with a large employment of active purgatives, abridge this more or less as their experience is matured by time.   No physician, indeed, as I have before said, can rightly relinquish the benefits of this treatment, boldly and vigorously employed, in cer-tain cases of disease; but the limitation of such vigour to actual disease is that which a wise experience will teach, as the general rule of practice.   It is a rule, indeed, like all others in medicine, with many needful exceptions.   One of the most frequent and reasonable of these regards the use of laxatives with direct reference to the prevention of disorder; as in those cases where, from con-stitution or habits of life, there is strong tendency to accumulations, morbid or otherwise, in the vascular system, and to various forms of deposit in the body.   Here full purging, at certain intervals (and these may often most usefully be made periodical) is the best safe-guard we have against great contingent evil.   The gouty tempera-

---

* Even as respects the practice of bleeding in acute inflammations, there is something yet to be learnt as to the relative fitness of the remedy at different periods of the disorder. We may wholly put aside the limitation of Hippocrates to bleeding on the fourth day in inflammation of the lungs, and yet acknowledge that one time for such remedy is fitter and more effective, as regards the given quantity of blood removed, than another: and further, that there may be specific inflammations of different organs, in which the rule materially varies.

ment, when strongly marked, may be taken as an instance in point. But here too the same principle must be kept in mind, and forbearance be blended with our vigour; otherwise the prevention of one mischief becomes the source of many.

Nor can the need be doubted of aiding the natural action of the bowels in many cases where there is habitual costiveness, either from particular temperament or the casual condition of life. But I have already pointed out the great abuse by excess in this part of practice, and the importance of giving more scope than is usually done to the natural powers of the organs in retrieving any such casualties. I advert to the subject again, as well to enforce this, as also to suggest the value in these cases of the direct combination of tonics with aperients; a form of prescription which might well be brought into more general use. In the greater number of instances of this kind, weakness in the proper action of the bowels is the cause of costiveness; and in seeking to remove the effect by means which act through irritation only, we do but add to the mischief.

The tonic, conjoined with the aperient, enforces its action, without weakening the organs. These, in fact, are the cases in which, if there be no irritation of the mucous membrane, bark will itself often act as a laxative. I have known many instances where calomel, colocynth, and gamboge, in large doses, have had little other effect than that of injurious irritation; but where a few drachms of infusion of senna, with decoction of bark, have been amply sufficient in producing the desired action.

This practice is of more especial value in those languid and strumous habits in which strength and good digestion are so carefully to be maintained; and where an irritation, habitually repeated, often becomes the source of active and permanent disease.

———⬥———

CHAPTER IX.

ON METHODS OF PRESCRIPTION.

The simplification of medicine, and of methods as well as principles in the treatment of disease, ought ever to be present to the mind of the physician. The more complex the objects before him, the stronger the motive for adopting and maintaining this rule. Even with all the curtailments and sounder views of modern practice, it must be admitted that more might yet be done in furtherance of the object. We have long abandoned those preposterous compounds, of which the number of ingredients, or the secret method of admixture, formed the sole science: but the error is still frequent of aiming at a greater number of objects than can be reached at once, or by any single combination of remedies; thereby forfeiting the good to be derived from simpler and more explicit means. Secondary and subordinate symptoms are apt to usurp a place in prescriptions, due to such only as are essential to the character and course of the malady. And it is not too much to affirm that the judgment of the medical man upon a disorder is often warped by the reflection of his own practice. He is apt to look at the symptoms through his own previous treatment of them, as well as through the false opinions of those around; and the trifling or casual symptom of one day gains undue weight the next, from its needless admission among the objects for which he has prescribed. All this is natural in itself; but undoubtedly a serious error in practice. In no way can it better be obviated than by carefully simplifying the character of prescriptions; and avoiding ambiguity, as far as possible, in the intention we assign to their several parts.

It may be alleged, and must be fully admitted, that combinations have often effects not resulting equally from any of their ingredients. This is true as respects many vegetable medicines of powerful action, whether narcotic, purgative, diuretic, or alterative. It is especially true as regards chemical medicines, where changes of combination may occasionally be calculated upon, favouring the effects desired; though much more frequently the facts by which their use is determined are merely empirical in kind. The observation of these facts is obviously one of the most important objects to the practitioner. But it must be added, one of the most difficult also; for even in the simpler combinations we can rarely obtain that precise estimate of effects, which is so essential to the success and certainty of practice;—still less can we do so in those of complicated kind. Each new ingredient added to a medicine increases in a higher ratio the chances of error, and obscures the evidence by which such error may be detected and removed. And the application of other science to this subject, though never to be lost sight of, is made so uncertain, by being subjected to vital actions, that it must ever be admitted with caution, and subordinately to experience. Several compound medicines, of undoubted efficacy, contradict chemical laws even in the points where it might seem of greatest moment to maintain them.*

The best general rule seems to be, to define in every case, as far as can be done, the main object of present treatment,—to make this the basis of prescription,—and to admit, subordinately and under limitation, all such means as apply to collateral symptoms. This rule ought especially to be kept in mind, when a new medicine, or new applications of an old one, are on trial in our hands. Com-

---

* It is an opinion, not infrequent among medical men, that the multiplication of medicines in our hands adds in the same ratio to the power and facilities of practice. This view is admissible only in a very qualified sense. It is, in truth, as correct to say, that the addition of new medicines or preparations, which do not expressly accomplish new purposes, or fulfil more advantageously those already attained, becomes an incumbrance to the practitioner, and an impediment to the progress of the science.

plexity here, especially that which arises from the admixture of new agents in the same prescription, disguises that which it imports us most to know, and which is always learnt with difficulty amid the many conditions tending to obscure the effect. In adding to these the uncertainty of combination, which is itself in most cases an experiment, we wrap one doubt within another, and play false with every just principle of medical research.

Such recommendations may seem trite and trivial; yet are they justified by the rarity of a principle of prescription, consistent with itself, and giving due proportion to the objects in view. The fitness of a man's understanding for medical practice can in no way be better estimated than by looking to these points. The physician who allows his attention to be distracted by secondary symptoms, and hampers a powerful medicine with petty appendages, directed to subordinate objects, shows a quality of mind adverse to sound practice, and incapable of attaining any valuable truth.

Not in prescription alone, but also in the examination of symptoms on which it is founded, much may be gained by a rule of inquiry. Vague and inconsecutive questions, whether from timidity in the young practitioner, indifference in the older one, or irregular habits of thought in either, are not merely useless, but often positively hurtful. They defraud the physician of his own judgment, and put the mind of the patient into the state least apt to give right information. In the adoption of particular methods to obviate this, every one having discretion should exercise his own choice. A man of sound understanding, and who holds good faith with himself, may discover (and it is fit he should seek to do so) in what points his faculties are oftenest at fault; and this ascertained, he is in case to determine how the correction may best be made.

Rightly used, and not allowed to become too technical, a certain rule pursued in questioning the sick will strengthen, by disciplining, the powers of observation. Nor is there much danger lest this should cramp that higher and rarer quality (derived either from long experience, or from quick natural perception) which enables some men to comprehend at the first glance, to seize by a sort of intuition, all that is most needful to be noted in the diseases before them. These instances are not so frequent as to form a rule; nor can the faculty, though an eminent one in itself, ever preclude the necessity of further research. The persons thus gifted, moreover, cannot really be fettered by methods; and will use them only so far as they are actually conducive to good.

It is a frequent error in young practitioners to allow themselves to be betrayed into hasty diagnosis or prognosis of disease, either by their own nervousness, or by the importunity of the patient and those around him. The fault is serious;—not merely as a source of embarrassment, but often by impairing integrity in practice, from the desire to redeem a wrong opinion thus given. It concerns greatly the reputation and usefulness of the profession that every caution should be exercised on this point. Forbearance in words, till the judgment is well decided, is therefore in some sort a duty, as well as an act of prudence. And it further behoves the physician to acquire as much mastery and readiness as possible in the observation of those symptoms which distinguish a disease or foretell its probable event,—another phrase, it may be, for medical experience; yet with the advantage of being more explicit as to a very important part of practice.* If mistakes in judgment be still made (and this will occur to every one), though their avowal is not always needful or desirable, yet I believe the character of the profession, as well as of the practitioner, to be best sustained by truth;—spoken as a man of sense and integrity will speak it. This is a point of medical morality to be impressed upon all who are still young·in their professional career.

Not only in the examination of symptoms, but also in describing them, it were much to be wished that something like a determinate method could be devised, admitting of being carried into general use. Such method, if attained, would render practice itself more exact, and the record of cases more intelligible and useful to others; besides facilitating greatly the study of those general relations of disease and remedial means, upon which the progress of medicine, as a science, mainly depends.†

In the treatment of disease, it is not a bad rule to look first to the external remedies befitting each case, before determining those for internal use. This also may seem a trifling suggestion. Yet such technical arrangement, if involving no practical error, is generally useful, and especially to the young practitioner; who is often painfully harassed, not only by the responsibility of instant judgment, but by the number of objects and methods present to him for consideration. Nor is it the technical aid alone which is of value· here. It is well that every practitioner should keep in mind the expediency of attaining all that is possible by external remedies;— a discreet preference, strongly sanctioned by modern research, and in nowise incompatible with the bold and sufficient use of internal means, when called for by the more urgent necessities of practice.

The physician who leaves the bed-room of his patient, especially in cases of fever or acute disorder, without attending to more than the prescription of medicine and diet, has very imperfectly fulfilled his office. He is bound further to look to temperature and ventila-

* There is reason for affirming that neither diagnosis nor prognosis (particularly the latter) have attained all the exactness of which they are capable, even on our present knowledge. It is worthy of note how much more the ancient physicians deal in the prognostics of disease, and the mutual relation of symptoms, than do those of our own time. Perhaps the very progress of physical knowledge, and of methods of experimental research, are concerned in this change. When physiological science scarcely existed, these particular signs had a more especial value in the interpretation of the course and results of disease. It might be curious, and not useless, to collect all the προρρητικα and κρισεις of Hippocrates, in comparison with the results of modern observation on the same points. A vast number would be found affirmed by him of which we have no present note; some wholly groundless, but many others true and of useful application.

† Dr. Todd, of Brighton, published some years ago a short treatise containing some excellent suggestions on this subject.

tion; the fit state of the patient's bed; his posture; the needful changes of clothing; the proper use of water for cleanliness or coolness; and the maintenance of quiet.   These things, contributing alike to the comfort of the patient and to the chances of recovery from disease, are often, it must be allowed, passed over or too hastily dealt with, in the hurry of practice;—an omission the more important, as many of them are expressly the subjects of popular prejudice and mischievous error.   The ability and good faith of the practitioner are equally put to test in these less ostentatious parts of his science, as in those to which common opinion assigns a higher value.   And it is a further reason for the use of certain regulated methods in these details, that nothing may be omitted, where so much is to be considered and done; and this under circumstances the least favourable to collectedness of thought, or exactness and sufficiency of direction.*

CHAPTER X.

ON GOUT, AND THE USE OF COLCHICUM.

ARETÆUS has said of gout—Αιτιην δε ατρεκεα μεν ισασι μουνοι Θεοι, εοικυιαν δε ανθρωποι—and even now, with the lapse of nearly eighteen centuries between, it would be difficult to state our knowledge of the intimate nature of this disease in very different terms.   The greater part of that which is either ascertained, or strongly to be presumed, may, I think, be comprised under the following general heads:—

1. That there is some part of bodily organization disposing to gout, because it is an hereditary disorder.

2. That there is a *materies morbi*, whatever its nature, capable of accumulation in the system,—of change of place within the body,—and of removal from it.

3. That though identity be not hitherto proved, there is a presumable relation between the lithic acid, or its compounds, and the matter of gout; and a connexion through this with other forms of the calculous diathesis.

4. That the accumulation of this matter of the disease may be presumed to be in the blood; and its retrocession or change of place, when occurring, to be effected through the same medium.

* The medical scholar will recollect the various precepts of Hippocrates as to the methods fitting to be observed in a sick room, as well as his more admirable maxims touching the moral demeanour of the physician in his professional life.

If it should seem that the remarks in this chapter (a small part of so wide a subject) are either too familiar or made too much *ex cathedrâ*, I must plead my conviction from experience of their importance, and my hope that they may be useful to some, who need guidance in details in the earlier and more difficult stages of practice.

5. That an attàck of gout, so called, consists in, or tends to produce, the removal of this matter from the circulation; either by deposits in the parts affected; by the excretions; or in some other less obvious way, through the train of actions forming the paroxysm of the disorder.

6. That there is intimate relation between the condition of gouty habit, and the functions of the kidneys and liver, both in health and disease.

7. And that the same state of habit, or predisposition, which in some persons produces the outward attack of gout, does in others, and particularly in females, testify itself solely by disorder of internal parts, and especially of the digestive organs.

To these heads others might be added, in relation both to the predisposing and exciting causes of the disease, but less definite than the foregoing. I am aware that several even of these points are liable to dispute; and as regards more especially the existence of a material cause for gout, formed and circulating in the system, and eliminated from it by the gouty fit or in other ways, that there have been high authorities opposed to this belief. Nevertheless I see cause to suppose that the opinion, now entertained by many,· will in the end be generally adopted. All the facts and analogies furnished by recent inquiry, some of these form unexpected sources, come in evidence of it ;—and though the proofs be yet insufficient for its establishment as a physical fact, there are on the other hand no arguments to attest its being either impossible or improbable ; nor any different view proposed, so well capable of solving the difficulties of the question.

In the observations which follow, I have kept this principle mainly in view ; convinced that in every discussion as to the origin, nature, or treatment of gout, the condition most essential to be maintained is, that of its being a malady of the general habit; capable of showing itself in various ways, and of affecting, directly or indirectly, almost every part and function of the body. Little ambiguity now exists as to these points:· and their better determination leads us to attach less importance than formerly to the actual fit of gout; regarding this as one only of a series of changes taking place within the system ; though perhaps the most characteristic· and interesting, in its obvious effect of relieving the constitution for the time from the causes of the malady.

This distinction is in every respect of much moment to the true pathology of gout. It solves some of its most singular anomalies ; and furnishes the principle to which we may best resort in all difficulties of practice. Any future progress that is made in the knowledge of the disorder, will probably depend on such mode of viewing the subject, in connexion with a material cause.—And if so established by reasonable proof, this disease becomes the index and interpreter of many obscure and anomalous affections, which have hitherto perplexed research ; as well as of numerous relations with other diseases, the thorough development of which is singularly important to medical science. The proper theory of gout is in every sense an object worthy of the most sedulous research; and to this some aid may be given, even by new methods of arranging and considering the facts best ascertained in its history.

Looking first to the hereditary character of gout, it may be inquired whether this diathesis consists in the tendency to form or accumulate the matter of the disease, by secretion or retention, within the system? or whether what is transmitted is some peculiarity of texture in solid parts, and particularly in the fibrous membranes of the joints, rendering them liable to inflammation of a peculiar kind, and to occasional deposition of this morbid principle, when abounding in the body from other causes?

Though it is not easy to answer these questions unequivocally, yet the whole history of the disease makes it probable that the former opinion is nearest the truth. If the latter were correct, gout, in its most general sense, would be simply a disposition from the peculiar texture of certain parts, to show topically, what in other cases, from difference of structure, produces no like effect. This view cannot well be admitted, in contravention of the many proofs that there is some peculiar substance generated within the system, which, either by its morbid nature or morbid excess, gives cause to the active phenomena of the disease. Without speculating at present upon the nature of this matter, it is presumably the same, whether there be hereditary predisposition, or not;—it affects the same textures and in similar manner, as respects both the kind of inflammation, and the nature of the deposits which occur;—its metastases and irregular effects are seemingly alike in each case.

We have no reason then to regard hereditary gout as more than a disposition to generate a certain morbid matter within the body; in effect of certain circumstances of structure, either favouring its formation, or preventing that excretion of it from the system, which is essential to a healthy state. Or in other words, gout as an hereditary disease, may depend upon some transmitted peculiarities either in the organs of assimilation, or in those by which certain parts are separated from the mass of blood. And we must further admit (which analogy allows us readily to do), that the same peculiarities may exist from other and independent causes;—in explanation of the many cases, where gout is present in the habit, cannot authentically be traced through the parents or families on either side.*

This question of relation between hereditary gout and that generated in the individual, is obviously of much moment to a right theory of the disease. It connects itself closely with the important distinction already noticed, viz., that the fit of gout in the joints is but a local declaration of a disorder of the whole habit, or more especially

* Sir C. Scudamore, in his valuable work on gout, states that, out of 213 cases, 84 only did not admit of being referred to hereditary predisposition. The liability to error is chiefly, perhaps, that of making the latter class too numerous; from the frequent difficulty of obtaining proof, even where the fact exists.

of the circulating fluids. And, considered alone, it involves merely the inquiry why this particular texture should be so prone to give an active and outward shape to the general malady of the constitution.

Under this view, as well as from other considerations, we may fairly receive into the class of gouty affections, those indolent swellings, and permanent thickenings of joints, which are evidently constitutional in cause, and admit of little relief but by constitutional treatment.—The habits in which these swellings occur; their connexion with urinary derangements; the textures they affect; and the nature of the deposits; all prove a similarity if not identity of origin. In fact, there is very little difficulty in conceiving that the same morbid material cause, which in some cases produces the sudden and acute attack, may in others act by a slow process of chronic inflammation, making its deposits as gradually in the parts affected. There is not less diversity of form in other diseases, from the same cause acting upon different temperaments or textures.

These views are the more important, inasmuch as it is certain that the greater or less tendency to deposition, whether depending on structure or not, is an essential circumstance in the pathology of gout, influencing the whole course and character of the disorder. Though this tendency seems in part to depend on the frequency of the previous fits, and is perhaps augmented in rate by articular deposits already begun, there are many cases where it shows itself in the earlier occurrence of the disease; and where the gouty virus, after producing a few acute inflammatory attacks, seems to expend itself chiefly in these deposits, with comparatively little activity of any other kind.

Another point of great interest in the pathology of the disease, is the singular frequency with which its morbid actions are shifted, rapidly and without apparent reason, from one place to another. In the degree of this tendency, gouty inflammation differs remarkably from all others. Though ignorant for the most part why such translations take place, or how their direction is determined, we may presume that very slight causes are capable of producing them; from the readiness with which we can bring gouty inflammation into a joint by trifling external provocation; removing it from another before affected. This facility of translation cannot be due alone, or even chiefly, to the texture of the parts concerned. It is more probably connected with the peculiar nature of the morbid matter of gout, in its relation to the general mass of blood, and to the secretions and excretions taking place within the system. We do not indeed by this supposition obtain any actual solution of the difficulty: but we connect it with the general causes which lie at the root of the disease; and to which all its variety of aspects, as well as every question of treatment, must more or less be referred.

It is to be noticed here, that some authors of eminence have considered the translation of gout to depend altogether on the agency of the organic nerves; deriving argument for this from those cases, where the reciprocal shifting of the disease from one joint to another, or between external and internal parts, is seemingly instantaneous as to time. Admitting, however, the frequent suddenness of these changes, it is probably never greater than may be supposed possible through the blood; seeing the rapidity with which other changes, indisputably occurring through this medium, are effected. And as we have every reason to presume the morbid cause of gout to be present in the blood, and that all ordinary transferences of it are thus made, it becomes improbable that another agency should be concerned in the cases just referred to; unless, indeed, we begin by asserting every local determination of gouty action to be due to some nervous condition of the part;—a view which, though it seems to carry us a step forwards in explanation, is too vague to be admitted as any real addition to our knowledge.*

I have often heard curious description from old martyrs to gout, of the sort of perverse course of the disorder, as it wanders among the several joints before fixing itself upon a part; the sensation in each being generally that of sudden pain, followed by as sudden sense of local weakness, after the translation has occurred to another part. Or I have known it thus to affect several joints within a few hours, and then recede altogether, without leaving other obvious effects than this weakness in a very singular degree. These conditions chiefly occur, where the attacks have been already frequent, and many joints become the subject of the disease. It would seem that a part often affected with gout has less power of resisting any fresh access of the disorder, and perhaps also less capacity for locally retaining it: and hence, smaller accumulations of the morbid cause testify themselves in the joints, in patients long thus afflicted; but with symptoms generally less acute and distinct, and with intervals between the different attacks shorter and less regular. The deposits and thickening about parts frequently affected may be concerned in these modifications of the disease, as diminishing the power of healthy resistance to its morbid actions.

Connected, it may be presumed, with the same causes, is the fact, that the precursory symptoms of gout in the constitution are usually more severe and protracted before the earlier attacks of the disease in the joints; and often affect organs and functions which are afterwards less prone to be disordered by this cause. Irregular actions of the heart, hypochondriacal depression, as well as the more common symptoms of dyspepsia and disordered secretions, frequently antecede by months the first appearance of gout in the extremities; and occasionally give serious alarm even to those who look with medical eye upon these ambiguous cases. I have known instances where disordered action of the heart (such in degree, and so long

---

* The singularity of the electrical states of the body, noticed by some Continental observers to exist during attacks of acute rheumatism, could scarcely be taken in evidence here, even were the same shown to be present in gout also. In our actual knowledge of the subject, changes in the blood may be deemed as likely to produce, as to be produced, by variations in this agency.

continued, as to lead to a thorough conviction of disease in this
organ), has at once ceased upon the first fit of gout, and never again
returned.* Other cases have occurred to me, where severe attacks
of hypochondriasis, of many weeks' duration, have so distinctly
alternated with fits of gout, that the occurrence of one in the course
of the year has wholly superseded the other. In fact, the external
appearance of gout not only explains, by suspending them, the
cause of these symptoms; but in opening, as it were, places of outward deposit for the disease, seems to render its effect on internal
organs less in duration and degree. This view may appear too
mechanical a one for changes, even of morbid kind, in the living
system. Yet it is probably that which conforms most closely to
the facts of the case, and best explains the anomalies which are so
frequent in this part of pathology.

A point of equal difficulty in the history of gout, and seemingly
at variance with the condition just stated, is the frequent attack of
some joint with gouty pain and swelling, without any well marked
symptoms to give warning of its approach. We have here to
explain how the matter, capable by accumulation of producing the
attack, should have been dormant up to the time of seizure? and
why, latent thus long, it should suddenly show itself in an acute
form of disease? These questions cannot be answered explicitly
on our present knowledge. But it may be asserted, that there are
few, if any, cases, in which some token of approaching gout may
not be discovered upon due observation, though often marked only
by irregular and fluctuating symptoms, or occurring in parts remote
from those affected with gouty inflammation. And further, that the
same difficulty occurs in other instances of disease; where active,
or what may often be termed, critical symptoms, suddenly show
themselves without obvious ailment beforehand; sometimes even
with the aspect of better health than usual. Although quantity of
the morbid matter is doubtless concerned in some of these effects,
it is probable that they depend in many cases on changes taking
place in its quality also. A certain definite degree of such change
may be required, before the disorder can put itself into an active
shape, or affect the external parts. There is strong presumption
that both these conditions, of quantity and quality, have several or
combined effect in producing the varieties of the disease.

To render any hypothesis as to the nature of gout tolerably complete, it must be made to show some cause why the disorder should
seldom occur in an obvious form before the age of thirty-five? why
its appearance in the joints should be so rare among females? and
why the disease should be so much limited to the wine-drinking
classes? We are still far from any complete answer to these questions. The general limitation here stated as to age and sex, may
partially be explained on the view before alluded to, of a peculiar

* This is a point well deserving notice at the present time, when disordered
actions of the heart are not only more closely studied by medical men, but have
become the subject of much greater attention and anxiety to patients themselves.

texture in some of the solid parts, prone to take on what is called gouty action, when a certain quantity of the morbid matter is present in the system. We have reason, however, to suppose peculiarities beyond this ; and one especially, having relation respectively to each of these cases ; viz., the state of the sexual functions. That there is some connexion between these and the causes and course of gout in the system, is an old opinion, and probably a just one. Little can be presumed as to the nature of this relation ; but probably it is subordinate to the causes, which more directly determine the presence and qualities of a morbid matter in the body. All changes, gradual or sudden, in the great functions of life must modify more or less the production of this ; and none, perhaps, more importantly than those taking place in the sexual state.*

We have no just reason, however, to presume that the gouty diathesis is absent from the female constitution, because not showing itself in similar or recognised shape. The presumption, as derived from the hereditary nature of the disorder and other observations, is widely different. And it is matter of curious inquiry, not yet adequately pursued, what are the particular indications of such temperament in the female sex ? how far it is modified by menstruation ? or by what other causes in female life ?

In answer to the question why gout should be so much limited to the wine-drinking classes, we have to refer, first, to the hereditary nature of the disease, tending to make it permanently prevalent in any class, where circumstances have originally produced it ;— and secondly, to-the direct influence which habits of diet have in changing both the quantity and quality of the circulating fluids ; and to the many instances where even a single excess or deviation from rule in a gouty habit, will bring on an attack in the joints. It must be admitted that this is illustration rather than explanation. Looking to the effects of various modes and articles of diet, it is impossible to conjecture regarding any one, why it should have this influence. Our knowledge of organic chemistry, improved though it be, is still unequal to the details of such a theory. We can proceed little further than to affirm, that certain kinds of diet do produce distinct changes in the blood, and in the secretions thence derived ;—that these changes consist either in the addition of new ingredients, or in the excess of those which healthily exist in the blood ;—and that they may depend either on faulty assimilation, or on deficient action of the excretory organs.

I am led by various considerations, to believe that the latter is the more frequent cause, and having greatest influence in the production of gout. Though somewhat less obvious than the direct formation of morbid matters in the blood, it is certain that the want of due separation and removal of its excrementitous parts must have equal effect in producing a disordered state of this fluid. And while

* The statement of Hippocrates regarding the infrequency of gout in women is well known. Γυνη ου ποδαγρια, ην μη τα καταμηνια αυτη εκλιπη· Though correct as a general rule, particular exceptions often occur to it.

admitting that wine, as the article of diet having seemingly closest relation to gout, may act directly by engendering the materials of the disease, I think it more probable, that its chief influence is in altering the secretion of the kidneys; the functions of which organs are obviously of the highest importance in all these phenomena.*

The question here respecting the production of morbid states or ingredients of the blood,—whether it be directly by faulty assimilation, or indirectly by deficient excretion,—is one deserving more attention than it has yet received. We may view this distinction in reference not to gout only, but to other diseases where there is presumption of a material cause, generated and circulating in the body. The inquiry is rendered difficult by the complexity of the agents concerned, but it cannot be doubted that more definite results will hereafter be derived from this source.†

The various points that have been touched upon in the theory of gout, all conduct us to the question regarding the nature of the morbid matter, which has been thus presumed to give origin to the disease. Future observation, the "longioris ævi diligentia," is still required for the solution of this difficulty. Yet the course of recent research, applying itself to the various conditions of the blood, and to the composition of the secretions, as well in morbid as in healthy state, offers a fairer chance than at any former time of attaining this knowledge. It is probable that the discovery, if made, will show it to be,—not a matter alien to the system, and wholly morbid in kind,—but rather the excess, either from superabundant formation or undue retention in the blood, of some material, a certain amount

* In many habits it appears that the attacks of gout have relation to the amount of animal food used in diet. I am seeing at this time a very intelligent patient, in whom even a moderate meal for three or four consecutive days never fails to bring on painful swelling of the joints; a fact so well assured to him by some years' experience, that he rarely allows the risk to occur, except with view to ascertain the continuance of the habit. Such exciting cause of gout is perhaps more intelligible than the action of wine, seeing the predominance of nitrogen as an element in the secretions which are so abundant in this disease.

† Amongst the diseases having kindred with the gout, there can be little hesitation in giving foremost place to acute rheumatism; including the fibrous and synovial varieties of this disorder, and what may more especially be called rheumatic fever; but excluding certain neuralgic and other affections which are often classed under this name, injuriously as respects the clearness of pathological distinction. Setting aside slighter analogies, the three great relations,—of hereditary character,—of frequent and sudden translation from the joints to internal organs,—and of the peculiar disorder of the urinary secretions,—are sufficient to show, not indeed identity of disease (for this is fully disproved by observation of the symptoms in detail,) but a cause of analogous kind, in which the constitution at large is concerned, and more especially perhaps the state of the blood; and of which the local inflammation and fever, as in gout, are but indications of excess in amount.

I have made various notes on this disease in the course of practice, but they are wholly superseded by the complete and valuable treatises on the subject which have appeared of late years, both in England and France. Dr. Macleod's Gulstonian Lectures (1837) may especially be mentioned for their excellence as a history of rheumatism. We owe to Dr. Chambers some important practical distinctions in a disease where such are singularly needed.

of which is compatible with, or even necessary to, the health of the body. Or this view may be modified in part, by supposing that, though generated in the body, it is so, only as an excretion needful to be removed, and hurtful in its retention or accumulation there. I have already alluded to what at present is the most plausible conjecture on this subject. Without venturing to antedate our future knowledge, by expressly defining the matter of gout to be either lithic acid, or urea, or one of the lithic or purpuric salts, or any other highly azotised principle, it is impossible not to suppose that there is produced in the blood some animal principle having close kindred with these, and morbid either in kind or by excess;—a matter in the separation of which the kidneys are largely concerned, and the retention of which in the system is the cause of various disorders, according to the age, sex, temperament, or other peculiarities of the persons affected.

The true theory of gout clearly lies in this direction. It is here that we may look to obtain more intimate knowledge, not merely of the causes of the disease in its active form, but also of its connexion with other local or constitutional disorders, with which it is associated by some common morbid action. Modern observation has led us to recognise some of these relations under the names of gouty headache, gouty ophthalmia, and gouty bronchitis. My own experience would lead me to add certain forms of asthma to the number. But many more undoubtedly yet remain to be determined; and not the least important, those which subsist between gout and the system of the brain and nerves. Reference has already been made to hypochondriasis; and it is highly probable that other disorders of the same class, still less generally viewed under this connexion, will hereafter be submitted to it.

The relation of gout to the functions and disorders of the liver, is another point of much interest in pathology,—clearly attested both in the active systems of the disease, and by those which are common under other forms of the gouty temperament. Its connexion with cutaneous diseases is an additional topic, yet almost unexamined; though I cannot doubt, from my own observation, that certain of these disorders occur as effects of the habit in question. I have so often seen psoriasis, for example, prevailing in gouty families,—sometimes alternating with acute attacks of the disease, sometimes suspended by them, sometimes seeming to prevent them in individuals thus disposed,—that it is difficult not to assign the same morbid cause to these results, however unintelligible its mode of action under such different forms.

But the kidneys, as already stated, are evidently the organs of the body, upon the disordered or deficient action of which depend those changes in the circulating fluids, which have closest relation to all the phenomena of gout. These functions, it is important to observe, undergo variation at successive periods of life, independently of actual disease. By such variation they serve in part to the destined changes of the body at these respective periods; this influence being attested by an altered state of the secreted fluid, both in the nature and proportion of several of its ingredients. That period which begins the decline from perfect manhood, is marked generally by an excess, if it may so be termed, of the lithic acid, which continues more or less through after life;—testifying itself with greatest safety, and often remedially, by large habitual discharges of this substance from the kidneys ;—becoming a source of grave and various disease where this separation is insufficient or suddenly interrupted. Much certain discovery for the future (perhaps even as respects the causes and phenomena of fever) may be affirmed to lie in this particular path of physiology. And much more of practical caution might be drawn, even from our present knowledge, as to interference with these important functions, whether in health or in the treatment of disease.*

Organic chemistry has taught us how readily the elements out of which all animal matter is formed, are displaced from one combination, and enter into others; and how very slight frequently are the differences, indicated by analysis, between substances eminently noxious to the system, and those indifferent or beneficial to it. We owe further to recent experiments the explicit proof of what simple observation had partly shown before,—the remarkable effect upon the whole mass of blood of minute quantities of certain matters brought into the circulation ; leading to the inference of analogous effects from an increased proportion of one or other of its principles accumulating, or being unduly retained, in the body. Applying these circumstances to the secretion from the kidneys, we have here complex chemical processes constantly going on (in some small part capable of being imitated artificially), by which changes are manifestly made in the total mass of blood ; the partial arrest · of these processes by disease inflicting speedy injury on the system ; and where this has been more complete, from palsy or other cause, rapidly producing a fatal event ;—unless relieved, as sometimes happens, by a vicarious discharge of the same principles through other organs. In the instance of urea, which has been detected in the blood, these noxious effects are more expressly ascertained ; and there is no reason to doubt the same result from the other constituents of urine ; particularly those which occur in the form of the lithic acid and its compounds.†

* I might specify many cases where practice is directed (often on slight or single examination) to correct sediments in the urine, which are actually relieving the system by their free and abundant discharge ; or which in other instances depend solely on a lessened proportion of the liquid to the solid ingredients, without any increase in the quantity of the latter. I have known persons in perfect health, in whom a warm bath, or copious perspiration, produced for many hours afterwards a sediment of amorphous lithates, in effect of this altered proportion. Such changes are frequent; and arising from various causes in diet, weather, exercise, and even from mental emotions and affections of the nervous system.

† Modern inquiry in the great field of organic chemistry, has made much advance as respects the products of the urinary organs. The able and successful

These circumstances, now familiar to us, do certainly not identify the material cause of gout with any of the animal excretions just named; but they tend to concentrate our views towards them, and give a much more specific direction to future research. The assured connexion of the gouty with the calculous diathesis,—the chemical nature of the concretions and deposits in the former,—and the evidence that these deposits often become in part a substitute for the more active forms of the disease,—all concur in further sanctioning the same general view. If we cannot affirm that urea, the lithic acid, or other animal compounds circulating in the blood, give cause to the phenomena of gout, neither can we on any sufficient grounds deny the possibility of this. And under the most cautious reasoning we are at least entitled to assume, with some confidence, that these matters, secreted from the kidneys, are the equivalents to gouty matter present in the system; that they have certain proportion of quantity to each other; and that upon this balance depend all the essential characters of the disease,—its modifications being determined by various causes, some of them topical, some belonging to general functions implicated in the effects of this common cause.*

researches of Dr. Prout are well known, in their relation both to theory and practice. The more recent experiments of Wöhler, who has actually formed urea by combination of cyanic acid and ammonia; and of Liebig, who has obtained allantoin from uric acid, and also directly by the decomposition of cyanogen and water, —possess great interest, as the first examples of animal organic substances artificially formed; and further, as showing the intimate connexion among all the chemical compounds of this class; and the facility with which, by slight causes of chemical change, they may take place of each other, even within the living body.

The relation of urea to sugar in anatomical composition, and the gradual change which appears sometimes to take place from one secretion to the other, as in certain cases of diabetes, may well be reckoned among the more interesting of these facts. The researches of Dr. Bright have given new importance to all that concerns the presence and proportion of albumen in the urine. And Dr. Prout has justly remarked, that, although without any express evidence on the subject, we have every cause to regard the separation by the kidneys of phosphorus from the blood, as an important condition to the health of the body; the occasional excess of this element, or its several compounds in the urine, showing its connexion with other functions in the animal economy.

Dr. Bostock, to whom we owe much in this and other parts of physiology, has suggested an excellent tabular form, as a means of recording with greater precision and uniformity the several physical characters of urine, both in health and disease. (*Med. Chirurg. Trans.*, vol. xxi., p. 25.) A method of this kind is almost essential to the successful prosecution of an inquiry, in which the elements are so numerous and intricate.

* I find in my notes the narrative of a case remarkably illustrating these views, the principal points in which I may briefly cite. In a young man, about twenty-two years of age, painful inflammatory swellings occurred of the feet and ankles, having every apparent character of gout, and considered as such. These attacks were two or three times repeated in the course of twelve months, during which time he was gradually becoming more feeble and reduced in health. When I first saw him, the emaciation was great: a general state of oppression and febrile anxiety was present; with dyspnœa, a labouring and generally slow pulse, and much drowsiness. The urine was very copious in quantity, of colour like water having soap-suds diffused through it, and without the proper urinous smell. It yielded, on evaporation, a large quantity of albuminous matter (resembling

This, as far as I can judge, is the step upon which we at present stand in our approach to a more complete knowledge of gout. We have reason, on fair grounds, to deem it almost certain that such knowledge will hereafter be attained. And it is important again to observe, that there are few examples in medicine where the right theory of a disease bears so obviously and immediately upon its treatment as in the one before us.

—————

Without entering at large into this subject of the treatment of gout (one that has been much and ably discussed by modern writers), I may subjoin a few remarks, founded on my own experience of the use of colchicum; the most remarkable, certainly, among the φαρμακα μυρια, which at all times have been applied to practice in this disease.*

The first question occurring is, whether colchicum can rightly be deemed a specific remedy in gout? and in what sense, and under what manner of operation, it is to be considered as such? Its first and most obvious action, that moreover which originally gave it the fame of a remedy in this disease, is simply the removal of gouty pain and inflammation from a joint, or the abridgment of their duration and severity. Does this operation consist in destroying the matter of gout, by some specific change? or in withdrawing it

what Dr. Prout has termed *incipient albumen*,) which coagulated into a gelatinous mass; yet flaky in parts, and showing in others a somewhat granular texture. In some portions of urine the proportion of this matter was nearly an ounce to the pint. There existed much thirst, and considerable craving for food, with other symptoms of diabetic character.

The progress to a fatal event was rapid. The oppression of breathing, drowsiness, and debility increased. Four days before death an epileptic seizure occurred, followed by frequent but less severe convulsive attacks, and with a state of partial stupor, passing by degrees into perfect coma, which continued to the end.

A post mortem examination showed the kidneys to be the only organs obviously diseased. They were scarcely half the natural size; the texture semi-cartilaginous and extremely hard; and resembling in various other particulars the third form of disease of this organ so well described by Dr. Bright. In the cavity of the chest there were two pints of serum effused, but without any disease of the heart or lungs. The only peculiarity about the head was, that the bones of the cranium were more compact, and the dura mater more closely adherent than usual.

Looking to the history of this case, there is every reason to believe that the disease of the kidneys was the first in order; that the swellings of the joints; called gouty, were the effect of the altered secretion of urine thereby produced, that a more advanced stage of this organic disease led to the large separation of albumen from the blood; while a yet further and final change produced the obscure inflammation of the lungs, the effusion of serum into the chest, and the cerebral symptoms, which closed this melancholy case.

* We have some curious testimonies in ancient authors as to the multiplicity of remedies employed in gout. Lucian, in his Τραγοποδαγρα, mentions more than fifty substances, animal, vegetable, and mineral, which were used as external applications only.

from the part affected into the general circulation?—or yet further, in procuring its removal from the system, through some of the excretory organs? Each of these suppositions may be possible; and collectively they seem to include all the modes in which the medicine can act; unless indeed we admit the improbable opinion, that its influence is upon the nervous system alone. Though our present knowledge does not carry us to certainty on the subject, there are various presumptions, clear enough to be of important application to practice.

The first of these, and that which best justifies the term specific, is the fact, that the action of colchicum is not limited to the removal of gout from the joints or other textures usually affected; but extends to the relief of the disease when present in parts differently composed, or when assuming the most irregular and changeable aspects. The proof here is wholly that of experience, and, it must be admitted, of recent date; but nevertheless sufficient to authorize the view just stated. We have not indeed much evidence applying to the acute forms of what are termed retrocedent and misplaced gout; and in such cases, other and still more instant remedies are often required by the urgency of the symptoms. But in all chronic forms of the constitutional disorder, the influence of colchicum is striking and well defined. We find it relieving, for example, the peculiar ophthalmia of gouty habits, where other remedies, local or general, have been of little avail. I have used it in a particular class of headaches, which I doubt not to be connected with this diathesis, and have obtained equal proof of its efficacy here. The same, though less explicitly, in gouty bronchitis. These and other instances clearly show that colchicum is not merely a local remedy for the disease. Its power of removing gouty inflammation from the joints, is subordinate to its action on the matter of gout throughout the system; and it is to the latter that we must look for explanation of those effects which may be thus deemed specific, in every just sense of the term.

Such explanation would be impossible to our present means of research, were we obliged to suppose any direct action of colchicum upon this material cause of the disease. But the supposition is not necessary, nor is it even probable. What we seek, is more likely to be found in the action of the medicine on some organ, the function of which is expressly connected with the morbid conditions of gout. And pursuing this course of inquiry, we again come to the kidneys, as the organs seemingly concerned more than any other in these changes, and at the same time most readily and extensively affected in their functions by extraneous agents.

While allowing that there is much ambiguity on the subject, it will, I think, be found that the action of colchicum upon the kidneys is better marked, and more considerable, than on any other part; and this too in case where no gouty action is presumably present at the time. Though I have given some attention to the subject, and feel assured that the medicine has effect in altering the urinary secretion, independently altogether of disease, I have never been able to obtain results free from ambiguity, or constant enough to satisfy me of the precise nature of the change.   It is obviously not one of mere quantity of fluid, (though this appears to be generally increased,) but involving, if the inferences be just, an alteration in the nature or proportion of the animal compounds excreted through this channel from the blood.   I have already alluded to that remarkable class of urinary ingredients which, in some one or other of the various changes they undergo, have manifestly closest relation to the phenomena of gout.   The complex nature of these agents, and the facility with which such chemical changes take place, from their actions on each other, as well as on the other animal or saline ingredients of the urine, render this inquiry one of singular difficulty, and only to be pursued by experiments expressly made, and repeated so as to obtain a large average of results.   I cannot doubt, however, that knowledge will hereafter be acquired, resolving these questions sufficiently to afford a principle for that which is now matter of empirical practice.*

The intimate connexion between gouty action and alteration or disorder in the secretion of the kidneys, is certainly an argument that colchicum owes its virtue in the disease to a specific influence upon this secretion.   It may be objected, that were this so, we should have some more marked testimony; seeing the extent and suddenness of the effect upon gouty swellings.   But this objection, it will be seen, applies equally to all different views regarding the action of colchicum.   And further, we must recur here to the fact before noticed, of the singular proneness of gouty inflammation, even from the slightest causes, to change its seat from one joint to another, or suddenly to recede within the system.   A change of action induced upon the kidneys, as the immediate effect of the medicine, may be sufficient to check or withdraw the inflammation from any given part; and such result is perfectly compatible with the analogies we derived from other sources.   The instances are frequent and familiar in the animal economy, where a new action begun, or an irritation suddenly given to another organ, will at once alter or remove morbid actions before existing; and the principle is one upon which we act largely in the treatment of disease.†

The case before us, indeed, is in no way more difficult to conceive, than that a single excess in diet should be capable of bringing the gout into a joint; and the one fact is not only an illustration, but an

* Knowing, as we do on good authority, that the average of solid contents in the urine passed in twenty-four hours, and of the common specific gravity, amounts to nearly two ounces;—and that part, perhaps the largest proportion, are matters the separation of which from the body is essential to health,—it is easy to conceive the influence on the system of alterations in this function, and the importance of all medicines which expressly act upon it.

† It is worth while here to advert to the fact, that the kidney is the organ in the body which receives the artery of largest size in proportion to that of the gland; and which, further, according to the recent statement of Lippi, has absorbent vessels entering its pelvis.

argument for the other.   If the use of the colchicum be suspended here, the matter of the disease, thus drawn into the circulation, and not provided with any further or sufficient egress, may be presumed ready to show itself in fresh attacks of local inflammation.   If, on the other hand, the altered action of the kidneys be sustained by the continued use of the medicine, it may be capable of removing the gouty matter from the system altogether; or that surplus of it at least which becomes a source of active disease.

This general view, more probable perhaps than any other, will explain many seeming anomalies in the effect of colchicum; and indicate, if correct, the best methods of its use.   In particular it shows, why three or four large doses, which may often suffice to remove gout from the extremities, do not so rid the body of it, as to prevent recurrence after some short interval of time.   The draining away of gouty matter is begun, enough to withdraw a local inflammation ever ready to be displaced; but the action needs to be sustained for its more complete removal from the system.

No point is so important as this to the right estimate of colchicum as a remedy in gout.   A suspicion has existed, (formerly, as well as since the recent revival of the medicine,) that though capable of relieving the present paroxysm, it renders the attacks of the disorder more frequent.*   This, if generally true, would be a serious impeachment of its value; and might warrant, in most cases, the older method of treatment by sufferance of the local inflammation to the end.   On my experience, however, I believe this opinion to be justified only where the medicine has been used imperfectly; or without other precautions, which are more or less essential to its success.   I can scarcely doubt the expediency of carrying its employment beyond the mere relief to the local inflammation of the disease.   The remedy, with due care, may be made preventive as well as curative of gout; and, as far as I can judge, with no less safety to the patient.

We may reasonably then, if this view be just, extend to its use as a medicine the remark before made regarding the pathology of gout, viz., that too exclusive attention is given to the external part of the disease, and the value of the remedy in the constitutional forms of the disorder, too little regarded.   Larger experience is making a gradual change in this respect; but there is still a tardiness and timidity in its application beyond the mere fit of gout, which is not warranted by any ascertained risk.   It has happened here as in other instances, (and especially in the case of new remedies,) that the medicine has borne the ill fame of events in which it had no concern.   The ordinary incidents of a gouty habit, as well as casualties from other sources, have been carried to its account, by a mode of reasoning common in such cases, and very embarrassing to the physician.   Where the morbid actions are so various, and

* Admitting the hermodactyl of the ancients to be the colchicum, as is reasonably supposed, we find Alexander Trallianus making this statement respecting the action of the medicine.

our knowledge of their causes so obscure, it is difficult rightly to discriminate the latter, or to rescue any particular agent from the charge of becoming such.   Future experience may remove these difficulties, but meanwhile they press unfairly on the reputation of the remedy before us.

The faulty employment of colchicum also, as already noticed, has doubtless added to the distrust of its expediency in gout.   Given solely to remove the local inflammation, and with scarcely a definite view beyond this, there is often great neglect of those evacuations, which may be deemed most needful when the matter of the disease is thus suddenly thrown back into the system.   Seldom ought colchicum to be employed for this express object, without the combination of other means, fitted to act freely on the bowels; and calomel, though not perhaps essential, may for the most part be preferred for this purpose.   The action of the remedy thus aided, if not more rapid, is certainly more secure.   In sustaining fully all the excretions, (for though that of the kidneys be most important, it is not solely effective,) we gain the best guarantee that the morbid matter removed from the joints is carried out from the circulation,—a due and timely attention to which point would probably remove from colchicum the reproach it has incurred of producing more frequent attacks of the disease.

All these considerations give cause to believe that we are still only partially informed of the value of the remedy, or the variety of the objects it is fitted to fulfil in that peculiar temperament, of which gout is the most distinct manifestation.   Its efficacy in the most obscure and irregular forms of the disorder, must be allowed as strong proof of its specific character.   And as bark, by curing, associates together many intermittent affections under the presumption of a common cause, so may colchicum furnish similar inference regarding various affections, seemingly remote in situation and symptoms.

This method of inference, hitherto very limited in its application, may hereafter be extended much further.   It is one of singular value, as closely connecting the treatment with the theory of disease, and rendering them mutually corrective of each other.   While in thus expounding the relation to a common cause, of symptoms, differing wholly in aspect and in the organs affected, it at once enlarges and simplifies our views in every part of pathology.   For the connexions here are so intimate and various, that each fact well ascertained, is fruitful of results far beyond those which directly appear to the view.

I have already noticed the use of colchicum in a class of headaches which I doubt not to be connected with the gouty habit; and my experience furnishes me with much proof of its efficacy in such cases.   These, indeed, are instances where it merits a free and fair trial.   Our practice has been hitherto so much at fault in certain varieties of this disorder, especially such as have a periodical character, that we are bound, for the credit of medicine, to look elsewhere than to old and inefficient means for their relief. I think it almost certain that some kinds of headache are produced by the same morbid cause in the circulation which brings on, in other persons or at other times, true gouty affections of the joints. With due attention to the family temperament, to the individual habit, and particularly to their connexion with certain states of the urinary secretion, it is for the most part easy to discriminate them; and thus attested, colchicum will generally be found to act as a safe and efficient remedy.*

The action of this medicine in rheumatic and other inflammations of the joints, is certainly more ambiguous than in gout; though the old epithet of *Theriaca articulorum* seems to have been applied under this more general view of its use. Wherever active and beneficial in such cases,—and it is certainly so in many,—a similar principle of operation may, perhaps, be presumed; and as respects acute rheumatism, probably with some analogous relation to the morbid matter producing the disease. In cases of this kind, where no febrile action is present, the combination of colchicum with bark will often be found very beneficial; the latter medicine obviating any injury that might arise from the continued use of the former.

It is a question of interest regarding colchicum, what those effects are, which contradict or check its employment; and show themselves injuriously or dangerously, when the medicine is given in excess. That they are not so well defined as might be desired, is partly owing to the causes before mentioned, viz., the frequent attribution to the remedy, of symptoms which really belong to the disease; and the actual difficulty of discrimination in many cases, even to those who have greatest experience. Other cases, however, occur, where this application will not apply; and where there is proof that the colchicum itself is injurious, either from idiosyncrasy in the patient, or from its own peculiar properties. Its influence in gout attests the amount and singularity of the latter. It cannot, from analogy, be thus efficient for good, without the power of inflicting ill; and in the nature of its alkaline ingredient, closely related to veratria, we have an explanation of its general sedative effects, as well as of the more immediate disorder of the stomach following large doses of the medicine. Though there is strong presumption

* This relation of headache to the secretion of the kidneys, is often very strikingly marked. A remarkable case has occurred to me, of a gentleman, who from about the age of forty (which Dr. Prout has well remarked to be a common period of the commencement of lithic-acid deposits) had been subject to very frequent attacks of gravel, with constant sediments of the same nature in the urine. At the age of fifty-five, when I first saw him, this tendency had suddenly ceased; and he became affected by acute headaches, so severe as to produce urgent expressions of pain; and continuing, with scarcely the interruption of a single day, for five or six months. Symptoms of chronic bronchitis then supervened, with copious expectoration. The headaches were gradually relieved as this fresh disorder gained ground; but death ensued about two years afterwards, from a more active form of pulmonary disease. At the time when this case occurred to me, colchicum was little known as a remedy, or there would have been explicit reason for employing it.

that much of the specific effect of colchicum depends on this active principle, the question still needs farther examination. Its solution might contribute greatly to render our employment of the medicine more beneficial and secure.

The proofs of injury, indeed, from wrong or excessive use, even if much more numerous than they are, ought not to affect its character as a remedy. The case is common to all other powerful agents in medicine; and further experience will teach us how to obviate these evils, or to correct any which may be inseparable from its use.

In these remarks I have treated of colchicum generally, without reference to the several preparations now in use. Among these, I I know none more certain in effect than the acetous extract, or better capable of fulfilling the peculiar purposes of the medicine.* There may be greater convenience sometimes in employing the wines of the root or seeds; but I am not aware of any superiority they possess, unless possibly it be a somewhat more rapid action. I have given this extract, in moderate doses, every night for three or four weeks, without a single manifestation of ill effect. Its combinations with calomel and other purgatives in the outset of an attack of gout,—with morphine or other sedative, and with occasional laxatives, in the progress of the malady,—and with alkalies and stomachic bitters in sequel to it, and for the prevention of its recurrence,—furnish us with the greater part of what is needful in this disorder, as far as medicine merely is concerned. Limiting the present remarks to one point of treatment, I do not enter on the question—discussed and disputed from an early period—regarding the use of active antiphlogistic remedies during the attack. The rules of diet and methods of life befitting the gouty habit, form another part of the subject; upon which, though much has been written, there is yet scope for more exact inferences, and a steadier application of these to practice.

CHAPTER XI.

ON SOME SUPPOSED DISEASES OF THE SPINE.

It has happened to me in practice to see a great number of these singular affections; in which certain morbid states of the nervous system, or occasionally visceral disorders, assume every character of spinal complaints, and are medically treated as such. The large majority of these cases occur among females; and though the com-

---

* The powder of the root of colchicum, if properly prepared and preserved, is also, I believe, a valuable form of the medicine, and deserves further trial in practice.

plaint is now better understood than formerly, yet I doubt not the instances are more frequent than is imagined. The simulation of serious disease of this nature, independently altogether of the will, is often so remarkable, that we may fairly presume many such fictitious disorders to remain undiscovered to the last.

A common cause of deception in these instances is the existence of pain, sometimes fixed, sometimes fluctuating, along the course of the spine; and this pain, according to the assertions of the patient, very often relieved by local bleeding, blistering, moxa, and other similar applications. There is frequently, moreover, weakness or numbness of the lower extremities, sometimes such in amount as to be construed into paralytic affection,—pain from exertion, relief from recumbency,—tendency to muscular spasms,—and often difficulty in emptying the bladder. Yet all these, and other symptoms, may arise from nervous or hysterical state of the constitution without any local affection; and in many cases are best relieved by remedies which have no relation whatever to the spine.

It is, in truth, one of the ill effects of the misunderstanding of the complaint, that its symptoms are often greatly aggravated by the means designed for their relief; and spinal disorders even produced, when not existing before, by the muscular debility due to long confinement, recumbent posture, and local depletions. I have seen cases, well worthy of notice, where patients having no nervousness or infirmity of mind, but suffering from topical nervous pains in some part of the spine (the result often of sympathy with internal organs), have been reduced by various treatment to a state of almost total inability of the lower extremities. The proof of the real cause is that afforded by their recovery in very few weeks, from symptoms which have had duration for months or years;— and this recovery derived, not from remedies applied to the spine, but from steel, bark, ammonia and valerian, cold salt-water bathing or washing, and exercise of the limbs sedulously persevered in and extended. In those instances, by no means infrequent, where some mental infirmity is added to the physical condition producing this state, the moral remedies which the judicious practitioner may employ will greatly aid the success of the treatment.

I allude to these cases, not from any novelty they have to men of professional experience, but because it is important to press that due notice of them, which may exempt the young physician from the chance of error, and equally protect the patient from the mistakes of mere ignorance, and from the maltreatment of quackery and fraud. It well merits attention, in relation to the history of such disorders, how very large a proportion of those affected by them are females. As there are no causes which can adequately explain this degree of disparity between the two sexes as to actual spinal complaints; and as there are many peculiarities in the female constitution tending to produce the deceptive appearances of these, we have here a practical proof of the frequency of the latter, and of the importance of being well prepared for their recognition.

Both firmness and experience, indeed, are greatly required in treating these anomalous disorders. Our first steps are often embarrassed, not only by the fluctuating nature of the symptoms, but by the condition of the patient's mind and nervous temperament; a state of constitution generally concerned in producing the malady, and almost always aggravated in its progress. These are cases in which, if our foundation of practice be well laid, we need in nowise be disconcerted by seeing failure in the outset. Some of the most remarkable instances I have seen of complete eventual success, have been those in which the contrarieties in the early part of treatment were most numerous and discouraging.

Ambiguous cases there no doubt are, where the topical symptoms of pain, fulness, or irritation upon some part of the spine are sufficiently distinct to call for local remedies, on trial at least of their effects. In such instances, and equally so where cause is found for the continuance of these means, I think leeches are generally to be preferred to blisters, caustic, or other irritating applications. The symptoms, as already noticed, are most frequent in habits where there is a morbid sensibility of the whole system ; and any active irritation, or even one so slight as hardly to affect other persons, will frequently be found to excite disordered actions, and disturb the whole progress of cure. I have often seen the most obvious and immediate good from removing an issue or open blister ; which had effect only in aggravating the symptoms they were intended to relieve.

In cases of this nature, opium might be used much more extensively as an external application than is usual in practice; and, according to my experience, with great benefit. That very condition of the nervous system, which renders a slight local irritation of the cutaneous nerves a source of disturbance to the whole body, gives power and value to this means as an antidote. Where true inflammation has not existed, or has been removed ; and where irritation and nervous sympathies are the source of the distress thus attached to the spine and limbs, it is singular what good this application will produce :—not used, however, in the careless and inefficient way which is common with external remedies ; but sedulously, and with sufficient proportion of opium in the forms employed.

These cases of supposed spinal disease are further interesting, as they belong to and illustrate an important class of diseases, which, though much more closely examined than heretofore, have scarcely yet been defined in their whole extent. I allude to the various forms of hysteria ; and especially to that frequent and curious variety of the complaint, where there is disorder of the sensations, or perhaps it may better be said, of the sensorial functions involving the former. The pains upon or along the spine, in the cases already referred to, often belong to this condition ; as does also the inability to give proper action to the limbs, which is so marked a symptom in these disorders. Sir B. Brodie (with whom I have seen many examples of them) has made the observation, that in hysterical paralysis the muscles are not incapable of obeying the acts of volition, but the function of volition is not exercised. In the truth of this observation, all that I have seen leads me fully to concur. In fact, the whole series of symptoms in these cases, whatever the remote causes, is independent directly upon sensorial derangement, affecting irregularly certain classes of sensations, and impairing the state and action of the voluntary powers.

Many of the anomalies just noticed are expressly due to a depraved state of the sense of touch; testified not solely by the increased irritability already noticed, but in other instances by the sensibility being unnaturally blunted. And these singularities are increased by what is often observed of their partial occurrence and frequent change of place,—phenomena which belong to the general theory of sensation, as well in healthy as in morbid states of the body.

In some of these cases the patient may be said to live in a sort of cycle of disordered sensations, displacing and replacing each other in the most singular way; but all removed for the most part when a real pain supervenes, the result of inflammation or other true diseased action. I have known a toothache, or a slight catarrh, or the irritation of a sprain, completely to banish, for a time, morbid impressions of the most distressing kind and long duration in the habit; all recurring when this cause of interference had subsided. The intellectual and moral faculties frequently partake, in greater or less degree, of the same infirmity; producing some of the most singular perversions of feeling and action which it falls to the lot of the medical man to encounter; and these sustained occasionally during a long period of time.* But, as I have remarked, there are many instances where the bodily symptoms alone exist, without any such conjunction; and it is to these chiefly I seek to direct attention in the present chapter.†

We are further indebted to Sir B. Brodie for the first description of that very remarkable hysterical affection of the joints, which has close kindred with the disorder now under consideration. They are, in fact, corresponding effects of a common cause, and require for the most part similar treatment for their relief.

Looking generally to the cases associated together by this common character, they may be considered as amongst the most curious and instructive in all pathology. Like insanity and intoxication, they illustrate many points in the connexion of the mind and bodily

---

* Such cases, of which I have seen examples quite as remarkable as any I find recorded, give aid in explaining some of those anomalous phenomena which have perplexed even thinking men, and furnished in all ages large material for wonder to the credulous or uninstructed.

† In the latter cases we may perhaps best seek for a cause in the reflex actions of the nervous system of the spine, which have recently been the subject of so much able research by Dr. Marshall Hall in this country, and Professors Müller and Stromeyer in Germany. To Dr. M. Hall we owe the earliest distinct exposition of this class of facts, and of their application to the phenomena of spasmodic diseases; a very important step in the progress of medical science.

organs, which are not equally obvious in the healthy state: and they instruct us, moreover, in the history of insanity itself, by displaying various partial hallucinations of mind, often traceable throughout their whole progress, and forming links, as it were, betwixt reason and madness. It is a sort of natural analysis afforded us of conditions too complex for examination, when they are fully formed and established.

CHAPTER XII.

ON THE BRAIN AS A DOUBLE ORGAN.

I AM not sure that this subject of the relation of the two hemispheres of the brain, has yet been followed into all the consequences which more or less directly result from it. Symmetry of arrangement on the two sides of the body is common indeed to all the organs of animal life.* But the *doubleness* of the brain, like all besides pertaining to this great nervous centre, offers much more of curious speculation than the same constitution of other parts. That unity of consciousness in perception, volition, memory, thought, and passion, which characterizes the mind in its healthy state ("illud quod sentit, quod sapit, quod vult, quod viget"), is singularly contrasted with the division into two equal portions of the material organ, which more immediately ministers to these high functions. Yet, on the other hand, in almost exact symmetry of form and composition of each hemisphere; in their relation precisely similar to the organs of sense and voluntary motion on each side of the body; and in the structure of the nervous connexions subsisting between them; we find argument, not merely for the correspondence of functions, but even for that unity or individuality, of which consciousness is the interpreter to all. This unity, indeed, as it actually exists, is of necessity compatible with the conformation of the brain as a double organ, even had we no such presumption to refer to.†

Here it must be admitted, we are close upon that line, hardly to be defined by the human understanding, which separates material

---

* The distinction established by modern physiologists between the animal and vital organs, as respects the symmetry of the sides, is an important one, and well sanctioned by facts.

† Though the nervous system in all its parts, with the exception of that belonging to the great sympathetic, is subject to fewer anomalies than any other organs of the body, yet are these deviations more frequent in man than in many of the mammalia most nearly approaching to him in structure; an observation made originally by Vic d'Azyr, and confirmed by later physiologists. It is further to be noticed, as an anatomical fact, that in the brain and spinal marrow, the external parts on the two sides are less exactly symmetrical than those within; the surface of the brain showing this perhaps more distinctly than any other part. —See *Meckel's Handbuch der Menschlichen Anatomie*, vol. i., ch. 3.

organization and actions from the proper attributes of mind,—the structure which ministers to perception from the percipient,—the instruments of voluntary power from the will itself. Our existence may be said to lie on each side this boundary; yet with a chasm between, so profound and obscure, that though perpetually traversing it in all the functions of life, we have no eye to penetrate its depths. If we sometimes seem to obtain a show of further discovery (and human thought has exhausted itself in the effort), this arises generally from the deception of language, which gives the appearance of advancing, when in truth we are but treading in our former steps.

While approaching these limits, however, in the subject before us, it may be pursued to a certain extent within the boundary. Many of the questions of greatest interest here have not more concern with materialism, than have the facts which connect dreaming and intoxication with certain physical changes occurring in the body. The intellectual existence, of which consciousness and personal identity are the simplest expressions, but which spreads itself out into the endless varieties of thought and feeling (μη χωριστη κατα μεγεθος, αλλα κατα λογον), has been given us, subject to external agents from the first moment of our being; both in the functions of health, and under the various circumstances of disease.* And any results we

---

* I know no happier expression of personal identity, and its relation to the nature of mind, than that of Mr. J. Smith of Cambridge. "Mere matter could never thus stretch forth its feebler force, and spread itself over all its own former preëxistences." The same argument (for the force of the remark renders it such) may be followed into the future, as well as fetched from the past; and still more remarkably, as respects the intellectual existence of man. By facts already attained, and methods of thought previously acquired, the mind becomes capable of passing beyond its actual knowledge, and gaining what may be deemed certainty as to the result of combinations which have never yet existed; or, if existing, have never before been the subject of human observation. Physical science abounds in examples, where predictions thus made have been verified in the event. The conversion, by two reflections in glass, of the plane polarization of light into the circular, is an instance of the highest class of such generalizations directed towards the future, and realised in the progress of research. The undulatory doctrine of light offers other examples no less remarkable, in the anticipation, by a profound theory, of complex effects, wholly unknown as facts, and even in seeming contradiction to all the analogies of the science; yet which experiment afterwards established as real, and in harmony with the other laws of light. The loftiest attributes and objects of a philosophical spirit all lie in this direction. Here it is, in passing from " the region of facts to that of laws " that man takes his peculiar position in the scale of created beings; and here, also, that the intellect of one man stretches furthest beyond that of another.

Under the same light (for all the higher views in science associate themselves into principles of common truth) we may best view the great argument regarding causation,—the "selva oscura" of philosophy, as it has been ever rendered by the inefficiency or ambiguity of language applied to the subject. The frequent misuse of the term *final causes* (perhaps even the adoption of the phrase at all) may be cited as one of the chief sources of error. No proof of efficient and intelligent causation, as distinguished from the bare sequence of events, is more complete and convincing than the power we possess of predicating results which have never occurred to us before; but which arise out of laws so fixed and general, that we can safely anticipate the unknown from what we already know. In pursuing science along this path, (the happiest exercise of man's divination,) we

may obtain from the inquiry are but further examples of this essential condition of our existence in the present state.

If making a single comment here upon the question of materialism, it would be that the advocate for an immaterial principle is often unjust to his argument, in his assiduity to rid himself of those facts which attest the close and constant action of matter upon mind. They are too palpable, not merely in matters of sense, but also as regards the purely mental processes, to admit of any evasion. His true doctrine lies beyond this, in asserting a principle submitted indeed to these influences, but different from them,—capable of independent changes and actions within itself,—and above all, capable of self-regulation in those functions of thought and feeling, to which external agents minister in the various processes of life. The ministering agents may become disturbing ones, and such they frequently are to a singular extent: but in this we have no proof of identity. Whatever of reason we can apply to an argument insuperable by human reason, is against it : and the record of such instances is wholly comprised within that one great relation, which pervades every part of our present being ; but the intimate nature of which is a sealed book to human research.

We may then as fairly reason upon the states or changes of mind depending on the brain as a double organ, as we do on the effects of palpable injury or disease, affecting it directly or indirectly through other parts of the nervous system. And, indeed, in the doubleness of the nerves and other organs of animal life, we obtain a series of phenomena which variously interpret these more obscure disturbances in the mental faculties ; and make it probable that some, at least, depend on changes in the relation of parts, to which a strict unity of action belongs in the healthy state.

Paralytic affections, whether of the organs of sense or voluntary motions, are the most distinct and familiar example of morbid results, connected with this doubleness of structure. However numerous the facts now collected, there is still much to be learnt as to these affections ; and particularly regarding the parts of the brain or spinal marrow with which they are severally associated, and the nature of the diseased changes on which they depend. Modern anatomy has, with much reason and great success, been directed especially to those portions of the nervous system which form, by decussation, the commissures or bonds of union between the two sides ; as well as to those which seem to connect the sentient and motor nerves in their course and functions. These are manifestly parts of singular importance to the whole animal economy. On the connexions they afford depend, it may be presumed, the unity

obtain certainty of an intelligent cause from a source hardly separable from the consciousness of our own intellectual existence. And in thus making the highest efforts of the human faculty the interpreters of the principle of divine causation, we bring our conception of moral cause into closest relation with the physical, and gain not only elevation, but distinctness and stability to all our views on the subject.

and completeness of the functions of this double organization, as well as the translation of morbid actions from one side to the other;—and any breach in the integrity of the union, and of the relations thus established, may no less tend than disease in the respective parts themselves, to disturb the actions of the brain and nervous system. It is probable that many phenomena of sensorial disorder have their origin in these connecting parts more especially, as the seat of disease. The decussating fasciculi of the anterior pyramid, for instance, are a portion of such structure, where any morbid cause might be likely to produce peculiar effects; and to which, in fact, we must look for one of the most remarkable conditions in hemiplegia. The relation of the two eyes in natural vision, and under disease, offer some curious evidences on this subject; and here the facts are more distinct in certain other animals, as birds for example, than in man. But it is probable that minute anatomy, in its connexion with pathology, may hereafter furnish us with many more proofs to this effect than we at present possess.*

Without actual paralysis, however, or any obvious default of the external organs, there is a frequent dissimilarity or inequality of the two sides of the body as regards their nervous condition; testified by differences in sensibility and voluntary power; and also, though more ambiguously, by liability to morbid affections, connected with

* We have reason, as is well known, to attribute to some morbid cause affecting the commissure of the optic nerves, where the semi-decussation occurs, the singular phenomenon of *suffusio dimidians*, where one-half only of the field of vision is perceived by the mind. That the interruption causing this deficiency takes place here, is made more probable by its being usually a transient occurrence. I have known a patient, suffering under various symptoms of diseased brain, who frequently saw only half his face when looking into a glass. Very recently I have met with an instance where a father and daughter had each the liability to this affection. The case of Dr. Wollaston is known from his own description, and was too well explained by the circumstances of cerebral disease, which closed the days of this extraordinary and excellent man. During the latter period of his life, when the existence of such disease, and the certainty of its event, were alike known to him, he was accustomed to take exact note of the changes progressively occurring in his sensations, memory, and voluntary power. He made daily experiments to ascertain their amount, and described the results in a manner which can never be forgotten by those who heard him. It was a mind unimpaired in its higher parts, watching over the physical phenomena of approaching death; and, what well deserves note, watching over the progressive change in those functions which seem nearest to the line separating material from intellectual existence.
In a paper by Dr. Alison, "On single and correct vision, by double and inverted images on the retinæ," (*Trans. of Royal Society of Edinburgh*, vol. xiii.,) will be found some striking and original views on this curious subject. His reasoning in favour of the doctrine that single vision by two eyes depends on the *partial* decussation of the optic nerves (a phrase he prefers to semi-decussation);—his views as to the connexion between the decussation of the pyramidal bodies and that of the optic nerves, in reference to the single or separate vision of different animals;—and the explanation given of erect vision by inverted images, upon anatomical facts which indicate that impressions made on the retina do really reach the cerebro-spinal axis in the same order as those conveyed by the sense of touch;—all deserve great attention, though still leaving difficulties which belong to the metaphysical part of the question.

some of the proper functions of organic life.   The observation of
such inequality, whether connate or proceeding from changes in the
progress of life, is often made by patients themselves. I have known
a case where blisters, and all other external stimulants, acted more
powerfully on one side of the body than the other.   Andral mentions an instance where perspiration occurred only on one side of
the body; and I have seen a singular example of such limitation to
one-half of the face; under the circumstances, however, of this
perspiration being morbid in kind and degree.* Hemicrania is one
of the most familiar forms of headache, and it is well known with
what exactness the pain often follows the median line.   I have
recently seen a case where, in hemicranial headaches, occurring
generally every fortnight, there has been for nearly a year past a
regular alternation of the two sides; so that the patient has got the
habit of reckoning with assurance which side is next to be affected.
It has been observed that deafness is more frequent in the left ear;
but this, if it be true, depends probably on some external cause.†
The instances, however, are numerous of disparity of certain kind
or degree in the sensibility of the two sides; connected occasionally,
it may be, with the external parts serving to sensation; but sometimes, there is cause to believe, with inequality in the corresponding
parts of the brain which more directly minister to the perceptions
of the mind.   The effects of injury or disease show this most distinctly; but it may occur as a consequence of original deviation
from equality in the two hemispheres.

   Differences in the voluntary power of the two sides are so far
subordinate to the disparity of power and use in the two arms, that
it is difficult to appreciate the influence of other causes, unless
when they reach the extent of actual disease.   Whence this disparity itself proceeds, and how it acquires such uniformity, are
points still uncertain:—that some organic difference is concerned,
must be inferred from the exceptions to the habit being occasionally
congenital, and frequent in the same family. Meckel, indeed, affirms
that a great majority of cases of mal-conformation occur on the
left side of the body; and, as far as my observation goes, the remark
is well founded.‡   Whether it be so or not, the frequent difference
in the two sides, as respects liability to morbid actions and sensations, cannot be denied; and there is much cause to attribute it to
variation in the two hemispheres, and perhaps also in that part of
the system of the spinal cord which is most directly associated with

   * The patient here was a gentleman about thirty-six years of age, and of good
health, save that, on the slightest exertion of speaking, eating, or emotion of
mind, sweat broke out profusely in drops from the right side of the face, strictly
defined by the median line, the other side remaining in its natural state.   As far
as I could see, there was no similar affection of the right side of the body.   The
complaint had existed four or five years, coming on without any recognised cause.
I lost sight of the case afterwards.
   † Perhaps on the common habit of sleeping on the right side, thereby leaving
the left ear more exposed.
   ‡ Handbuch der Menschlichen Anatomie, vol. i.

the sensorial functions.* One side of the brain is often found more affected with atrophy than the other, and this cannot exist without showing itself in some corresponding inequality throughout every part of the body.

Bichat is the author who has dwelt most explicitly on the symmetry in the organs of animal life, and the effects of default in this, either from natural conformation or disease. The relation of the symmetry of double parts to unity of action and individuality of result, is so important in all the economy of life, that every deviation from it deserves careful notice; and especially where it is associated with some definite injury of the nervous system. Hitherto I have spoken principally of the effects of such disparity upon the senses and voluntary power. But must we not look to the functions of memory and association also, as probably affected in various ways by unequal or incongruous action in the two hemispheres of the brain? These faculties (if indeed we can rightly define them as separate) are manifestly dependent on organization, and only partially subject to the intellectual being. Their unity of action is as needful as that of the senses and voluntary powers, and may be presumed as closely connected with symmetry of the two sides of the brain. Without referring, then, to those more striking consequences of accident or disease, where these functions are suddenly altered or impaired, we must admit the likelihood of analogous effects from slower, slighter, or transient deviations from equality. It is difficult to conceive such to exist without the occurrence of some change, however obscure to observation from the complexities which surround it.

* Or, looking to the reflex nervous function as one distinct from the true cerebral, and depending on an especial organization in the spinal cord and certain other nerves, disparity of the two sides may equally exist here, and influence the respective actions both in health and disease.

The inquiry, indeed, may be pursued in connexion with the doctrine, now held by some of the best anatomists, that all the organs of the body are symmetrically double in their earliest state, even those which subsequently form cavities or continuous tubes. Pathology follows and supports the same view, in the general fact that, where organs are symmetrical as regards the median line of the body, or contain a median line in their own structure, there is a tendency in all morbid actions to terminate at these lines; a tendency often hidden or obscured by other circumstances, yet obvious enough to form a principle of frequent application in the treatment of disease. The general symmetrical arrangement of the nerves and blood-vessels of the two sides is doubtless directly concerned in the phenomenon; but we must look beyond this secondary cause to the more general one just mentioned for its full explanation.

It would be worth while, as a curious point in pathology, to collect the various cases in which diseased action or structure terminate or undergo change at a median line in the organs affected. Many such are familiar to the most common observation, where the difference exists not merely in the sensations, but also in the texture and intimate functions of the two sides. I might name as an example (more singular from a tube being concerned), certain inflammations of the larynx and trachea, in which the vascular injection is perceived in one-half only of the circumference of the tube, the other half preserving its ordinary appearance. Andral states that he has made the observation in several cases where one lung only was diseased, and this on the same side as the affection of the trachea.

It has been supposed indeed by some, in relation to the mental faculties, that each side of the brain is separately capable of fulfilling the functions, whatever they may be, in which this organ ministers to them; and this view has been applied, although somewhat vaguely, to explain the alleged fact that every portion of the brain has been found in different cases the subject of disease, without obvious disturbance of the faculties of the mind. The evidence here, however, is insufficient in nature and amount. And were we even to admit the assumption that a given portion of one hemisphere could minister to a certain function in all its completeness, the action being suspended of the corresponding part on the opposite side, yet is there no proof that such substitution can immediately take place, and still less any presumption that it is likely to occur where the functions of the affected parts are not suspended, but merely altered and deranged. The distinction in the latter case is manifest; and it is only partially obviated by referring to those phenomena of sensation where the organ of one side appears under certain circumstances to perform all that belongs to the entire function. The instances are as frequent of disturbance to the common action of both, from morbid changes in which one alone is originally concerned.

The considerations already stated bring us immediately to the question, whether some of the aberrations of mind, which come under the name of insanity, are not due to incongruous action of this double structure, to which perfect unity of action belongs in the healthy state? When the functions which directly place us in relation to the world without are liable to so much disorder from this source, it is to be conceived that the intellectual part also may suffer change; the result either of disturbed perceptions, of irregular associations, or of some unequal consciousness or exercise of voluntary power. The subject is very obscure, and all proof of difficult attainment; but I think it more probable than otherwise that such inequality may be a cause of some among the many forms of mental derangement. Obvious lesion or active disease are concerned in numerous cases; and these also, when affecting one side of the brain only, may produce effect by disturbing the proper correspondence, or unity of action, of the two sides. But there are presumably other cases where, without manifest injury of structure, there may be inequality enough in the actions of the two hemispheres severally, to disorder and derange the trains of thought for longer or shorter time, and in every variety of change and degree.

It has been a familiar remark that in certain states of mental derangement, as well as in some cases of hysteria which border closely upon it, there appear, as it were, two minds; one tending to correct by more just perceptions, feelings, and volitions, the aberrations of the other; and the relative power of the two influences varying at different times. Admitting the general truth of this description, as attested by many curious examples, the fact may be explained in some cases by the coexistence before the mind of real and unreal objects of sense, each successively the subject of belief;—a phenomenon possibly itself depending on the doubleness of the brain and of the parts ministering to perception, though we cannot obtain any certain proof that such is the case. But this explanation will not adequately apply to the instances where complete trains of thought are perverted and deranged; while others are preserved in sufficiently natural course to become a sort of watch upon the former.* Here, indeed, we may still seek for explanation, by supposing the two states to be never strictly coincident in time;—and this view is in part sanctioned by what observation tells us of the inconceivable rapidity with which the mind shifts its state from one train of thought or feeling to another; a fluctuation and rapidity much greater in reality than we recognise by language or in our common contemplation of the subject. Articulate speech, in fact, is often unable to keep pace with such changes; nor have we any means of measuring by time these momentary passages of mental existence, crowding upon each other, and withal so interwoven into one chain, that consciousness, while it makes us aware of unceasing change, tells of no breach of continuity. If the latter explanation be admitted, then these cases come under the description of what has been termed *double consciousness;* where the mind passes by alternation from one state to another, each having the perception of external impressions and appropriate trains of thought, but not linked together by the ordinary gradations, or by mutual memory. I have seen one or two singular cases of this kind, but none so extraordinary as have been recorded elsewhere.* Their relations to the phenomena of sleep, of somnambulism, reverie, and insanity, abound in conclusions of the deepest interest to every part of the mental history of man.

Even admitting, however, that these curiously contrasted states of mind are never strictly simultaneous, it is still a question whence their close concurrence is derived. And, in the absence of any certainty on this obscure subject, we may reasonably look to that part of our constitution, in which manifest provision is made for unity of result from parts double in structure and function. This provision we know in many cases to be disturbed by accident, disease, or other less obvious cause; and though we cannot so well show this in regard to the higher faculties of mind, as in the instance of the senses and voluntary power, yet it is conceivable that there may be

---

* It is remarkable how distinct an expression to this effect may occasionally be had from patients themselves. I have recently seen a case of which the most marked feature was a frequent and sudden outbreak of passion upon subjects, partly real, partly delusive, but generally without obvious or sufficient reason at the moment; these excesses attended with loud screaming, execrations, and acts of violence in striking or breaking things within reach. Here the patient himself described to me the sort of separate consciousness he had when these violent moods were upon him ; his desire, but feelings of inability to resist them ; his satisfaction when he felt them to be passing away. It was a painfully exaggerated picture of the struggle between good and ill. " Contra miglior voler, voler mal pugna."— *Dante.*

† One of the most remarkable cases of this nature is that narrated in Mr. Mayo's Physiology, 4th edition, p. 195.

11*

cases where the two sides of the brain minister differently to these functions, so as to produce incongruity, where there ought to be identity or individuality of result.

It is not easy to carry this argument beyond the form of mere question; yet there are other points connected with it of much interest to the physiology of man. For example, we have cause to suppose that there is in infancy a progressive education of the organs of sense, correcting the original perceptions they afford; defining the relations of the several senses; and giving unity of effect to impressions made on double organs. In like manner the education of the voluntary powers may be said not merely to extend the influence of the will to new muscular movements, but also to concentrate and individualize the powers of the mind in acts of volition, separating them more entirely from the involuntary actions of the same parts. And carrying the argument further, we may suppose that the faculties of memory and combination are subject to the like education; tending always to give more proper and perfect unity to these functions than belongs to them in the outset of life, and to establish more completely the conscious individuality of the being.

This view, if just in itself, is fertile in curious inferences; and serves better than any other to conciliate the phenomena of infancy with those of advancing age;—the progress from confused, or it may be double perceptions,—from automatic or ill-regulated motions, —from imperfect and confused associations and impotence of recollection,—to that singleness of perception, volition, and memory, which the mind attains in its healthy state, and which marks the intellectual character of man. This is, however, one of the many points at which human reason is forced to pause, before entering on paths too obscure for its further progress.

In the foregoing remarks I have spoken generally of the brain as a double organ, without referring to the several parts of this complicated structure, or to the effects of morbid changes upon these respectively, in altering the relation of the two sides, and the functions which are perfect only from their entire correspondence. The excuse for this want of detail must be found in the very incomplete knowledge we yet possess on the subject. Notwithstanding all that has been obtained from comparative anatomy, pathology, and actual experiment (and large has been of late years the gain from all these sources), there is still scarcely a single part in the structure of the great nervous centres composing the brain, in which we can affirm with certainty the connexion between particular function and portion of structure. The inferences drawn with seeming assurance from one experiment or pathological fact have been as expressly negatived by others. In a few instances,—such as the general facts that the lobes of the cerebrum have more express relation to the mental faculties; that the organs of speech depend on the anterior lobe; the motions of respiration on the corpora olivaria; the senses of sight, hearing, and smell, on certain tubercles or ganglia proper to each,—approach has been made to more certain knowledge; but still not without much ambiguity, arising from the complex nature of the functions themselves, as well as of the disturbing causes from which inferences are drawn. In the case of vision, for example, we have the perplexing fact of blindness, more or less complete, produced by injuries to remote and seemingly unconnected parts of the brain, and even by affections of the spinal marrow; and similar contrarieties exist as to other senses and functions.

One of the most singular proofs how much is wanting to our knowledge of the brain, may be found in the fact, that we are yet ignorant, or at least not assured, of the true functions of the cerebellum,—a part which, from its size, situation, and structure, must be judged to fulfil some one or more of the most important purposes in our being. That it is a source of, or determines the distribution and agency of some particular nervous power, may be deemed certain; but the contradictory opinions or confessed ignorance of the most eminent physiologists, as to the nature and actions of this power, denote it to be an object of discovery still unattained.*

That our knowledge of the respective functions of the cortical and medullary parts of the brain and spinal cord should be still mere surmise, is another striking proof how much we have to gain on this subject. We can affirm almost with certainty that the functions must be different; but whether the first be a structure for generating power, the second for conveying it,—or whether, as others have supposed, the cineritious part has to do with motive power, the medullary with sensation and volition,—or whether the distinction is to be sought for in some less obvious source,—are questions yet open, the solution of which will singularly enlarge our knowledge in every part of physiology.

In treating thus generally of the brain under its condition as a double organ, there has been no occasion to refer to the doctrines of phrenology. This system indeed, in recognising separate organs, perfectly alike and equivalent to each other, in each hemisphere, is bound more especially to suppose that any casual disparity between the corresponding organs of the two sides must have the effect in disordering the faculties therewith connected. But the course of argument just pursued is independent of these particular assumptions. And, while affording a foundation on which to rest future knowledge of these parts, it does not profess more than to trace one great condition of the cerebral structure,—that of doubleness of parts,—into some of its probable effects on the sensorial functions and the general economy of life.

* Even the minute and delicate anatomy of Reil has failed of reaching this discovery. The inferences derived in common from the researches of Magendie, Flourens, and Hertwig, are probably those which approach nearest to the truth. Seeing the uncertainty which hangs over this subject, there is much interest in the late discovery by Mr. Solly of direct nervous communication, through the restiform bodies, between each lobe of the cerebellum and the sentient and motor nerves of the same side. And to the researches of Sir Charles Bell, fruitful in so many great discoveries, we owe much that bears upon this obscure point in physiology.

CHAPTER XIII.

ON SOME POINTS IN THE PATHOLOGY OF THE COLON.

I DOUBT whether all the functions and disorders of this bowel have obtained proper attention in practice, or their influence in producing disorder elsewhere been sufficiently regarded. The colon is often viewed merely as a part of the alimentary canal, with the office of simple transference through it, after the more important stages of digestion have been completed. It is certain, however, that there is much beyond this, in its actions both of healthy and morbid kind. Its peculiar situation, connexions, and flexures,—the great extent of internal surface, multiplied by the bands, folds, and other inequalities of the lining membrane,—its liability to unequal distension, contraction, or stricture,—and the variety of secretions from the glands and vessels of its inner surface —all concur in giving great importance to this intestine in the animal economy. From its continuity with the rectum, many circumstances are common to the two portions of the canal, and to these the following remarks will equally apply. But each part has its peculiarities; and those of the colon, for obvious reasons, have hitherto engaged less than their relative share of notice.

The nature and amount of change in the alimentary matters, as they pass through this part of the canal, are yet not wholly known; nor are we assured as to the opinion lately propounded, on the authority of Dupuytren and other accurate observers, that the large intestines are peculiarly concerned in the digestion of the vegetable part of food. That there is power of absorption into the system through some part of their structure seems certain; and, equally so, that this power may be much augmented by especial circumstances. But as a general fact it is probable that this portion of the intestine is much more an organ of secretion than of absorption; and, further, that these secretions are not merely subservient to changes in the matters passing through, but useful or necessary in removing other excrementitious or hurtful parts from the system. It cannot be doubted that much of what is healthily voided by the bowels is, in fact, a secretion from the follicles of the lower intestines, and not simply a residuum of food. Under this view, the colon becomes one of the excretory organs in a more direct sense; and, admitting such double natural function, the study of its morbid conditions is one of much interest to the medical practitioner.

I shall not here speak of the disorders or diseased states of the colon, more familiarly known:—spasms, acute or chronic inflammation of its mucous membrane, dysentery, the various forms of ulcerated or gangrenous intestine, induration or thickening of its coats, &c.; but confine myself chiefly to a few points less recognised in general practice.*

Many morbid states attributed, with the too frequent vagueness of medical language, to the stomach and liver, are chiefly, as I believe, connected with the colon as their seat and source. This remark applies alike to disorders of secretion, and to those in which the symptoms depend either on nervous sympathy, or simply on the mechanical effects of juxtaposition and attachment of parts. As respects the first of these cases, it cannot be doubted that many of the various egesta from the bowels, usually termed bilious, and treated as such, have no other relation to bile than that of mere admixture. They are separated from the vessels or glands of the larger intestine by exudation or secretion,—act upon the contents of the bowel, as well as upon the living parts of the system, according as they deviate in quantity or quality from the healthy state,—and, in the excess of such deviation, indicate a state of the glands and secreting membranes, or it may be of the system at large, con-

* It is difficult, however, to mention ulceration of the colon (connected, as so often happens, with similar state of the adjoining membrane of the ileum), without adverting to the singular and sudden influence which this state of bowel seems occasionally to have on the system at large,—the condition of typhoid fever and sensorial disorder speedily brought on, and often with fatal issue. I have known this termination so rapid in some cases, even within a few days of the first seizure, and with so little severity of local symptoms, that it was difficult to consider the ulcerated state of the intestine as other than a partial effect of the constitutional disorder. This view, however, is not equally warranted by other cases; and we have still much to learn on every part of the subject. The value of research directed to it is well indicated by the statement of Andral, that, out of ten cases of acute malady occurring in other parts of the body, there is an average of eight in which derangement is found either in the texture or functions of the alimentary canal. This statement may be too precise for the many ambiguities depending on our ignorance of the primary seats of disease, but it is nevertheless true to a remarkable extent.

The whole subject of gastro-intestinal disease has additional interest in its connexion with the modern doctrine of some pathologists (of whom Broussais is the most conspicuous), who regard all the varieties of continued fever as merely symptomatic of certain morbid states of inflammation of these membranes, or their follicles and glands. This opinion, were it true, would go far to decide that still unsettled question which lies at the root of all pathology, whether there be any true idiopathic fever wholly separate from local irritation or lesion of texture? But, besides that the arguments for this doctrine are manifestly too exclusive in their direction to the intestinal canal, they do not furnish any adequate proof that the affections of its membranes are really prior in date to the febrile symptoms, even in some of the fevers to which the term of gastric seems especially applicable. The uncertainty arising from this source is best denoted by the fact, that almost every argument employed to prove the derivation of fevers (and especially those of typhoid type) from disorders of the intestinal membranes may be equally directed to show their immediate origin in affections of the brain. The parity of weight, in reasoning thus differently applied, gives strong presumption that neither opinion can be really just. And adverting to all the circumstances in the history of fevers,—their varieties, origin, course, and termination,—it is impossible not to find in the changes of the blood itself a source equally probable as those just mentioned, though perhaps as little to be determined by any precise evidence. No author has better treated this subject than Dr. Alison, in his Outlines of Physiology and Pathology.

nected with some of the most important diseases of which we have knowledge.

The peculiar matter, resembling coffee-grounds, which sometimes comes away in such large quantity from the bowels is often described as disordered bile, though I believe it to be separated in great part in the lower intestines. Those secretions also which resemble chopped grass or spinach have probably the same origin; and even of the liquid which is called green bile it is doubtful what proportion may come from the liver. The colour of what passes from the bowels is often the effect of changes taking place within the intestine itself. This may readily be conceived, looking to the many materials present for chemical combination, both in the egesta and secreted fluids; and to the facility with which colour is changed from very slight causes, such as a small excess of acid, in matters thus composed. We know from experiment that such changes are readily effected by artificial means, as well in the urine as in the matters passing from the bowels; and, though not having certain knowledge of the same chemical agencies going on in the body, many that are analogous may fairly be presumed to exist.[*]

The liver in fact, important though its functions and diseases be, is often charged with more than belongs to it; and the provocation of mercurials applied and continued under this view, in cases where the coats of the intestines are chiefly or exclusively the seat of the action which it is sought to remedy. In some instances benefit may arise from the practice, though founded in error as to the direction of treatment. But if the appearance of the matters separated from the bowels be made, as it often is, the exclusive argument for persistence in these medicines, they may be carried to an injurious extent, and interfere with the natural course of actions really salutary to the system.

In like manner, those other secretions which have the character of minute specks of blood disseminated through a fluid; or sometimes of a black matter almost as deep as ink in colour; may be considered chiefly owing to exudation from the mucous membrane of the bowels.[†] These secretions or exudations, which contain elements of the blood and partake much of its nature, may be extravasated, it would seem, from the membrane of any part of the intestines. But I have seen instances where products of this nature, coming away in large quantity before death, have been found on examination everywhere lining the coats of the colon, without any appearance of similar kind in the smaller bowels.

Secretions, having certain of the characters of blood, do in fact show themselves in every grade of change from pure blood to appearances widely different; with certain evidence that they are

---

* The researches of Tiedemann and Gmelin in Germany, and those of Dr. Prout in our own country, afford many valuable results on this subject.

† Andral describes the separation of this black matter (*mélanose*) from the coats of the bowels by the phrase " la membrane muqueuse la laisse suinter." —*Anatomie Pathologique*, vol. ii. Perhaps there can be none better than this.

separated from the intestine itself, whatever name be given to the process by which this takes place. It is important to distinguish these from mere bile, and to note their various appearances; partly as concerns questions of treatment directed to the membranes; equally so, because these secretions are often the index to changes taking place in the system. In some cases they precede and indicate a fatal event; depending here, it may be, on a particular state of the exhalants, akin to that which produces cold sweats upon the skin; or possibly in still greater part on changes in the state of the blood itself. In other instances it would seem that these large discharges of dark grumous fluid (of different quality doubtless from the preceding) actually relieve the blood from some morbid matter, loading and disordering the whole system, and particularly perhaps the chylopoietic organs and venous circulation. The apparent relation of certain of the matters, so removed, to the morbid products which have been classed under the name of melanosis, is one of the results derived from recent examination into diseases of the blood.

The alteration in general health, which often follows these discharges, undoubtedly justifies our placing them among the various actions (whether assuming the aspect of disease or not) by which important changes are made in the mass of the circulating fluids, and through these on the various functions of the body. I have seen many cases of hypochondriasis of long duration, many also of protracted disturbance in the action of the heart, speedily and wholly relieved in this manner. We have other authority for this view in the peculiar quality of some of these excretions; rendering them, if retained, exceedingly noxious to the body in which they are generated. And there is further evidence here in the analogy to those curious fæcal excretions from the roots of various plants, poisonous more or less to the vegetable life by which they are produced.*

The treatment of the cases mentioned above is not without many difficulties, and we have reason to believe that mischief is often done by a mistaken practice. To deal with these instances as with common diarrhœa, by opiates and astringents, may injuriously interfere with actions beneficial or needful in their results. On the other hand, irritation, by medicine or otherwise, to the vascular surface which is the source of these peculiar excretions, may inflict mischief of another kind, and equally prevent a salutary issue.

These difficulties, in truth, are common to cases of diarrhœa of more ordinary kind, arising out of the complication of the causes

* The observations of Macaire on these remarkable excretions from the roots of plants are valuable to agriculture, as well as interesting in the analogies they afford to animal life. On the latter point I have notes of several instances, showing the noxiously sedative influence of some of these matters generated within the body, and thus separated from it. One case is now before me, where, in a vigorous young man of two-and-twenty, the pulse, habitually about seventy, was brought down below forty, and rendered very irregular, by the passage through the intestine of a large quantity of that peculiar secretion resembling black oil; the pulse rising again immediately after it was removed from the body.

concerned ;—the various ingesta received into the stomach,—the different secretions poured into the alimentary canal, as well from the large glandular apparatus of the liver and pancreas, as from the innumerable mucous follicles in every part of the canal,—and further, the great extent of vascular surface from which fluids may be separated by exudation or otherwise. In effect of this, a great variety of division and nomenclature has arisen as to these disorders ; adding much to the embarrassment of the student, and increasing the chances of error in practice. It will probably be admitted by all who give honest expression to their experience, that even in these very familiar complaints the rule of treatment is less certain and consistent than in most other disorders, fluctuating perpetually between the doubt whether the diarrhœa present is to be checked by direct means, or allowed to proceed on its course ?— whether medicines should be given with intent gradually to alter the secretions; or, with a bolder hand, to remove at once such as may be disordered or hurtful? This uncertainty of practice in bowel complaints, as they are termed, can only be obviated by experience, and the careful observation of what is mere mechanical irritation,—what vitiated secretion from other topical causes,—what the separation of noxious matters from the blood through the liver or intestinal membranes. Technical rules here may be too minute, as well as too general and vague, to be useful in practice. At all events, they can never supersede individual discrimination.*

Some of the remarks just made relate to disorders of the small intestines as well as to those of the colon ; but the cases are so numerous in which this bowel is especially affected, and to which these questions of treatment directly apply, that it is impossible not to notice them as an essential part of the subject.

The disturbances produced in the body by what may be called the mechanical conditions of the colon are deserving of notice, particularly as they are sometimes mistaken for more serious disorders of other organs. The whole subject, indeed, of the sympathetic and reflex actions produced by unequal distension and change of place in the parts of the intestinal canal, is curious and instructive in various points of pathology. Their influence upon the nervous

* In all general reasoning on the disorders of the abdominal viscera, it is needful to estimate fairly what is still wanting to an adequate knowledge of the healthy functions of these organs. The stomach is now perhaps best known ; but chiefly through researches of recent date. The progress in the minute anatomy of the liver, for which we are chiefly indebted to Mr. Kiernan ; and even the valuable experiments of Tiedemann, Magendie, and others, expressly applied to its physiology, have left us yet in doubt as to the uses of the bile in the animal economy ;—whether specific for certain purposes in digestion,—or as an agent in the separation of carbon or other elements from the blood,—or for both these objects in conjunction. The functions of the spleen are still matter of vague conjecture. Numerous questions remain to be solved as to the especial functions of the several parts of the alimentary canal. And though much more has been done towards the history of the kidneys both in sound and diseased state, yet the relations of the urine, in its quantity and properties, to the various changes occurring in other parts of the body, still offer singular difficulties to the physiologist.

system, even as connected with the common processes of digestion, is familiar to us in every moment of life. It is more strikingly shown in different states of disease, especially in the female habit; as well as during the period of infancy, when the nerves are more sensitive to all automatic impressions, and less under the control of those functions of the brain which afterwards govern so large a part of the muscular system.

As respects the colon, these effects manifestly depend on the contiguity or attachments of the intestine to other parts, making the latter liable to be affected by the distension which so often occurs in the whole or parts of this bowel from temporary causes. Its peculiar course through the body renders some of these connexions very important in pathology; since not only the stomach and other parts of the alimentary canal, but also the action of the heart and the respiration, are liable to great disturbance from this cause. The latter effects are more especially produced when the transverse arch, as so often happens, is distended throughout; forming a tight girth across the body, and pressing directly or indirectly upon the diaphragm, stomach, duodenum, and even the large vessels underneath. Though there is often ambiguity from the distension of the stomach itself, yet in many cases it is obvious that the colon is solely concerned; either through air confined in the bowel, or from more solid matters compacted in some part of it; and it forms one of the various circumstances in digestion by which the heart's action is disturbed, so much frequently as to alarm the most experienced practitioner.

Irritation to the stomach is often produced by distension of the transverse arch of the colon; and many states of disorder supposed to belong to the former organ are really due to this cause. The distress so common to dyspeptic patients in the course of the night, and obviously connected with the bowels, seems frequently to belong to this part of them especially; the recumbent posture giving more effect to all such irritations as depend on its distension and pressure on adjoining parts.

The close attachment of this portion of the colon to the stomach and duodenum has doubtless also the effect of exciting sympathetic irritation in these organs; and we may look to such connexions as explaining many of the symptoms of disordered digestion, and the morbid sensations or actions suddenly spreading between distant parts of the alimentary canal. A distended state of the colon may disturb an earlier stage of digestion, either mechanically by pressure on parts nearer the stomach, or indirectly through the system of nerves by which these various organs are associated in one common function.

Disturbances in the colon are not unfrequently mistaken for complaints of the kidneys; and there is the greater liability to this mistake from the influence they really have, (either mechanically, or by some cause of sympathetic irritation, or by changes in the circulation,) in disordering the state and secretion of the urinary organs.

12

Whencesoever it arise, so close and frequent is this connexion, that we may always expediently begin the treatment of apparent disorder of the kidneys by full evacuation of the larger intestines; secure that we shall obtain alleviation in this way, if not entire relief. Few of the means especially directed to the urinary organs are so effectual as those which operate upon them through this part of the intestinal canal.

Many pains in the back and loins, which pass vaguely under the names of lumbago and rheumatism, are distinctly to be referred to the same cause. The effect of treatment here is usually the most certain proof; purgatives and injections relieving these symptoms speedily and effectually in some cases, failing in others. The very peculiar pains in the same parts, which attend the whole course of acute dysentery (and which are by no means sufficiently indicated in the common descriptions of this disorder), give further evidence how remarkably the morbid state of these bowels affects the adjoining textures.*

Cramps, and other spasmodic and painful affections of the lower limbs, are a frequent effect of the mechanical distension of different portions of this bowel: perhaps, also, of disordered secretions lodged within or passing through it. Of the latter we obtain proof in the very common occurrence of these symptoms with dysentery or ordinary diarrhœa. The acid also, which, according to recent observation, is for the most part predominant in the larger bowels, may be in such excess as to produce various disturbance by sympathetic irritation. The cœcum, for obvious reasons, is the part most liable to distension; often from solid matters accumulated there in extraordinary quantity. Its effects when thus loaded, even upon distant organs, are so various and considerable as to require discrimination in practice. I have seen more than one case where pains were produced in the right leg, severe and constant enough to suggest the idea of more permanent disease in the joint or limb.

There is some difficulty in understanding the cause of those circumscribed swellings, to which all parts of the intestines seem liable, and which are sometimes so contracted in extent as to convey to examination the idea of hard, well-defined tumours, occasionally deceiving for a time by the resemblance. These swellings, as well as all other distensions and inequalities of the bowels, are more frequent in the female habit, and seem in certain cases connected with the peculiarities of the hysterical temperament. As the passage along the intestine, though impeded, is not generally closed in these cases, we must suppose that its coats are distended into a sac out of the direct course of the canal; originally, perhaps, from air generated suddenly or detained in this part of the intestine, or from

* Those physicians who consider that dysentery expresses not so much a state of the intestinal membranes, as a more general disorder of the chylopoietic viscera and of the portal and mesenteric circulation, may find somewhat different explanation of these pains. It is probable, indeed, that they are derived from different sources.

the irritation of other more solid matters producing partial contractions, with relaxation of the intervening membrane and loss of power in the muscular coat. The sudden and unequal distension of the bowels from certain articles of food, or during the action of irritating medicines, illustrate the nature of these more circumscribed swellings. They are often relieved by a single active purgative (with which creosote or cajeput oil may beneficially be combined) : but the habit of using frequent laxatives, by weakening the canal and rendering its motions irregular, increases the tendency to such disorders.

The whole subject of tympanitis, to which these circumscribed tumours have relation, is under some obscurity. It is certain that there occurs occasionally a powerless or palsied state of the intestine through more or less of its extent, concurrently with which tympanitic swellings come on;—whether as cause or effect is not well ascertained. I think it probable that each supposition may be correct in part. The distension of any portion of the canal beyond a certain point clearly impairs or destroys its power of action; and still further distension may thereby be produced. But we have reason to suppose that this state of intestine (especially when general throughout the canal), arises from other causes, such as belong either to the nervous system of these organs, or to the effects of inflammation on the surface of the lining membranes. It is not easy to discriminate among these cases of mutual action, nor is it often attempted, though some points of practice might be founded on the distinction.*

The various distressing sensations and disturbance to other parts, which thus arise from undue distensions of the canal of the colon, almost defy enumeration. They form part of the sufferings of the dyspeptic, affecting all parts of the nervous system; and are unhappily aggravated in general by the means which such patients are prone to employ. I have elsewhere spoken of the importance to the healthy state of this bowel and of the rectum, that there should be a proper and equable distension by the contents passing through them ; and of the evils arising from habitual or frequent purging, in reference to this point, as well as to the state of the secretions from the coats and glands of the canal. I again allude to the subject from persuasion of its importance in practice. I may add further that the habit in question seems occasionally to be chargeable with that opposite state of the colon, equally distressing in its results,—the permanent contraction of the canal for more or less of its extent, particularly along the transverse arch.†

* Dr. Abercrombie, in his work on the Diseases of the Abdominal Viscera, relates one or two cases in which large tympanitic swellings were speedily removed by the use of electricity.

† In two of the most remarkable instances I have seen of this organic disease there had been a long habit of using large and very frequent doses of salts ;—in one of these cases to a greater extent than I have ever before known it. This may have been casualty, but it is worth noticing.

I have often sought to ascertain what are the appearances of the tongue especially indicating disordered states of the colon. Such have been described, and it is likely that they exist, seeing how variously and delicately this organ gives testimony to changes in the long tract of internal membrane, of which it is one of the terminations. But so many are the complications here present, chiefly from the state of the intervening parts, that I have never been able to satisfy myself with having obtained any well-defined knowledge from this source alone.*

I do not enter here into the treatment of disorders of the colon, which, in their more distinct forms, receive ample notice in all medical works. I will merely remark that, in many painful and spasmodic affections of this bowel, more aid might be got from external applications over the back, whether stimulating or anodyne, than is usually done. I have often found them greatly more effective here than on the abdomen, where they are generally used from regard to convenience; and this remark especially applies to the complaints of children. The remedy so employed, comes nearer in many places to the actual seat of disorder, and has more diffused effect on parts continuously affected. Where opium cannot be given internally, its employment in this way by embrocations is often very beneficial, provided these be adequately used. And even where such means are not effectual alone, they at all events come greatly in aid of those which are administered within.

* Among the external indices of change within the body, the tongue is perhaps the most valuable. Constantly as it is referred to in practice, we are still only partially informed of all the diagnostic marks it affords. Scarcely can the pulse compare with it in the extent, variety, and accuracy of these indications; which are not limited to disorders of the membranes and secretions of the alimentary canal, or to the presence of fever in its several forms, but extend also to the nervous power, of various states of which it affords very correct evidence. The sensibility, the voluntary powers, and even the more intellectual functions are often exactly thus interpreted. (Αι τρομαδεες γλωσσαι σημειον ουκ ιδρυμενης γνωμης. —*Hippocrates.*) No one can doubt this who is familiar with the appearance of the tongue under great debility; slowly and with difficulty put out of the mouth; withdrawn with equal effort; tremulous the whole time; its surface parched from stoppage of all secretions; its sensations blunted or depraved. There are various parts of morbid anatomy which less merit the care bestowed on their representation than do the disordered states of this organ. The fugitive nature of the appearances, and their less fixed relation to disease from the variety of parts they represent, are the obstacles here. But the opinion may be repeated that the physician cannot better study any set of signs than those afforded by the tongue, the palate, and fauces; the terminating portions of that inner surface along which so many actions are carried on both of health and disease. The Observations of Dr. Beaumont on the precise and uniform relation between the tongue and stomach, in the case of St. Martin, might well justify this remark, were it needful to seek other authority than that of daily experience.

CHAPTER XIV.

ON THE EPIDEMIC INFLUENZAS OF LATE YEARS.

In the whole history of disease, there are few subjects of greater interest than those epidemics, which, under the familiar name of influenza, have prevailed so frequently of late years;—with certain common characters not to be mistaken, and identifying the disorder with others which stand on earlier medical record. In a former chapter, I have mentioned the singular relation of these epidemics to other forms of disease; particularly to some of the exanthematous, intermittent, and continued fevers.* These connexions, though in no case sufficient to establish identity, yet are intimate enough to suggest some community of cause, and a closer correspondence in every part than is expressed in our nosological tables. The pathologist and practical physician may both draw knowledge from this source. While to the more general observer, the epidemics in question are matter of deep interest, in their sudden appearance, in their wide but successive diffusion over vast tracts of the earth's surface, in their very general yet unequal influence, and in the amount of mortality they inflict.

Little can be added to the many exact descriptions we possess of the course and symptoms of this malady. What I have to say chiefly regards the question as to origin; some particular points in the pathology of the disorder; and a few others, having reference to the principle and methods of treatment.

The first of these topics is one of exceeding difficulty, and upon which scarcely any certain knowledge has yet been obtained. The only opinion which can be stated with any assurance, is, that there must be some peculiar virus of the disease, whatsoever its nature, which, like the virus of measles and scarlatina, is capable of spreading or communication under certain laws; and probably of remaining in the body a certain time, before evolving the more active symptoms of the malady. It seems hardly possible to avoid such conclusion, looking at the whole course and history of these epidemics. It is the only view under which we can explain their identity at different periods of time, and in distant places, during the course of the same epidemic. Sir G. Baker's narrative of the influenza of 1762, or Huxham's still earlier reports of the epidemics of 1733 and 1743, might be taken throughout as a description of those of 1833 and 1837. That which occurred in 1675, and is recorded by Sydenham, equally corresponds with our recent experience. The history of the disorder at Copenhagen and Berlin will serve with little variation for its course and character at Lisbon

---

* See Chapter VII. On the Connexion of certain Diseases.

12*

and Malta. This uniformity can scarcely be explained but by identity of physical cause; and for such identity it is difficult to look to other source than some material virus;—recurring, we know not why, at different periods,—and capable, through certain unknown laws, of being widely duffused, without change of character or loss of power.

It is true that some authors, and in concurrence with common opinion, have attributed these epidemics solely to atmospheric changes, and the influence of extraordinary seasons upon the human body. And it must be admitted on behalf of this opinion, that certain of the seasons during which they have prevailed, have been remarkable and anomalous; and further, that in common catarrh, arising from obvious causes of atmospheric change, many of the symptoms resemble the lighter and more transient forms of the disorder in question. But there is something manifestly beyond this relation, and independent of it. A disease which has appeared and spread at different seasons, in the middle of summer as well as in the depth of winter;—which has been found traversing whole continents, continuing this course through many successive months, and often assuming even a definite direction of progress;—which affects contiguous places in different degrees, and at different times;—which frequently continues in the same place for several weeks or months, under every appreciable variety of atmospheric state;—and which often affects, almost simultaneously, large masses of people living on the same spot, while others in adjoining localities are exempt;—such disease cannot be considered as due to any of the known qualities or variations of the atmosphere, to which the term weather is applied. If changes in the air are at all concerned, they can scarcely be conceived to act in other way than as engendering, or giving greater intensity, or readier diffusion, to some material virus, the active cause of the disorder. Even this is difficult to suppose under the diversity of conditions just noticed; while beyond this we cannot go without contradicting some of the most assured facts which enter into the history of these diseases.

The argument and inference here may best be established by taking a single epidemic; tracing, as closely as the report of facts will allow, the manner of its spread both as to time and localities; and removing all the conditions which we can thus prove not to be concerned. The influenza which spread over every part of Great Britain and Ireland during the spring of 1833, (after having previously appeared in Russia and the northern parts of Germany, inflicting great mortality in every part of its course,) might well be selected for such illustration; were it not that the similar epidemic of 1837 was even yet more marked in its characters and progress, and attested by more various record from the countries it traversed. I have given below certain facts regarding this epidemic; chiefly illustrative of the points just referred to, and in so far aiding towards the general history of the disease.* Some of these facts may bear the aspect of atmospheric causes being directly concerned; but when it is considered that these states of weather were similar and

* The influenza of this year made itself distinctly known as such in London, the first week in January; the weather during the four months preceding having been singularly wet and stormy. On the 29th of November a hurricane occurred from the S.W., of almost unprecedented violence in this country : on Christmas-day a storm of wind and snow, simultaneous over the whole of the west of Europe, snow falling even in the streets of Lisbon and Palermo; in such quantity in England as for some days to impede all intercourse throughout the country. What is more remarkable, from the remoteness of the locality, snow fell at Canton on the 8th of February, never before seen by the oldest inhabitant of that place. As another singular event in this widely spread storm, the French army marching upon Constantina suffered severely under three days of incessant snow. About the same period violent hurricanes prevailed over every part of the European and American seas. It might seem as if the earth, in its movement through space, had been exposed to other than the ordinary periodical causes acting on its atmosphere or surface. And it is yet for philosophy to say, whether some of the more general conditions to which we are thus subject do not arise from various agents, wholly external to itself, with which our planet comes into contract or proximity while sweeping along its orbit? Some sanction is given to this idea by the periodical meteoric appearances which have recently been the subject of observations, with results so remarkable in their nature and details.

Succeeding to the Christmas snow in England was a severe frost for some days; then a thaw the first week in January, followed by very uncertain and fluctuating weather till the middle of February, this being the period during which the influenza chiefly prevailed; the winds variable and from every quarter; the barometer high and low; the thermometer ranging from 25° to 55°; fogs and clear atmosphere, though tending to the former; rains and dry weather, though the former much more frequent. It was a remarkable peculiarity in London, which I noticed also during the last weeks of 1836, that the heaviest and most continuous rains occurred with a high barometer; the longest courses of dry days with the barometer below 29°. Succeeding to the period of the influenza the cold was again very severe, with heavy falls of snow all over England, from the 20th of March to the middle of April, and the thermometer as low as 10° or 15° below the freezing point during the latter days of March. Even in May the temperature was several times considerably below 32°.

The duration of the influenza in London might be stated broadly at six or seven weeks. I saw no new cases after the 16th of February, but the tendency to relapse continued a long time afterwards in one form or another. The greatest severity of the disorder was from the 20th to the 24th of January. Including the slighter cases, it would be no exaggeration to rate the number attacked at half the population of London, (perhaps few escaped the influence altogether,) while the ordinary ratio of mortality during this time was nearly doubled. The valuable report of Dr. Clendinning from the Marylebone Infirmary, and Dr. Heherden's Analysis of the Bills of Mortality during the epidemic, may be consulted on this part of the subject.

As respects the local progress of the disease, the following are a few of the facts I have noted, but which might be easily rendered much more numerous from authentic sources. The epidemic appeared in Russia, Sweden, and Denmark, during the month of December; two or three weeks, as it would seem, before its occurrence in London. In Copenhagen, according to the memoir of Dr. Otto, at least 30,000 persons were under the disease at one time early in January. In Scotland, also, it was observed earlier than in England; and generally in the northern and eastern parts of England before the southern and western. It had been prevalent about a fortnight in London before it became so at Brighton and other parts of the southern coast. It was from a week to a fortnight later than in London before it appeared in Lancashire, Cheshire, Gloucestershire, and the

simultaneous over vast tracts of continent, while the disease made its progress by steps, having a certain course of general direction, but very irregular both as to space and time;—that it appeared at Madrid about three months later than in Scotland, and in Malta six weeks still later;—and that various intermediate towns and tracts of country seem to have been wholly exempted;—we cannot reasonably look to weather as a direct cause, whatever its influence in giving action or diffusion to other materials of disease.

Amongst other particular proofs to the same effect, the following may be cited as especially remarkable. The influenza of 1831 began in London about the middle of May, and continued during June and a part of July, under very hot though damp weather. While that of 1837, still more violent in degree, appeared during the first days of January at the close of a severe frost, and prevailed till towards the end of February, followed again by weather of singular severity. Again, with respect to this latter epidemic, we have the fact of its raging in England and the northern parts of south-western counties. Though very general over the island, yet were there places seemingly unaffected, even in the contiguity of others where the disease greatly prevailed.

The epidemic showed itself in Paris about a month later than in London, having previously appeared at Calais and other intervening places. I saw patients who, on their journey from Paris to London, had come upon an infected town, and been suddenly seized with the malady. At Paris it was stated to have affected at least half the population, but seemingly with less mortality than in London. The epidemic spread gradually over other parts of France. About the end of February it affected the northern coast of Spain, the more conspicuous there from its influence on the events of the civil war, then raging in Biscay and Navarre. Almost at the same time it appeared at Lisbon,—a new occurrence in that city,—spreading *successively* to the several towns which lie upon the Tagus, even to the Spanish frontier. Dr. Leitao, who has narrated its progress in Portugal, seeks to show that it is contagious, and was brought directly from England to the British squadron in the Tagus, in the vessels of which it first appeared. The same idea prevailed in Biscay as to its manner of importation. The disease reached Madrid about the end of March, and prevailed there the whole of April.

In Germany the influenza appeared at Berlin in January, affected Dresden somewhat later, and Vienna and Munich a fortnight after Dresden. At Hamburgh, where it appeared in the first days of January, Dr. Rothenburg states that more than half the population was attacked. I do not possess any information as to its progress in Italy. In Malta it first showed itself about the 1st of June.

A remarkable fact is, that an epidemic, having the characters of the influenza of the northern hemisphere, prevailed at Sydney and the Cape of Good Hope in the latter part of 1836; the time thus corresponding with its earliest appearance in the north of Europe, though under a date of *season* wholly different. Sir John Herschel informs me that the weather was warm and apparently genial, at the time when almost every individual in the Cape District was suffering under the epidemic. The malady spread up the country as far as Gnadenthal, producing there considerable mortality in the Hottentot population.

The influenza of 1762 is first recorded at Warsaw about the end of February; over the north of Germany it spread about a month later. At Hamburgh and in London it appeared about the same time. Paris, and the greater part of France, were wholly unaffected. Venice appears particularly to have suffered. In the month of July the disease appeared in the English fleet in the Mediterranean. Beyond this time we have no record of its progress.

Europe during the depth of winter; while its prevalence in some southern countries of Europe was extended to the latter end of May, or the beginning of June.

Recurring to a former period, the influenza which spread over England in 1782 during April and May, had been noted in the East Indies during the latter months of 1781; had prevailed in Russia from December to February; and did not reach Italy and Spain till the autumn of 1782, three months after its prevalence in England.

It is impossible to look fairly at these circumstances, and not to see that the known conditions of the atmosphere, as we estimate them by our instruments, are inadequate to their explanation. Perhaps the more than common prevalence of easterly winds, with a hazy atmosphere and dense fogs, during the seasons of these epidemics, are the facts most favourable to the hypothesis in question. The latter circumstance in particular has been noted at many different periods of their occurrence. And, though correct observations are much wanting on the subject, something may be assigned to the electrical state of the air, manifestly disturbed during some of these periods, and possibly becoming in this disturbance the cause of the phenomena just noted. Still these circumstances are too partial, and too often occurring without like concomitant effects, to justify the belief that they act as direct causes of the disease. The most summary statement then of the argument is this:—that all obvious conditions of weather being the same in a certain number of places, the disease appears in them at very different times, or in some not at all;—and secondly, that it occurs in various places, or in different years at the same place, under states of season and weather wholly opposed to each other.*

Arguments of the same kind, somewhat modified, apply equally to the notion of what has been vaguely termed terrestrial influence, —an undefined agency proceeding from unknown source within the earth itself. In one instance, the simultaneous appearance of a similar epidemic in the northern and southern hemispheres might seem to give sanction to such hypothesis; but this instance, as far as we know, is a single one, and cannot be placed in opposition to the many facts attesting the slow and irregular progress of the disease

---

* Sir G. Baker, though relating certain singularities in the winter and spring of 1762, yet is wholly opposed to the view of these being directly concerned as the cause of the epidemic. Amongst other objections to this, he states the fact that places within two miles of London were attacked much later than London itself. He remarks further, what well merits notice, that the disorder appeared in the metropolis before it was known in any other part of Britain. It began here the first week in April, in Edinburgh a month later, in some parts of the north of England not before the end of June.

Before quitting this subject, I must refer to a very valuable memoir by Dr. Black of Bolton (see *Seventh Report of the British Association*), on the epidemic of 1837, as it appeared in that town. This paper, besides other important statistical details, contains a meteorological register for the first three months of the year; from which, however, no especial inference can be drawn in relation to the periods or peculiarities of the disease.

even through adjacent localities, under conditions apparently the most inconsistent with this idea of its origin.

I have dwelt so far in detail upon these questions, not merely from their intrinsic interest, but from the connexion with many other important points in the history of disease. Whatever the causes of influenza, it is clear that they are closely associated with conditions which operate in producing or giving greater frequency to other disorders also. It is most important to estimate the nature and extent of these connexions through the illustrations which they mutually afford. And no disorder furnishes such explanation more remarkably than that of which we are now treating.

It is impossible that the relation to the Asiatic cholera should escape notice here. Independently of some singular concurrences as to time, the question regarding dependence on atmospheric causes is so much alike for the two epidemics, that any argument admits of being directly translated from one case to the other. The symptoms are less analogous than the manner and extent of diffusion of these erratic disorders : but even here there are certain resemblances in the suddenness of invasion ; and the rapid or sometimes instant prostration of power which ensues. All the proofs we possess of a virus peculiar to the cholera equally apply to the epidemic influenza ; and the need of such specific agent to explain the facts is scarcely less than in the case of scarlet fever or measles, though there is no evidence of contagion here as complete as in the latter diseases.

I have already noticed the argument to this effect from the identity of the disorder at different periods of its occurrence, and in distant countries ; and the force of this becomes more apparent on consideration of the various details of time and locality given above. On careful comparison of my notes during the several influenzas which have occurred since 1831, and extending the comparison to those best described of former periods, I cannot doubt that every essential character of the disorder is the same ; and that there must be identity of material cause to explain this fact. It seems impossible to suppose any series of circumstances, really different, yet thus capable of producing and disseminating the same exact character of disease ; and under conditions which needfully imply a continued and fresh production of the morbid cause. The near equality as to periods and duration of the disorder in each given place is a strong collateral argument ; a correspondence extending even to the period which it has generally occupied in passing over the different countries of Europe. Were other arguments wanting to establish identity of cause, it might be found in the remarkable sequelæ of the disease, to which I shall afterwards advert.

While admitting, however, as almost necessary, a specific virus or matter of the disorder, we are scantily provided with facts to indicate its manner of generation and spread,—why it should be produced at periods so irregular as to interval,—and the precise nature of its action on the human body. Still these difficulties are not greater than occur in the case of the contagious exanthemata ; where but for the familiar view of infection (an explanation itself of recent date in some of these disorders, and which gives the aspect of more knowledge than it really conveys) we are equally ignorant of the nature of the animal poisons concerned, or of their manner of action. That the virus, if not generated by certain conditions of atmosphere, derives activity or power of diffusion from them, must be admitted as probable ; and it is under this view that states of weather may be considered to have influence, and not from changes in the obvious qualities of the air operating directly on the body. The distinction here is obvious ; and best accords with the facts already noted in the history of these epidemics. It is moreover more satisfactory to reason than the vague phrase of an epidemic constitution of atmosphere, which can be understood only by referring to the points on which such distinction is founded.*

Without speculating on the nature of a material agent, which if existing, is yet removed from all direct research, the question may fairly be entertained, whether this disease of epidemic influenza is contagious in the ordinary sense ? and also whether the virus, when received, has a period of incubation, like the infectious matter of some other diseases ?

On the first of these questions, the opinions of medical men have been for the most part negative; though without much inquiry directed expressly to the subject. This is singular, seeing the many points of analogy between the manner of diffusion of this disorder and of cholera ; and the active controversy that has existed as to the contagiousness of the latter. Any proof respecting the influenza is indeed made difficult by the greater and more rapid diffusion of the malady ; by the resemblance of its lighter forms to catarrh, and the connexion of those of graver kind with other diseases ; and by the greater effect of idiosyncrasy and collateral 'causes in modifying the whole course and aspect of the disorder. Little more can be affirmed on the subject than that we have no distinct proof of infection from one person to another; but at the same time no evidence directly against the opinion, and some presumptions for it.†

To the world at large it seems strange that this and similar questions should remain in state thus equivocal. Those accustomed to

* In another chapter I have stated the arguments which may be alleged for the hypothesis of animalcule life as the source of the Asiatic cholera. It is obvious that many of these arguments, if valid, must apply equally to the epidemic influenzas now under notice. But I do not repeat them here ; it being enough to state once what is still speculation without proof; and the cholera furnishing a better instance than any other on behalf of the hypothesis.

There seems sufficient evidence that, among other animals, horses and dogs at least are subject to a disorder resembling influenza, during the period of its prevalence in any given locality.

† The scantier and more tardy intercourse between distant places in 1762 made the evidence at that time more explicit than at present. Sir G. Baker remarks that at several towns, Norwich, Lincoln, Leicester, and Exeter, the first cases occurring of the disease were persons recently arrived from London.

deal with medical evidence in practice can alone understand the difficulty of attaining results on such subjects, free from ambiguity. If the point be better determined hereafter, as regards influenza, it will probably be found that the atmosphere is the medium in spreading the virus; and that modifications are derived as well from changes in this medium, as from concentration of the virus in particular situations. The latter condition brings us nearest to the view of personal infection; and the kind and amount of evidence are much the same as in the case of certain fevers of typhoid type, to which these influenzas are in so many ways closely related.

It is, from similar causes, no less difficult to ascertain unequivocally whether the matter of the disease be dormant for a time after received, like that of certain other infections. The impression I derive from a comparison of many instances is in the affirmative. It must be owned that there are various cases from which an opposite inference might be drawn. Such, in particular, are those where the disease seems suddenly to attack persons arriving at a place in which it is already prevailing;—those also, well attested, where in a prison, barrack, or hospital, a large proportion of the inmates sicken almost at the same time;*—and, further, the remarkable examples, frequent during the more severe of these epidemics, where the patient, seemingly well at one moment, is at the next laid prostrate under the disorder; a seizure scarcely less rapid than that of cholera, though less dangerous in kind. The former cases, however, are somewhat ambiguous; and, for the latter, analogy may be found in many conditions of fever and exanthematous disease, where the onset of the symptoms is equally sudden, though an interval of many days has succeeded to the action of the exciting cause.

We have further argument for this view in the length of time during which liability to recurrence of the disorder exists in the constitution; either with the same symptoms as in the first access of the malady, or more frequently under some of the modifications already adverted to, and particularly that of intermittent fever, with various local affections of anomalous kind:—the intervals between such recurrences, though rarely perfect, yet well enough marked to denote explicitly the changes taking place. A peculiar form of angina, a sort of dusky red band stretching across the tonsils, and giving a sense of constriction and difficult deglutition rather than pain, is one of the symptoms most prone to return; and this disposition may often be taken as an index of the time during which the patient is under the influence of the malady. At the period when it tends most to an intermittent form, I have known the angina

* In one of the London prisons fifty or sixty persons fell ill on one day. The same thing happened with respect to regiments both in London and elsewhere. I have often, in private practice, known six or eight persons seized in a house within twenty-four hours. Still all these instances may be reconciled to the supposition that a certain time is required for the disease, actually received, to evolve itself in an active shape.

to come on at stated times every day, for many days together, with intervals of almost entire disappearance between.

It is a question full of curious import in what this disposition to recurrence consists. If analogy could solve it, we might find this, very closely in every sense, in the phenomena of common ague; equally recurring at repeated and often distant periods from the time of the original attack. But, intimate though this relation be, it rather extends the difficulty than solves it. We are totally unprovided with facts in either case to show the nature of this singular liability of the body. Looking to the great and sudden prostration of power, which is so frequent a symptom of influenza even in its earlier stage, it might be conjectured that there is a state of the nervous system, giving proneness to return of the disorder. Or it may be that the relapses, whatever form they take, are due to the virus of the disease still present or recurring, and acting on the body under modifications, either in its own nature, or derived from changes in the media of communication. Still these are terms too vague to advance us much in real knowledge. We must regard the question as one among the many to be committed to future research; aided perchance by the discovery of new relations between external agents and the body, which may illustrate the phenomena both of health and disease.

Their long persisting influence upon the constitution is certainly a remarkable point in the history of these influenzas. When the disorder has been severe, the state is often distinctly continued for many months. But even where so slight as scarcely to be defined at any one time, there yet is frequently observable a condition of body, prone to various ailments and disturbances, all having relation more or less to the same general cause. These slighter cases, testified chiefly by such liability, and lasting sometimes for a considerable period, are instructive in many ways. It is the same virus of disease ; enfeebled in its action, either by lesser quantity or intensity, or by the difference of bodily constitution to which it is applied. Each of these modifying causes must in fact exist; and both are doubtless concerned in some of the singular varieties which the disorder assumes; connecting it with other maladies by relations which deserve the most sedulous observation. Several of these relations I have pointed out in the chapter on the Connexion of certain Diseases, to which reference has already been made.

The amount of virus (expressing in this term what may be due to concentration as well as quantity) is obviously a very important circumstance, and not enough regarded in common reasoning on the subject. We may argue here almost as securely as if we knew the actual nature of the material cause. Whatever it be, quantity and intensity must, according to every analogy, have their appropriate effect; and the modifications so produced, though they cannot be specified on our present knowledge, yet are certain in their existence, and form the proper objects of future research.

There is difficulty in discriminating as to the relative influence

of the two conditions mentioned above; viz., the individual susceptibility of the patient; and the amount of virus present and active
at the time.   One evidence, but this only of general kind, may be
found in the proportion of severe cases of the same character, existing at the same period.   When this is large, the inference may
be drawn that the material cause of disease is abundant and active
on the spot.   Where but few urgent cases occur in relation to the
extent of the disorder, there is fair reason (though obviously not
conclusive) to attribute these to the particular state of the individuals
so affected.   The same general rule may be applied in all diseases
where a specific virus is presumed to exist; qualifying it of course
by a regard to those local and partial concentrations of this virus,
which doubtless occur wherever it is present as the cause of disease.

Without going into any needless history of symptoms now so
well known, I may notice two or three points especially characteristic of these influenzas, and at the same time indicating their relation to other morbid states of the body.

Perhaps the most remarkable of these is the sedative influence of
the disorder; exceeding in degree what belongs to common fevers;
—testified in the graver cases by a sudden and often extreme depression of the vital powers, even as the first obvious symptom of
the malady, with rigors and congestion in the internal organs, and
feeble reaction succeeding to this state;—in other cases, less severe,
by a speedy passage of the early and more active febrile symptoms
into those of low fever, with something of a typhoid type;—in cases
slighter still, by a prostration of strength out of proportion to the
other symptoms present, and continuing after they are removed.
This depression in different degrees extends in remarkable manner
to the whole nervous system; and the mental functions and feelings
are impaired almost in the same ratio with those of the body.*   The
latter effects seem especially to occur where the attack of the disease is most sudden.   I have seen cases where there was rambling
and indistinct utterance at the very outset; others in which the
state was one of vague stupefaction; some attended with the consciousness of urgent danger at the moment of seizure.   Not unfrequently the symptoms came on suddenly in the middle of the night.

The tendency to the congestive or typhoid form has shown itself
especially, as I think, at the time when the epidemic was at its
greatest height in the number and severity of the cases; and when
therefore the virus might be presumed most active in its influence.   This warrants the conclusion that its direct effect is sedative upon the body; and such inference is confirmed more or less in
all the forms the malady assumes, and best explains its various anomalies, as well as the relations it exhibits to common fevers of the
typhoid kind.   Though identity of nature or origin can in nowise
be proved from these relations, and though the material cause must

* "In omnibus animi demissio, virium que defectus, major longe quam pro
morbi ratione."—*Georg. Baker Opusc. Med.   De Catarrho Epidemico* anni 1762.

be presumed really distinct, yet the analogies become more remarkable in proportion as they are closely pursued. This, moreover, is one of the cases where knowledge may equally be drawn from studying the differences and the resemblances of disease. The exact correspondence of some symptoms, the partial or entire deviation of others, afford a sort of practical analysis; capable probably of being reduced to a more definite form than has yet been given to it, and of great value in a science, where strict evidence is of such difficult attainment.

The reaction which in the influenza succeeds to this first prostration, though manifest in most cases, yet becomes so under the same general aspect of depressed powers. There is fever, often of some days' duration, and attended with great restlessness, sometimes with low delirium; but at the same time little vigour of circulation, and continued perspiration, with no obvious relief to the symptoms. The pulse speedily loses any quickness it has had in the outset; and may often be felt beating sixty or seventy in the minute in an adult, who is suffering at the moment under the violent paroxysms of coughing which attend the disease; with pain, constriction, laborious breathing, and every other symptom ordinarily marking inflammation of the chest.

This latter condition is another token of the adynamic state of the system; one scarcely capable of maintaining true inflammation of parts, yet simulating the character of it; if such phrase may be used, under ignorance of the true nature or proximate cause of the affection. The more common catarrhal symptoms of the disorder; the peculiar irritation of the fauces, windpipe, and bronchial tubes; the corresponding irritation of various parts of the alimentary canal, from the œsophagus downwards; all show the same generic character and type. The mucous membrane lining these passages seems to be the texture primarily, perhaps chiefly, affected. If a name were required to mark the nature of the inflammation, it might best perhaps be termed erysipelatous in kind, having manifest relation to some of the various forms of that disorder. But it is safer in our present knowledge to treat of it as specific; seeing the singular nature of the disease, the manner and extent of its diffusion, and the strong proofs of a specific virus as the source of the whole.

Few things about the influenza are more striking, than the contrast, just noticed, between the seeming severity of local inflammation and the actual adynamic state of the body; and none is more perplexing to the practitioner new to the disease, or inattentive to its peculiarities. The violent and painful cough attending it is the most striking example of this. And here we may best recur to the analogy of booping-cough; there being, together with some essential differences, certain points in which the disorders show curious relation to each other.* These are the cases where bleeding is either

* In the chapter " On the Connexion of certain Diseases," I have noticed the frequent prevalence of booping-cough concurrently with the epidemic influenza, and the difficulty in many cases of distinguishing the two disorders.

useless or directly injurious; and where cordials and quina are sometimes an effectual remedy for symptoms apparently the most opposed to their use.   The pulse, as I have already noticed, is the fairest interpreter here; and no material error can arise in practice, if it be adequately consulted.   Should we admit the term pneumonia, to describe some of the cases where the lungs are chiefly affected (and it is scarcely possible to avoid altogether the name), it must be taken with qualification annexed.   The condition is probably nearest akin to that form of pneumonia, called typhoid; which is generally concurrent with low fever, and in fact has been singularly frequent in the fevers of this type following the spread of the epidemic influenza.

Another point, already in part noticed, of great interest in the history of the disease, is the variation of the parts affected in different-individuals, or at different periods in its progress.   I have elsewhere adverted to the importance of this consideration in all our reasonings on the communication and connexion of diseases.   It is certain and obvious (though as a principle by no means sufficiently recognised) that the same virus, acting upon different parts or textures, from variations in its own intensity or manner of application, or from idiosyncrasies in those receiving it, may produce an aspect of symptoms very different in kind as well as degree.   In the earlier stage and slighter degrees of the influenza, the action of the specific cause seems to be chiefly on the membranes which are the seat of common catarrh, producing symptoms which in various ways resemble this complaint.   There is every reason however to presume that the relation here is not closer than that of the same surfaces undergoing irritation from causes specifically different.   The connexion with that singular form of catarrh (if so it may be termed) to which the name of Hay Fever has familiarly been given, is manifestly more intimate; and especially in what regards the tendency of the latter to intermittent character.   But in truth the whole subject of catarrh is perplexed by nomenclature, and by a confusion of causes and symptoms, justifying, even at this day, the phrase of *Catarrhi Deliramenta*, which Van Helmont formerly applied to it.

In a more advanced stage, or under exposure to a more active virus, or from difference of bodily temperament, (for it is not easy to fix the relative influence of these conditions,) the disorder extends over the membrane lining the air passages of the lungs, and down the œsophagus, more or less extensively, towards the stomach and alimentary canal; producing large mucous secretions, cough, and laborious respiration; and often that peculiar distress about the præcordia which we find in some eruptive diseases, before translation has taken place to the skin.   As these symptoms occur sooner in proportion to the severity of the illness, there is reason to attribute them to greater activity or a more diffused influence of the virus, rather than to mere spreading of the inflammation first induced. And the same reasoning will apply also to those singular cases where the constitutional effects of the virus are more sudden and complete; bringing on, almost without intervention of other symptoms, a typhoid state of the whole body. I have already alluded to the greater frequency of such cases at the period when the epidemic is at its height; and when therefore the material cause may be presumed in greatest activity. I have been led by observation to believe, that in these instances the more direct and extensive effect is on the membrane of the bowels; an inference according well with the many cases in which affections of this membrane bring on, or are blended with, fever of a typhoid kind.

The form of the malady last mentioned is by no means limited to the age, or those of feeble temperament. I have seen it quite as often, and equally severe, in persons of strong constitution and middle age; and hence may be found further reason for concluding that the variation is in the intensity of the cause applied. The sudden stupefaction or low delirium of these extreme cases is represented in those of slighter kind by the weakness, nervous depression, and great restlessness at night; all characteristic of the remarkable effect of the disease upon the nervous system.

The state of the tongue and fauces; the frequent occurrence of angina, with a peculiar kind of dusky efflorescence rather than any considerable swelling; the sense of heat or excoriation passing down the œsophagus into the stomach; are other symptoms indicating the direct effect on these membranes, not less certainly than on those of the respiratory passages.* And a like inference may be drawn from the eruption or efflorescence on the skin frequently attending the complaint; such symptoms, as well as the *herpes labialis*, being a very common index of translation of irritation from the internal membranes to the surface.

Of the disorders directly consequent upon influenza, if not indeed to be regarded as an integral part of the malady, one of the more frequent and remarkable is the tendency to neuralgic intermittent pains or morbid actions in different parts of the body; with periods often as regular as those of common ague, and sometimes taking the tertian as well as the quotidian type. I shall notice certain of these curious facts in another chapter, when treating of intermittent actions of morbid kind; and I need not further particularize them here, though they well deserve to be studied in the relations they express between different forms of disease. Beyond these general relations we have no means of proceeding. Little connexion, save that of priority and sequence, can be traced between the early and more familiar symptoms of influenza, and such partial intermittent affections. Whether they depend on idiosyncrasy of the patient, or on some peculiar application of the virus, or simply on liability given to be affected in this way by other causes, are points equally

---

* Both Huxham and Baker describe the white creamy mucus with which the tongue is covered in this malady, and the observation agrees with what we see in the more recent influenzas. But I do not find noticed by them, or others, the peculiar and vivid redness of the point of the tongue, even when thus coated elsewhere; a mark so frequent as almost to be discriminative of the disorder.

obscure. They seem to be more frequent when the epidemic is declining in any given locality; as the typhoid character of the disorder is more common and distinct when the influence of the morbid cause is apparently at its height. But, however these questions
be decided, a reference to them must enter into all our reasonings
on this part of pathology.

I have also noticed in another chapter the frequent occurrence
of dysenteric symptoms, (often a well marked form of this disease,)
during the progress of the influenza ; or, it may perhaps more justly
be said, in sequel to the ordinary course of the epidemic. The description by Sir G. Baker of the very severe dysentery which prevailed in London immediately after the influenza of 1762 is well
known.* The facts here are so well established by their repetition,
that it is difficult not to suppose a direct connexion, either in the
nature of the cause, or in a liability created by the prior disease to
be affected by the ordinary causes of the latter. I know no decisive
evidence on which to determine this point. The latter, perhaps,
may be conceived the more probable, seeing the apparently increased
liability to other disorders, also epidemic or contagious in kind,
which exists either during the prevalence of the influenza, or as an
effect of the state of constitution it leaves behind. The tendency
to gastric fevers, and other disturbances of these viscera, is, however, that especially marked ; and we have probably no record of
the epidemic influenza largely prevailing, without its being followed
speedily by some other epidemic of this character. I have already
sufficiently dwelt upon the importance of noting all such relations
in practice.

Any remarks on the medical treatment of influenza must be prefaced by the consideration, that we have here a disease depending
on a specific cause, to meet which we possess no specific remedy.
We are notoriously unprovided with any means to resist the access
of this cause ; or to remove it from the body, when received and
in action there. Nor is there any explicit proof that we have the
power of shortening the period of its action, or altering its course
and direction as regards particular parts. What alone can be
effected in our present knowledge is to watch over the symptoms
severally; to mitigate their excess; to promote a healthy and sufficient state of the natural excretions: and to obviate injury to any
particular organ or function.

These circumstances need to be kept before the mind of the practitioner. It is very important for the right conduct of practice, to
know as far as possible in each case the exact scope of our power.
Much fruitless or injurious interference is thereby prevented; and
a better chance afforded of attaining eventually the objects which
are thus clearly defined as wanting to us. While extending more

---

* I am led to infer from Sir G. Baker's narrative of these two epidemic diseases,
(if they may be spoken of thus separately,) that the influenza was less virulent
than those of 1833 and 1837, but the dysentery much more general and fatal
than any of recent occurrence.

or less to the treatment of every disease, the precept especially applies to those where there is a specific virus or definite course of
morbid actions, for which we yet know neither preventive or specific antidote. Here the officiousness of active practice is often a
source of much mischief; and the prudent physician will reserve it
chiefly for the conditions stated above, where alone it is justified by
reason and experience.

A question, however, may be raised regarding the influenza, whether the disorder does not admit of being stopped in the outset? and
common opinion, founded on cases where the symptoms speedily
subside after their first appearance, lean towards this belief. The
proof, however, is ambiguous, seeing the variations which may arise
from different states of the virus, or temperament of the patient;
and the frequency of such cases occurring under different remedies,
or where none whatsoever have been employed. If I were from
my own observation to name any remedy, having some pretension
to the effect, it would be an active emetic in the earliest stage of
the symptoms; but for the reason just given I am far from thinking
this an assured fact.

Whether so or not, vomiting is, I believe, the best means we can
employ at the commencement of the disease, as well as under different conditions of its progress. That it should have been so insufficiently used, in the treatment of the influenza in this country, must
be attributed to the same causes which have made the employment
of emetics comparatively so infrequent in modern practice. In
clearing the mucous linings both of the air passages and stomach
from the secretions which load them no remedy is of equal avail;
and none safer in its application, or more immediately attesting the
good that has been obtained.

The employment of purgatives in influenza is probably best regulated by the principles which direct their use in the exanthematous
fevers. Frequent and violent action of this kind I believe to be
useless, or positively injurious, in the disorder; having no specific
influence as a remedy, and tending to increase irritation and depress
the general powers. This is probably equally true when the pneu-
monic symptoms are most severe, and where the virus affects
chiefly the membranes of the alimentary canal. The cough which
is so peculiarly characteristic of the disorder, whether proceeding
from either or both these sources, is often manifestly increased
by the irritation thus given. While the bowels, under excess of
this practice, readily become tympanitic, and more fretful and disordered in their actions.

These comments of course do not apply to a better regulated use
of the remedy. The proper use of purgatives in influenza seems
to be to clear the bowels thoroughly in the outset; and subsequently,
by such as are simple and least irritating, to prevent accumulation
or disordered secretions. Nor does this view exclude the employment of mercurials to correct and maintain these secretions in
healthy state. However it may be at the beginning, the liver usually

gets gorged, and its functions disturbed, in the progress of the
malady; and this is true even in many of those slighter cases, where
the patient, though for weeks perhaps under the influence of a morbid cause, is never actually withdrawn from his ordinary occupations.   To relieve this state, mercurials are the speediest remedy ;
and often more effectual, generally less irritating, when uncombined
with other cathartics.   So employed, with the intervention of
stronger doses occasionally, calomel and blue pill act most beneficially, not simply in relieving present symptoms, but in preventing
many of the most distressing sequelæ of the disease. And this is an
effect which, in my experience, is by no means equally produced by
mere purgatives frequently or harshly employed.

I have never known any certain benefit from the treatment of
influenza by sudorific medicines. Ambiguous in use in other cases,
they are still less called for in a disorder of which continued and
copious perspiration is one of the most frequent symptoms. If antimonials are of any avail here, it is not, I believe, under this view,
or even as a common febrifuge, but solely as one means among
others of exciting vomiting, where this is desirable.

The same opinion may be fairly given as to the whole class of
expectorants.   I never saw any good obtained from them in the
influenza, unless when unintentionally they have acted more or less
as emetics.   The act of vomiting is in truth the most effectual expectorant in most cases where this action is urgently required.

It seems necessary to add opium to the list of medicines, from
which little certain benefit is to be had in this disorder.   The restlessness at night, which is so general a symptom, would seem to
require its use ; but from some cause or other it is rarely effectual
in giving much relief :—and, though the cough may for a while be
mitigated or suppressed by this remedy, it is doubtful whether the
good so obtained is an equivalent to the disadvantages in various
ways incurred.

The most important question of treatment in influenza doubtless
regards the extent to which antiphlogistic means may be carried,
or the fitness of employing them at all. And the point as to bleeding
is that which stands foremost here, and has chiefly embarrassed all
practitioners.   The most general precept on this subject is liable to
exceptions; but, collecting what on the whole is safest and most
expedient, it must be one which forbids bleeding as an ordinary
practice in the disorder.   The adynamic type throughout in the
greater number of cases,—the singular disproportion in all between
the seeming severity of the inflammatory symptoms and their real
slightness or nullity ;—the actual failure of bleeding in mitigating the
violent and painful cough which seems most expressly to require
it,—and the frequent success of remedies precisely the reverse of
this ;—all show a specialty in the disease, to which we must refer,
more or less directly, in every question of practice. Whatever the
cause or precise seat of irritation, it is certain that it has rarely the
characters of true membranous inflammation. In truth, the same

reasons which prevent or limit bleeding in hooping-cough apply no less to the peculiar cough and irritation of the influenza. We have rarely any authority for it in the state of the pulse ; which neither in strength nor frequency bears relation to these seemingly inflammatory symptoms. While the difficult or painful respiration, which often suggests the remedy, furnishes evidence against its fitness, by becoming frequently more laborious than before ; the effect of larger accumulation in the bronchial cells, and of diminished power.

These are all points of great interest in practice. It is less needful indeed to enforce them now, as the repeated experience in several epidemics, speedily following each other, has given general knowledge and warning on the subject. It is certain, however, that much injury resulted from the error, before this experience was obtained; and especially in the treatment of those of infirm habit or who were advanced in years.

Exceptions there undoubtedly are to the principle just laid down. In some habits, prone to inflammation, the first reaction of the disorder may pass into what is really this state, and require blood-letting for relief. There are other instances where the congestion on the lungs is such in degree as to demand the same remedy. And I believe on my own experience that these latter instances are more frequent than the former, and carry with them more distinct justification of the means employed. It is hardly necessary to add that, when used, it should be as early in the disorder as possible ; with a cautious regard to age, and with close observation of the effects on the pulse, cough, and respiration. When there is much doubt existing, blisters may expediently be tried first ; and especially where the cough is the symptom most urgent in the case. The epigastrium I believe to be generally the best place for their application.

The conditions which thus render bleeding for the most part improper, go further, in sanctioning to a certain extent the treatment which has for its express purpose to excite or sustain the vital powers. And accordingly cases are not infrequent where stimulants give immediate relief to symptoms which, on first aspect, and interpreting them by other diseases, would seem to require very different treatment. Here, happily, as I have before observed, the pulse is generally a more faithful guide ; and there are few cases where, if fairly consulted, and in immediate sequel to the means employed, it may not be relied upon for direction. If wine or other cordials give it force and steadiness, without adding to its frequency, and without exciting fresh cough, the inference may safely be drawn as to the treatment of the disorder in its future progress.

But watchfulness as to these tests is always needful, to guard against exceptions to the general rule, and excess in the methods so suggested. Stimulants may be used earlier, or to greater extent, than it is fit they should be ; and morbid actions brought on which would not otherwise have existed. It is well indeed to repeat here regarding the treatment of influenza, that the majority of cases require rather the forbearance of the physician than any strenuous use of active remedies, upon whatever principles adopted. Still it is important that these principles should be fixed as far as possible, and made capable of ready application to the more urgent, though rarer, cases which come before us.

The only other remark I have to offer regards the use of bark, or the sulphate of quina, in the influenza. Its value here is unquestionable; derived not simply from its quality as a tonic, but further, and more especially, from its specific power in various intermittent affections. Any inference that might be drawn as to its use, from the tendency in the disorder to these intermittent actions, is fully justified by the actual effects. It relieves them, when fully established, almost as speedily and certainly as the attacks of a common ague; and this whatever the part of the body so affected. This remarkable power over one of the conditions of the disease gives so far a specific character to the remedy, that it may rightly be adopted in prevention of a state which it is capable of curing. It is not easy to define an exact time at which its use should be begun. This must vary in different temperaments, and in different degrees of the disorder. But it is an inference from the reasons already stated, that quinine may be given safely and beneficially in many cases where there is still hard cough, with pain, oppression, and restlessness;—and experience confirms this conclusion. A soft feeble pulse, and moist skin, often occur with these symptoms, and furnish additional authority for the practice. If the cough itself, as frequently happens, tends to intermittent character, the security of the remedy becomes greater, and its effects more speedy.

It may seem that I have drawn upon my notes at too great length, regarding a disease not very frequently occurring, and the suggestions as to the treatment of which are rather negative than positive in kind. To this it may be replied, that we are wholly ignorant when, or how often, the epidemic may recur;—that the long lapses of time without appearance of it are quite as extraordinary as its frequent return of late years:—that the lesson of forbearance in some points of practice is as valuable as that of activity in others;—and that the best chance of reaching further knowledge on the subject is to define exactly the limits of that we now possess. Any excuse that may still be wanting for the length of these remarks must be found in the singular character and history of the epidemic, and in its relation to other diseases; points to which I have already sufficiently adverted, and which render the topic a very interesting one to the medical inquirer.

CHAPTER XV.

ON DREAMING, INSANITY, INTOXICATION, ETC.

DREAMING; insanity in its many forms; intoxication from wine or narcotics; and the phenomena arising from cerebral disease, are the four great mines of mental discovery still open to us;—if indeed anything of the nature of discovery remains, on a subject which has occupied and exhausted the labours of thinking men in all ages. These several states, singly and in their connexion with each other, unfold facts, and illustrate relations, which seemingly could have been known to us from no other source. By the curtailment or suspension of certain functions, by the excess of others, and by the altered balance and connexion of all, a sort of analysis is obtained of the nature of mind, which its waking and healthy acts cannot equally afford, either to individual consciousness or the observation of others.

The following remarks refer chiefly to the state of dreaming, intoxication, delirium, and insanity;—the conditions arising from obvious disease, though illustrating the others in many most important points, being in some respects better considered apart.

The relations and resemblances of these several states are well deserving of note, even in their most general aspect. A dream put into action (as in fact it is, under certain conditions of somnambulism) might make madness in one or other of its most frequent forms; and, conversely, insanity may often with fitness be called a waking and active dream. Delirium and intoxication may be considered transient effects, from temporary causes, of that condition of sensorium which, more deeply fixed and longer continued, obtains the name and produces all the aspects of mental derangement. It is obvious that there are circumstances in common here, not sufficient indeed to identify these various states—for how difficult to identify the several conditions of one only !—but enough to show that certain analogous changes occur as the cause and foundation of all.

Insanity, from having the characters of a malady, and this often of hereditary nature,—from its deep import as such to all the relations of human life,—and from the strange and painful forms it assumes,—has ever been viewed with more profound interest than any of the states thus allied to it. The feeling has led physicians and medical writers of every age to seek earnestly for some formal definition of madness;—a vain and unprofitable research! Its shapes and aspects are as various as those of the human mind in a sound state, and as little to be defined by any single phrases, however laboriously devised. Where such definitions are attempted, especially in courts of law, they fitly become matter of ridicule, or causes of contradiction and perplexity. Mental derangement, how-ever the name be used, is not one thing, nor can it be treated as such. It differs in kind not less than in degree; and in each of its varieties we may trace through different cases all the gradations between a sound and unsound understanding, on the points where reason is thus disordered.*

On this latter view we are entitled chiefly to rest in every inquiry as to the nature and cause of insanity. We shall find here a wider and more secure basis on which to found observation, than in any other mode of regarding the subject: and if such a phrase were per-mitted as "a just theory of madness," I know no principle so capa-ble of affording it as that which views all the forms of insanity, including delirum, in their relation to corresponding healthy states of mind; tracing this connexion through those intermediate grades, which are so numerously exposed to us in the various conditions of human existence. The diversities of the mind in what is accounted its healthy state,—the effect of passions in suddenly altering its whole condition, of slighter emotions in gradually changing it, and of other incidents of life in affecting one or more particular faculties, —its subjection periodically to sleep, and casually to the states of intoxication, somnambulism, and reverie,—its gradual transition in fever from a state where there is consciousness of vague and wan-dering ideas to that of perfect delirium,—all these furnish so many passages through which we may follow sanity into insanity, and connect the different forms of disordered intellect, as well with each other, as with the more natural functions of the mind.

Even looking to the broad distinction between congenital idiotcy (*amentia*), where there is simple deficiency of natural faculties; and active insanity (*dementia*), in its more various and formidable shapes, we find various connexions between them, best illustrated in those cases where a more active form of madness subsides by degrees into fatuity. The complexities of the mind in its healthy state are such, its natural changes so great, its relations to the body so various, and the causes of disordered action so obscure, that we must be satisfied by classing the facts generally, without drawing those arbitrary lines which nature does not recognise, and which observation perpetually belies.

Yet if it were an object to obtain a description of insanity which might apply to the greatest number of cases, I believe this would be found in the conditions which most associate it with dream-ing; viz., the loss, partial or complete, of power to distinguish be-tween unreal images created within the sensorium, and the actual

* As far as I can see, one of the most assured practical tests of insanity, par-ticularly in cases of difficult legal discrimination, is the sudden change of habitual judgments, feelings, or actions, without obvious cause. Many are the instances, indeed, where, from the less perceptible gradation of change, and its limitation to certain subjects, this criterion cannot be admitted alone. But it is manifestly more secure in general than the appeal to an imaginary common standard of reason, which scarcely two persons would describe alike.

perceptions drawn from the external senses; thereby giving to the former the semblance and influence of realities;—and, secondly, the alteration or suspension of that faculty of mind by which we arrange and combine the perceptions and thoughts successively coming before us.*

Though this general description will by no means apply to all that is termed mental derangement, yet, from the extensive influence of the causes denoted in it, there is reason for considering them more minutely: and particularly as they illustrate strikingly those grada-tions from the sound to the unsound mind, which I have mentioned as affording the best basis for every part of this inquiry.

A principal modifying cause, when tracing these relations between insanity and dreaming, will be found in the varying degree of ex-clusion of sensations from without. This exclusion is not marked by any single and definite limit, even in what may be deemed the soundest sleep. It varies presumably at every moment of time; and not only as to the degree in which the power of general perception is present, but even as to the ratio of sensation from different organs. One sense, in the plainest meaning of the expression, may be more asleep than another. In dreams this exclusion of external sensations is generally more complete than in madness, or the ordinary state of intoxication; and here, accordingly, the *excursus* of aberration appears to be widest. Cicero says, and justly, that if it had been so ordered by nature that we should actually do in sleep all we dream, every man would have to be bound down before going to bed:—"majores enim, quam ulli insani, efficerent motus som-niantes."†

Much has been written on the subject of spectral illusions, and not without reason, from their strange and almost mysterious nature; from the seeming warrant they give to the wildest tales of credulity; and yet further, from the link they form in the chain betwixt sound reason and madness.‡ Without repeating instances which have become familiar, I may remark that these singular phenomena, while connected on the one side with dreaming, delirium, and in-sanity, are related on the other, by a series of gradations, with the most natural and healthy functions of the mind. From the recol-lected images of objects of sense, which the volition, rationally ex-ercised, places before our consciousness for the purpose of thought, and which the reason duly separates from realities; we have a gradual transition, under different states of the sensorium, to those spectral images or illusions which come unbidden into the mind; dominate alike over the senses and reason; and either by their in-

---

* All the varieties which Dr. Arnold has brought under the general terms of *ideal* and *notional* insanity, would seem more or less distinctly referrible to the above heads.

† De Divinatione, 59.

‡ In the Zauber Bibliothek, a curious work by G. C. Horst (1825), will be found two or three striking narratives to which this interpretation manifestly belongs.

14

tensity or duration produce disorder in the intellectual functions, and in all the actions founded thereon.

In the gradations between these two states, the most remarkable is that in which the images of sensible objects, having no present reality, do nevertheless intrude themselves so forcibly that they cannot be put aside, although the person is fully awake, and conscious of the presence of illusion. Numerous instances of this fact are related. I have myself met with many singular examples of it; and more than one attesting that recorded by Dr. Abercrombie, in which the patient, though creating the illusion by an effort of will, had no equal power of removing it by voluntary effort. I recollect another remarkable case, where the patient, a robust young man, a native of Germany, suffering under various symptoms of cerebral disorder, was so severely affected by the continuance of these images of very painful kind, and the associations attending them, that his hair, in the course of about ten weeks, changed its colour from being nearly black to a grayish white; of which latter colour it grew again, after being shaved.*   In all these cases, we may affirm that the images are furnished solely by the memory of former impressions on the senses; although when reaching the degree of spectral illusions, they probably, like the dreams to which they are closely akin, assume combinations which could not occur in the healthy and waking state.†

It is not difficult to understand how some of the most singular incongruities of madness may arise from this coinage of the brain—this struggle betwixt spectral illusions and actual impressions on the senses; each severally credited, and each brought to bear upon action.   The combination of these conditions may be so various, the changes among them so rapid, as to explain every degree of such mental aberration, as well as the diversity of forms under which it occurs; from the simple reverie of the absent man, to the wildest incongruities of the maniac.

Nor is the application of this view limited to illusions in which sight is concerned.   As these images often assume the character of reality, so likewise are the impressions of sound, created by certain

---

* This gentleman spoke English well ; but during some weeks of his illness, though with English attendants around him, he spoke only German.   Suddenly one day, when I was with him, he resumed English with his wonted facility, and, though incoherent in sense, continued to speak it while he remained in London.

† Aristotle, in his remarkable chapter on Memory, which deserves to be more read than it now is, notices these spectral illusions.   Τα γαρ φαντασματα ελεγον ως γινομενα, και ως μνημονευοντες· τουτο δε γινεται, οταν τις την μη εικονα ως εικονα θεωρη. And again, more expressly, when treating of dreams—Διο και τοις πυρετουσιν ενιοτε φαινεται ζωα εν τοις τοιχοις απο μικρας ομοιοτητος των γραμμων συντιθεμενων· και ταυτα ενιοτε συνεπιτεινει τοις παθεσιν ουτως, ως αν μεν μη σφοδρα καμνωσι, μη λανθανειν οτι ψευδος· αν δε μειζον η το παθος, και κινεισθαι προς αυτα.

The phenomenon, having always existed, could not at any time escape notice. But it is interesting to mark these earlier notices of the fact, especially in the connexion given it with other mental phenomena, by one of the most remarkable observers of any age.

disordered states of the sensorium, such as to excite perfect belief in their exsitence from without. The noises of organs, bells, street cries, and " airy tongues that syllable men's names," are well known as frequent forms of these auricular illusions. Instances are common in cases of insanity, where the patient is so strongly affected by imagined voices, as to produce on his part earnest or passionate rejoinder. I have known these illusions of hearing such, in a case of delirium tremens, that the patient held a long and angry colloquy with an imagined person, whom he supposed (there being no illusion of sight) in an adjoining room. He allowed pauses to intervene, while his opponent might be presumed to be speaking; yet, amidst all this, answered immediately and with correctness every question I put to himself.

These illusions of hearing, like those of vision, may be traced through every grade, from the imaginations of sounds created by voluntary effort, or stealing upon us independently of the will, but felt to be without external source; to those which possess the mind with entire belief of their reality, and force it into action founded on this belief. A familiar example of what may be termed the first stage of insubordination to the will is that of certain musical sounds or airs coming unsought for upon the mind, and even tormenting it by their persistence, despite every effort to put them aside. Harsh sounds long continued, as of a carriage during a day's journey, will often continue to make similar though feebler impressions upon the sensorium, for hours afterwards. Some of these cases may depend upon changes within the organ of hearing itself; others, from their nature, must clearly be referred to the sensorium or percipient part. As this class of illusions has been altogether less noted than the preceding, I subjoin one or two singular cases which I find among my notes. They illustrate more particularly the gradations of states just alluded to, and the connexion between a natural and healthy function, and the morbid actions of the same part.*

* Mr. ——, at the age of eighty-five, in a feeble bodily frame, preserved a clear and acute understanding, great powers of humour, and a deep interest in all passing events. No affection of the brain had ever occurred in the course of life. A casual fall, on the 19th of May, threw his head with some violence against the edge of a sofa : a swelling was raised on the forehead, but no other obvious injury : some faintness ensued, but no stupor or sickness. An hour or two afterwards there came on a failure both in the memory and articulation of words. He could not remember the names of his servants, nor, when wishing to express his wants to them, could he find the right words to do so. The sounds he uttered, in seeking for speech, were not only unintelligible to others, but *consciously so to himself ;* a singularity he reasoned upon at the time, and recollected afterwards.

A restless night, with some vomiting, ensued ; but the following day the memory and speech returned to their usual state, and continued free from disorder on the 21st. On the 22d, when driving out in his carriage, for the first time after the accident, there came on the singular *lusus* of two voices, seemingly close to the ear, in rapid dialogue, or rather repetition of phrases, unconnected with any event of present occurrence, and almost without meaning. Mr. —— described himself as perfectly conscious of the fallacy of this, but as wholly unable to check or withdraw the perception of these voices, or to change the

We have instances, chiefly in cases of actual insanity, of corresponding illusions of the sense of touch, scarcely less remarkable than those of sight and hearing. Even the senses of taste and smell furnish intimations of similar kind. Hysterical affections, which, when highly aggravated, may be said to stand on the brink of insanity, abound in examples of disordered or illusive perceptions of touch, pain, and other feelings, which it would be difficult to define; the result of causes affecting all parts of the nervous system.

This struggle then, occurring in every form and degree, betwixt illusive and real sensations, affords perhaps the widest basis on which to reason as to some of the most frequent hallucinations of

phrases they seemed to utter. There was no nervousness on his part, but rather amusement in the strangeness of the phenomenon, and the absurdity of the speeches to which he felt himself listening. The same state continued during dinner. In the evening, while seeking to read, similar voices seemed to accompany him, as if reading aloud; sometimes getting on a few words in advance, but not beyond what the eye might have reached; sometimes substituting totally different words; the whole having the effect of distinct speech from without, and being entirely beyond control of the will.

These phenomena (of which I have notes made at the moment by Mr. —— himself) were almost wholly removed the next day, and never afterwards recurred. Their relation to some of the conditions of dreaming will be obvious; the main difference being the presence of that waking consciousness which receives real sensations from without, and regulates the course of thoughts within.

In another interesting case which occurred to me, there was a well marked passage from the state in which the patient (a gentleman about fifty-two, without any obvious disease), believed in and acted upon the reality of such illusive sounds and conversations, to the condition in which, having still similar sensations he recognised and treated them as delusions. The first state, which lasted many months, had the character of partial derangement, and thus impressed those around him. I saw the gentleman both at this time and soon after the change to the second state. On the latter occasion, I inquired from him, how, when the same articulate sounds still seemed present, he had learnt to regard them as illusions? He told me it was partly by his never discovering any person in the places whence the voices had come; chiefly by finding himself able on trial to suggest the words which were thus seemingly uttered by some one external to himself. To these reasons might probably have been added some change in the actual state of the sensorium, however incomprehensible its nature and cause.

In this instance there was no spectral illusion, the voices being always supposed in another room, and unassociated with any visual image. As far indeed as I know, these classes of illusions do not often coexist.

I may notice further respecting this case, that there was for the most part some obvious foundation in the thoughts or feelings at the time for the phrases which seemed to reach the ear from without. This fact abounds in curious inferences. It appears to make a breach for the time in the identity of the rational being. We have the strange phenomenon before us of thoughts and emotions rising within the mind, and arranged in the phraseology of words; which words, however, by some morbid perversion of the functions of the brain, are received and believed by the consciousness as coming from persons without. It is, if such expression be allowed, a sort of duplicity of the mind in its dealings with itself. Cases of this nature have kindred with some of the curious phenomena of somnambulism and trance. The madman of Horace, also, will be recollected here,—

" Qui se credebat miros audire tragœdos,
In vacuo lætus sessor plausorque theatro."—*Epist.* II. 2. 129.

insanity. While explaining the connexion of these phenomena with dreaming and reverie, it indicates a foundation for the whole in that natural function of mind by which we perpetually change our relation to external objects, even when all the senses are open and awake;—at one moment abstracting our consciousness from them altogether;—at another admitting some sensations, while others are excluded;—these unceasing changes, which in their series make up the chain or circle of life, being sometimes the effect of the will, sometimes wholly beyond its control. No attribute of the mind is more extraordinary than this; none which has such important connexion with all its functions, intellectual and moral, both in health and disease.

Though we thus find foundation for many modes of insanity even in a natural law of our constitution, more is required to explain the strange incongruities of thought which occur in these -cases of illusion, as well as in others where no false impressions on the senses exist. We cannot perhaps go further than to affirm, as matter of observation, that the same changes which impair the power of distinguishing between deceptive images and the realities of sense, do in like proportion impair that faculty of arranging and combining ideas, upon which the condition of man, as a rational being, depends. Here, as I have before observed, the relation to the state of sleep and dreaming is most distinctly marked. Let any one close his eyes, when in easy posture and quiet place; no strong impressions acting on the external senses. While yet retaining enough of waking consciousness to note the fact, images will be felt to steal upon realities, and ideas to blend more confusedly together, with less power of retaining them, or regulating their succession. A slight disturbance may recall the mind for a moment to itself; which being removed, it lapses again into the same state. This, carried further, becomes dreaming. The access to one sense is here in great part closed; the capacity of receiving impressions from the others is impaired; the powers of volition are diminished and misdirected; the consciousness of personal identity, essential as an exponent of reason in its sound state, is lost or obscured.

Let a similar state of sensorium exist from other causes, and for a longer time, but leaving free the action of the external senses and the power of volition, and we have a condition scarcely to be distinguished from many forms of mental derangement. Images and perceptions, real and unreal, coexist and confuse each other; while actions may result from both. From the same physical causes, presumably, the trains of thought become disordered, and ordinary associations are changed; or if they be in part coincident with the natural state, that power at least is lessened of retaining them before the mind as objects of thought, which seems an essential part of our reasoning existence. And as these causes, whatever their nature, may easily be conceived to affect one part of the sensorium more than another, and to vary in degree at different times, we have in such diversities the explanation, not indeed of the proxi-

14*

mate origin, but of the relations of many of the strange and anomalous forms of mental derangement.

The approaches of delirium in fever well illustrate many of these
phenòmena; often exhibiting, within an hour or two, every grade
from perfect reason to a state of wild or furious perversion of mind.
First, the wandering images or thoughts, which yet are known to
be unreal, and frequently described by the patient himself as *non-
sense*;—then, the vague rambling talk, from which, however, the
patient is still disengaged by being spoken to, by change of posture,
or other excitement;—afterwards, under further but gradual change,
the state of perfect delirium, where every function of the mind is
disordered by the unreal images and false combinations which possess it, uncontrolled by impressions from without.

In another chapter I shall have occasion to speak in detail on
that view of sleep, by which it is regarded as a series of ever fluctuating states; varying not only in general intensity, but even more
remarkably in the degree in which different mental functions are
under its influence at the same moment of time.   This view, which
more happily explains the phenomena than any other, is that also
which we may best follow in reasoning upon its connexion with
permanent states of mental disorder.

In various points, indeed, the phenomena both of dreaming and
insanity find more illustration from the waking moods of mind than
is generally supposed. Dreams appear inconsecutive in the series of
impressions and thoughts which compose them; and are so in fact in
different degrees, according to the varying condition of sleep. But
let any one follow with consciousness or immediate recollection the
ramblings and transitions of the waking state, when the mind is not
bound down to any one subject, and no strong impressions are
present to the senses, and he will often find these scarcely less singular and abrupt; though the effect of such irregularity is here
subordinate to certain regulating causes, which are absent during
sleep.*

---

* The admission of external sensations is amongst the most important of these.
Their influence in correcting aberrant trains of thought is marked in many
familiar instances. A person on the verge of intoxication feels confusion of
thought rapidly coming on him when he closes his eyes, which is lessened or
removed when opening them again. A patient under low rambling delirium will
pause from this when a question is asked him, or when any distinct impression
is made on the senses; passing subsequently again into the same state. Examples of this kind show how slight the line is, if line there be, which separates
the healthy actions of mind from those of morbid nature.

Milton, in a fine passage (though perhaps somewhat too abstruse for this
occasion), well describes this vague imagery of the mind, when external impressions are excluded:—
                    "When Nature rests,
           Oft in her absence mimic fancy wakes
           To imitate her; but, misjoining shapes,
           Wild work produces oft, and most in dreams;
           Ill matching words and deeds long past or late."
                                        Paradise Lost, book v.

In children, where the corrections of thought and experience are less matured than in adults, dreams often assume a very singular aspect in their passage to the waking state. · I have seen cases, where a child, waking affrighted by some imaginations of an unquiet dream, has continued for half an hour or longer in a state of agitation resembling delirium; the unreal images or ideas still possessing the mind, and being only slowly removed by actual impressions on the senses. Examples of this kind illustrate well the particular relations we are now seeking to examine.

Another connexion between these several states is that afforded by the curious phenomena of reverie, trance, or cataleptic ecstasy; where, with the external senses as much closed as in perfect sleep, it would seem that the intellectual and voluntary powers are sometimes exercised much more clearly and consecutively; yet not under the same relation to consciousness and memory as in the waking state. Though the evidence as to these extraordinary cases is much obscured by fiction, there is quite enough that is authentic to give them place among the most remarkable forms of sensorial disorder. Here, however, we may still follow out the connexion with the more common phenomena of mind. Reverie, in this medical sense, is probably but a higher degree of that which we call such in ordinary language; or what is still more usually termed absence of mind. And this again is but the excess of the condition, common to all and of constant occurrence, in which the consciousness is detached for a time from objects of sense actually present to the organs, concentrating itself upon trains of thought and feeling within;—a condition, in fact, which belongs to and characterizes man as an intellectual being.

I can scarcely doubt that to some of the states just described we may rightly refer what has been termed magnetic sleep; the sort of trance into which persons are occasionally thrown by the peculiar manipulations employed for this purpose. The effect, though more striking from the means being less familiar, is but one of the many modifications the mind may undergo even in its healthy state.* Here too the persons most frequently and powerfully affected are generally of a peculiar nervous temperament. The facts stated above show by close analogy how speech, or even partial conversations, may occur during such trance. But as respects the purport of the speech so uttered, what we find recorded by the disciples of animal magnetism must be set down to chance or cre-

* It must be admitted, however, on authentic evidence, that the state of trance thus induced is sometimes more intense than the condition of common sleep ; as proved by the more entire exclusion of external sensations. Stimuli, applied to the body in a way to awaken any person from ordinary sleep, appear in some cases to be unfelt by patients in this state. Though the difference is still only one of degree, it leads to some very curious inquiries regarding sensation, from the seeming fact that the sense of touch is that more especially affected in these cases, and that such experiments are chiefly successful in habits where this sense readily passes into morbid state ; as in females in whom the hysteric temperament is strongly marked.

dulity; as nothing but direct miraculous interposition could explain what is here offered to us for belief.

In extreme old age, again, the phenomena of dreaming and waking aberration are still more closely blended together. The two states of sleep and waking are severally more imperfect in kind; the distinction betwixt them becomes less marked; and the whole of mental existence seems as if contracted from both sides into a narrow space, and a lower scale of intensity. I have known instances of this kind, where, without any obvious disease of the vital organs, life had become a vague and feeble dream; scarcely broken into periods of time; and in which the capacity was almost lost of distinguishing between the real and unreal images which flitted unconnectedly before the mind. These cases, which cannot be looked upon without deep interest, undoubtedly depend on physical changes taking place in the brain; enfeebling and confusing all relations with the external world, and the associations and actions thereon depending.

There is greater difficulty in reasoning on the condition of the mind in infancy; yet this has doubtless its relation to the succeeding parts of life, and especially, as it would appear, to the cases where the intellect is disordered or permanently deficient. Idiocy, congenital sometimes, seems in other instances to be simply an arrest of the natural progress of the functions of the sensorium. The idiot retains the infant mind in an adult body. But as these functions may be thus morbidly checked at some point in their growth, so may they also, from physical causes, revert from a more advanced state to one of earlier life; and frequent examples occur, where both the deficiencies and hallucinations of insanity show close resemblance to the unformed intellect and character of the child. This connexion abounds in curious inferences, and well deserves more minute examination of its details.

I need scarcely dwell upon the application of the preceding remarks to the effects of alcohol and other narcotic substances, in their different modes of action on the brain. The states thereby produced are exceedingly various: for even intoxication, commonly so termed, differs much in kind as well as in degree. Still it will be found, upon close observation, that they all graduate more or less distinctly into one another; and that they are connected in common with the phenomena of insanity and dreaming;—not merely by vague resemblances of external aspect, but yet more by analogous changes in the sensorium itself, in its relation to external objects through the senses, and in those combinations within, which constitute trains of thought and become the causes of disordered action.

While seeking thus to associate together the several states of mental aberration, and to illustrate thereby the nature of each, it were vain to push inquiry far into the proximate cause of these phenomena. That changes, partial or general, transient or permanent, occur in the nervous substance of the brain, producing such states, is rendered certain by various evidence.* The most distinct proof, independently of that from actual observation, is furnished by hereditary insanity; which, however ignorant we may be of the particular structure affected, must doubtless be produced by some organization disposing to the disease, or to the series of changes which evolve it. How far these changes depend on the quantity of blood in the brain; on its local distribution; on the rate or manner of circulation; or on the varying qualities of the blood itself,—are inquiries of much interest and great difficulty. The history of all cerebral disease, and the examination of those instances where it has been fatal, show the remarkable influence of these several conditions; and particularly how small an amount of obvious change in the circulation, as in the slighter degrees of inflammation of the membranes, is capable of producing great disturbance in the mental functions. But still this is an influence only of indirect kind. Even in what seem the simpler of the cases before us, viz., those of dreaming, intoxication, or the delirium of fever, we must look to the nervous substance as the immediate source of the remarkable changes taking place. Its alterations, however produced, or in whatsoever consisting, are the causes which lie before us for discovery; but whether our present methods of research, or others yet to be devised, may hereafter afford us more complete knowledge, it is impossible to affirm.

In pursuing, indeed, any inquiry into the physical causes of insanity, it is well to define more exactly what is the right course, and what the presumable limit of discovery. In ascertaining the effects of altered circulation of blood through the brain, be it excess or deficiency, we are fixing a very important class of facts, and of great practical value. They are further of particular interest to the mode of viewing insanity which I seek at present to inculcate; as it seems certain from observation that the first effect of these changes of circulation is simply to excite or depress, without altering the nature of the functions in the parts thus affected. In slight inflammation, for example, of the upper surface of the brain, we find an unwonted irritation and restlessness of mind, excesses of natural temper, and a want of self-control; all which effects may terminate here, the inflammation being subdued. Or in cases of simple excited circulation, such as may be induced by emotion or by stimulants taken internally, but below the level of inflammatory action or intoxication, we often find an exaltation of the faculties and feelings, which may be deemed the first step of deviation from the natural state. These early gradations of change are frequently the sources whence discovery may best be derived.

---

* Sir W. Ellis, in his Treatise on Insanity, has stated, in evidence of the structural causes of this disorder, that out of 221 cases, male and female, examined after death, not fewer than 207 afforded proof of disease either in the brain or its membranes. It must be owned that the reports of Esquirol and Pinel are much below this estimate.

Still. as I have remarked above, this influence of the circulation, in relation to the intellectual functions, is wholly subordinate to the changes in the state of the nervous substance which intervene. And the same remark applies to alterations in the quality of the blood, whether consisting in different degrees of arterialization, or in the admission of substances foreign to its composition. From the nature of these causes, they have a diffused influence upon the intimate structure of the brain, by which certain of the sensorial functions are occasionally suspended altogether. Local congestions or extravasations of blood,—serous effusions into the ventricles or between the membranes,—thickenings of the cranium, or irregularities of its inner surface,—morbid deposits or tumours within the brain,—abscesses in its substance,—these and other deviations from natural structure, whether congenital or from disease, may be classed as causes affecting parts of the nervous substance, and therefore leading inquiry to the relation between these parts and the particular faculty or function affected in each several case. But they do not carry our knowledge beyond this point.

The question then ultimately and necessarily brings us to the changes in the nervous structure itself, thus variously acted upon by external causes, and producing in effect such remarkable alteration in the mental functions. The two morbid states of softening and induration of the brain, and its deficient development as to size, either altogether or in parts of its structure, seem to be some approach to a solution; and yet, if rightly estimated, carry us very little way towards it.* Not that we are to disregard such results of examination, as the medullary substance being softer than natural, or the cineritious substance darker. These alterations, though perhaps slight in degree, are presumably, from their nature and diffusion, more effective for permanent change and injury of function than many which are more obvious to remark. Looking, in fact, to what we know of the delicate and complex structure of some parts of the nervous system of the brain; to the impossibility of tracing the texture of other parts by the most minute research; and still more to the nature of the functions to which this system so closely ministers,—we must admit it as likely that the changes going on here, both in health and disease, will in great part be ever hidden from our knowledge.† Nevertheless, as these actions, however subtle and evanescent they may be, are still physical in their nature, the inquiry is fairly open. But it should be constantly so

---

* Meckel remarks, what doubtless is true, that in the brain the faults of conformation by defect are much more numerous and important than those by excess.

† To these reasons might be added the facts recently ascertained by Dr. Macartney and other observers, of the very small portion of true nervous matter in the brain, compared with its apparent size; proving further how exquisitely minute is the structure to which we are to look for results thus important. May it not be stated as a general presumption, that the configuration of the larger and more obvious portions of the brain is connected with the distribution and communication of nervous power, rather than with any absolute and independent function of these several parts?

conducted, as not to grasp at partial facts and hasty conclusions, where truth lies at such depth below the only surface exposed to our view.

Again, if the states of dreaming, intoxication, and delirium occur and pass away, without leaving traces behind on the brain, we may reasonably conclude that various forms of insanity, which we have seen to be so closely related to them, may exist, and even long continue, without permanent alterations of structure, or changes appreciable by the human eye. That organic differences do often exist as an original cause, must be presumed from the cases where the disorder is hereditary in the habit; and from the numerous instances where examination after death shows deviation from the natural structure. But even where there is proof that such organic changes have occurred, and that the derangement depends upon them, it is remarkable to what extent amelioration may for a time take place in the mental symptoms, though the original causes remain the same; giving further proof that the proximate cause resides in some part of structure to which our present means give us no access, and that to this we must chiefly look for the modifications of the disease.*

Viewing the question more generally, and in reference to the total mass of the brain, it may be stated as probable that where the intellectual and moral functions are chiefly disturbed, any physical disorder therewith connected will be found to exist in the cerebral hemispheres; consisting either in imperfect original development; or in softening or induration of substance; or in some more especial and local disease of structure. Our actual knowledge scarcely carries us beyond this; though some eminent physiologists have held the opinion that the cineritious neurine of the brain is the particular part relative to these functions, and the subject of the diseases which affect them. Every part indeed of this topic offers large scope to speculation. In another chapter I have ventured a suggestion as to the effect upon the mental functions of an unequal or incongruous action of the two hemispheres of the brain. As the variety of the disorder presumes a corresponding difference in its cause, another suggestion may arise, whether certain kinds of insanity be not the effect of simple excess or deficiency in quantity of that power (nervous, sensorial, or however denominated) by which the mutual rela-

---

* I recollect a case of mental derangement, where the post mortem examination showed great organic changes in the brain, many of them, from their nature, of long standing, and upon which it was next to certain the symptoms depended. Yet in this instance there occurred not long before death a lucid interval, so far complete, as to afford hopes of recovery where none had before existed, and where the event proved that none could reasonably be entertained. Other similar cases I find in my notes. The instances in fact are frequent and familiar, where the memory, affected manifestly, and it may be said permanently, by organic changes in the brain, does nevertheless at intervals, and without obvious cause, recover itself for a moment with singular clearness,—then pass under a cloud as before. An example of this, as it occurred in one of the most eminent men of this age, can never be lost to my own remembrance.

tions of mind and body are carried on? It is certain that such variation as to quantity exists;—certain also that it produces much influence on both these parts of our existence. If we might suppose that some maniacal disorders depended on morbid excess of this power, we should have an example of the case alluded to above—a derangement of mind proceeding from physical causes, but these involving only alteration in a natural function, and not any changes of structure leaving permanent traces behind.

Throughout the whole of the foregoing remarks I have used the term insanity in its most comprehensive sense; seeking to define its varieties chiefly by their relation to the healthy functions of mind; or to other states of mental aberration, either natural like dreaming, or at least frequent and familiar to us. It is one of those subjects in which the facts are so complicated, that truth may expediently be sought for simply by varying their arrangement. And this truth is likely to be best obtained when we can thus associate together the natural and morbid conditions by a series of intermediate steps, which bring no new element into our theory of mind, and at the same time best expound the strange and seemingly anomalous variety of these cases. Such gradations are most easily followed in all that regards illusions of the senses. But though becoming much less obvious as we advance into the inward recesses of thought, and seek for explanation of those states in which false combinations of ideas, and perverted passions and feelings, are chiefly concerned, yet we may still obtain illustration from the healthy habitudes of mind, especially as pursued through the intermediate phenomena of dreaming and intoxication.

In the most complete degree of melancholia, for example, it is often but the exaggeration and persistence of that gloomy mood of mind, which, in one degree or another, occurs occasionally to every person, overshadowing for the time all the thoughts and feelings of life. This may be the delusion of an hour, readily removed by change of place, occupation, or events; but it may continue longer under the character of hypochondriasis; or become permanent as a form of insanity; still depending on some common cause, however different the intensity and manner of operation.

A more difficult part of the subject, and that which we can least solve by any knowledge we possess, is what has been termed by some moral insanity; where no actual false perceptions exist, and the intellect in its ordinary sense is slightly affected; but where the feelings, temper, and habits are vitiated and variously perverted, sometimes assuming a character exactly opposite to that of the same mind in its healthy state, and seeming to alter the whole moral condition of the being.

It is needless to dwell upon the melancholy details of cases, which are so familiar to common experience. The attempt, moreover, is almost painful, of seeking explanation or analogy for them in the more natural conditions of human character. Yet such relations exist, and may be easily recognised in particular examples. In truth, we rarely meet with instances where this moral derangement is of sudden occurrence, or wholly detached from the prior life and habits of the individual. It comes upon the mind gradually, though often very unequally;—sometimes shown at first in the excess or misdirection of certain accustomed feelings;—these aberrations fostered often by the very circumstances they create,—acquiring the force of habits,—and in the same proportion losing the control of the intellect and will. The understanding, indeed, though exempt perhaps from any common hallucinations, is really perverted or enfeebled in most of those cases, and no longer gives that direction and balance which is essential to the healthy state of the mind. Even where a particular feeling or affection seems changed into one utterly opposite, a closer view will often show some relation to the previous temperament. While a more general regard to human character in its largest sense affords the proof that opposite extremes are not always so distinct or incongruous as at first sight they may appear.

All wonted methods of delineating character are, indeed, in some degree covenanted and artificial, and scarcely according with the reality of facts. We describe it as a unity, distinctly marked for each individual; and, in common sense, this is just. But there are few in whom the feelings and sentiments which compose it do not undergo fluctuations; as well under the influence of age and the greater events of life, as also more variously and incessantly from changes that belong to the day or hour;—the conditions of health,—the bodily sensations or instincts,—society,—and the many events which crowd upon every part of existence. Amidst such momentary changes, particularly in persons of a certain temperament, we very often recognise the elements of those future and more fixed aberrations, to which the name of mental derangement is needfully applied. The greater or less facility, indeed, of being thus affected, forms one of the most essential circumstances in character itself; and in few respects do individuals differ more widely than in their power of preserving habits, steady and unimpaired, under the circumstances ever pressing upon them. The highest exaltation of man lies in this direction; and the state of mind, moreover, which gives greatest security against every form of derangement.

These considerations, which might be pursued to much greater extent, obviously apply to the singular forms of madness which the French physicians have named *monomanie;* where we may generally discover connexion with some of the more ordinary states of mind; furnishing analogy, at least, in default of other solution. Most persons have felt at one time or other (oftenest perhaps during the " severa silentia noctis"), some dominant idea or feeling to possess the fancy; retaining its hold with a sort of malignant power, despite all efforts to shake it off; and by degrees distorting the subject, especially if it be a painful one, into a thousand false and alarming forms. If this train of thought be interrupted; and time, society and other objects come in between; the mind is felt as if passing out of a bad dream, which for a while had overshadowed it. But let there be a cause for the continuance of this state (and the duration of the impression is at least as explicable as its original occurrence), and we have an approach to monomania in some of its various shapes; nothing apparently wanting but the intensity, which is often so singularly testified in these cases by the actions induced, and by the length of period during which the delusion remains in force. Pinel, one of the best authorities on this subject, mentions instances where the same single insane impression continued without change for twenty or thirty years.*

In fact, the long persistence of the mind in one idea or feeling, not duly broken in upon or blended with others, is a state always leading towards aberration: and a common evidence of insanity, especially in its earlier stage, is that drawn from the dominance of a single impression, faulty perhaps only in the absence of those which should modify and correct it. It may be alleged that this reasoning tends to remove all distinction betwixt the sound and unsound mind; and to reflect madness back, as it were, upon the healthy and natural state of the faculties of man. But this is not truly so. The extremes are widely apart, and offer marks of practical distinction which can rarely be misunderstood. The existence of more doubtful cases, such as graduate between reason and insanity, is but a part of that law of continuity which pervades so generally every part of creation. It is attested by the actual difficulty often experienced in dealing both legally and morally with these cases; and by the observation of their progress, as well when first passing the limit of reason, as when reëntering it in the course of recovery.

Such observations, and founded on this basis, are the more important, as they bear directly upon every question of treatment. No principle of practice in mental disorders can probably be successful which does not recognise their relation to the phenomena of mind in its healthy state; and some of the more remarkable cures I have known, where physical causes of the infirmity did not exist, have been effected really, if not professedly, by a discreet application of this method. It is not my present purpose to speak on the treat of these disorders; but I am persuaded this will be found true as a general remark; and equally so the assertion, that from no other source can suggestions be drawn, of equal value in the prevention of them, when the predisposition exists in the habit.

Though the subject does not readily admit of separation, yet

---

* It must be admitted that these partial hallucinations, occurring often without obvious cause from without, and holding thus tenaciously on the mind, furnish argument to the phrenologists; and a reasonable one, as far as respects the opinion that there is a plurality of parts about the brain having connexion with different intellectual and moral functions. But phrenology points out no actual structure in the brain having especial correspondence with these functions, either in healthy or diseased state; and its indications from the form of the cranium are not yet authentic enough to be admitted as a system of facts. The doctrine, unless we admit this evidence by external configuration, does in reality carry us little further towards the theory of insanity than the point we had reached by other methods of inference.

having principally had in view to illustrate the connexions of insanity in its different forms with the more natural conditions of the mind, I shall not add much as to the predisposing causes of the malady. The influence of various kinds of mental excitement, whether with or without hereditary disposition to the disorder, has so often been discussed, that it is needless here to enter upon the subject.* There is one point, however, connected with it, to which, as having been less noticed, I may allude before closing this chapter.

It seems probable that certain cases of madness depend on a cause which can scarcely exist, even in slight degree, without producing some mental disturbance; viz., the too frequent and earnest direction of the mind inwards upon itself;—the concentration of consciousness too long continued upon its own functions. It would appear (if we may venture so to surmise) a design in the creation of this wonderful existence which we call soul, that while safely using the faculties with which we are gifted in exploring the world of nature without, through every part of the scale of being, we should find these powers to sink under us, when directed within to the source and centre of their own operations. In this matter every one may make experiments for himself. I believe it will be found that any strong and continuous effort of will to concentrate the mind upon its own workings; to analyse them by consciousness; or even to fix, check, or suddenly change the trains of thought,—is generally followed by speedy and painful confusion, compelling sooner or later the abandonment of the act. I doubt not that the long continuance or frequent repetition of such circumstances, from whatever cause, is sufficient to produce a temporary derangement in minds already predisposed to the infirmity. I have myself known more than one instance of aberration of intellect, which I had every reason to believe thus produced.†

These, however, may be termed excesses in the employment of a faculty which it is given us to use. The actual power thus to inquire into the mind and regulate the trains of thought, exist; is capable of cultivation; and, rightly exercised, becomes one of the highest professions of our moral and intellectual being. By no quality is one man better distinguished from another, than by the mastery acquired over the subject and course of his thoughts;—by the power of discarding at once what is desultory, frivolous, or degrading; and of adhering singly and steadily to that which it enlarges and invigorates the mind to pursue.

* The recent publications of Dr. Brigham, of Boston, on the influence of mental cultivation and excitement upon health, communicate some singular facts as to the effects produced by commercial, political, and religious excitement in the United States. The proportion of persons deranged in mind to the whole population is, according to his statement, nearly three times as great as in England.
† Even a simple difficulty of recollection, where the mind thus concentrates itself in inward search after some of its own former operations, becomes painful when long continued; and thought is often lost in utter confusion. In the chapter of Aristotle, περι αναμνησηως, will be found notice of this, as of many other curious facts connected with the subject,

CHAPTER VI.

ON MERCURIAL MEDICINES.

IT may seem that any remarks at the present day, on the principle or methods of using calomel, must be trite and altogether needless. Yet is this only in part true. One comment I would make is, that, in the ordinary use of this medicine as a mercurial, its good effects are often much impaired by admixture with other aperients. Such combination is doubtless most beneficial, where the object is to obtain large and speedy evacuation of the liver and bowels. But in the numerous cases where the proper mercurial action is desired, either on the mucous membrane of the intestines, or on the different secreting organs, or in arresting certain states of inflammation, calomel will generally be found to act most beneficially, and with greatest certainty, when given alone. Its combination with purgatives in these cases both obscures and impairs its effects; introducing at the same time causes of irritation, which disturb the body in other ways, and thereby check the course of recovery. The same remark holds good for the most part where the liver is the direct object of mercurial treatment. Even in cases of obstruction of the bowels, when there is threatening of topical inflammation, calomel adequately given, without the addition of other laxatives, will often be more effectual for relief than in any combination with them. Its single action is much less irritating to parts thus disposed; while there is generally more distinct and speedy exercise of its specific effect upon membranes already in an inflamed state.

To avoid irritation and pain, indeed, whenever this can be done without too palpable sacrifice of the objects in view, ought ever to be present as a principle in the treatment of disease. In all cases these are positive evils, counteracting or retarding more or less the good gained. In some habits their effects long continued, are mischievous even to the extent of danger and death. I doubt whether this principle is sufficiently regarded in the ordinary course of practice. We too often see methods of treatment, external as well as internal, usurping the name of remedies, and capable of acting as such in some constitutions; but which in others, by repeated irritation, have fretted the body into new disease more difficult and distressing than that which was the original object of cure. The proof here is the relief gained by intermission of the means; but it must be admitted that these are cases requiring judgment and discrimination.

When thus given in a simple form, and where there is no strumous disposition or idiosyncrasy in the habit, it is remarkable how much calomel may be borne without injury or inconvenience; and even without any such urgent effect on the bowels, as might be supposed from its effects in ordinary use. That the medicine is often needlessly and injuriously employed, as are many others, cannot be denied. But there is an abuse also on the side of timid and deficient employment, where its decided and speedy influence is required. This is often forfeited by using it in those small and scattered doses, which harass the bowels with fretful and irregular action, without being efficient for relief. If mercury be needed for its specific effect on the system, or even on a part of the body, the sooner, generally speaking, that it is brought into action, the better.* Or if exception be taken against this as a rule, its agency is at least important enough to warrant its being used singly and steadily; without the ambiguity of any combined means, other than such as may be wanted to support the system under its action, or to aid in directing it to any given part.

This consideration, of supporting the action of calomel by simultaneous assistance to the powers of the system, is often neglected; from some supposed incongruity, much greater than really exists, between its action and the functions which tend to repair or invigorate the body. In those cases where frequent repetition, or long use of the remedy is required;—or where the body, as often happens, is debilitated by disease, which yet needs the activity of this medicine for a chance of favourable issue,—the direct conjunction of calomel, or other mercurial, with tonics, is frequently not only the safest, but even the most effectual way of using the remedy. In such cases, of which some dropsical effusions may be taken as examples, the mercurial action in producing absorption seems quickened by the addition of bark or steel; and where no fever or irritation in the primæ viæ are present, these medicines may often be made beneficially to concur with every part of a mercurial course.

There is some cause to believe regarding mercury, as with respect to opium, that in certain conditions of active disease, where its agency is most beneficial and nearest to what may be termed specific, the medicine is capable of these effects, without any such action on other parts of the system as would have occurred under different circumstances. The truth of the observation is best attested in cases where it is given to subdue inflammatory actions in serous membranes; such inflammation as tends to effusion, unless speedily overcome.† May it be supposed that this arises from a more ex-

* This is a question of some interest in practice, and respecting which opinions will differ. Perhaps it may best be answered by reference to individual temperament, and the nature of the disease. My own impression is, as stated above, that when we seek to obtain the specific effects of mercury, it is for the most part expedient to get the medicine into the system as quickly as possible, with due regard to the other circumstances of the case; regulating afterwards the degree and duration of its action according to the symptoms.

† I find it justly remarked by Dr. Seymour, in his Treatise on Dropsy, that the quantity of mercury which may be beneficially used in cases where inflammation, ending in deposition of lymph, is going on in the pericardium, is almost inconceivable; and this without affecting the gums or producing other inconvenience.

press direction of the mercurial action to the kidneys in these and to similar instances? It is known that there are certain states of organic disease of the kidneys, in which mercury produces its constitutional effects more rapidly than usual. The fact, which is an interesting one, would seem to illustrate the supposition just made; and by showing the intimate relation of mercurial action to this function, will explain other anomalies in its effects on the system.

The remarkable influence of mercury in subduing certain inflammatory actions, both acute and chronic in kind, but particularly acute inflammations of serous membranes, is best explained by supposing its action to be on the capillary vessels, whether of membranous or glandular organs. Without assuming to define what is the particular state induced on these vessels as opposed to inflammation, I have always found this idea (long adopted by many eminent observers), to furnish the best clue to the various actions of mercury on the system. Its topical direction to particular organs (if indeed we rightly so interpret what in many cases may be only the different tendency in these organs to show the influence upon them) is subordinate, as may fairly be presumed, to this more general principle. And though it is difficult to understand how it should be a cause of specific inflammation in certain parts, compatibly with the other actions just stated, yet is this difficulty but part of our ignorance of the general theory of inflammation, attested still by so many differences both in opinion and the statement of facts. The whole subject is interesting, from the connexion it indicates between the action of a very powerful medicine, and the functions of that part of the vascular system which is now rightly looked to as the principal source and seat of disease.

I believe that a mistake is frequently made as to the manner of operation of calomel and other mercurials, in ascribing effects to their action on the liver, which are in fact chiefly due to their influence on the mucous membrane and glandular follicles of the intestines. The action, prompt and almost specific, of mercury upon the liver, cannot be doubted; but scarcely less in amount or importance is its effect upon the parts last mentioned. The secretions and discharges thence arising are often mistaken for those from the liver; and the treatment continued and pressed forwards upon this supposition. In many cases there may be no practical evil in this; in some it may even prove beneficial, mercury being the fit remedy, whatever the seat of the disorder. But in other instances the error is certainly of mischievous tendency; and at all events we are bound to seek for what is true as the basis of our practice.

In the employment of blue pill, as well as of calomel, I believe that the benefit is often lessened by combination with more active aperients; and this is especially the case, where it is used as an alterative for disordered secretions, or in certain cases of dyspepsia. In these instances, it will generally be found more advantageous to give it twice or thrice a day, in moderate doses and uncombined; than to limit it, as is usual, to one larger quantity at bed-time, with some purgative combination. I cannot affirm that I have seen any distinct effect from the very minute doses of the blue pill, recommended by some physicians; but I do not doubt from observation the benefit of small quantities, frequently repeated. This mode of using mercurial medicines is common in the complaints of children, but by some incongruity less frequent in those of adults. There is certainly no practical reason for the distinction, unless it be the seemingly greater power of resisting the mercurial action in the former; a point itself liable to some doubt.

I have no design here to enter into details as to the action or manner or use of calomel in different diseases. This is too large a subject to be otherwise considered than in its relation to each. If I might venture a general comment upon the present employment of the medicine, it would be, that it is too frequently used as a mere laxative remedy; and too sparingly and inefficiently, where relief to certain varieties of inflammation is sought for,—or the absorption of dropsical effusions,—or the separation from the system, principally through the liver and the secreting surface of the intestines, of certain morbid matters which, under one denomination or other, are largely thus excreted from the body. And I would repeat, that in pursuing some of these objects, particularly that of subduing inflammatory action, it is often much more expedient to give it alone than in any form of combination. The question of salivation is of less moment here than it might on first view appear. If the mercury, thus singly given, pass more readily into the body, it does for the most part accomplish more speedily the object sought for. And in the cases of exception to this, and of anomaly in the action of the medicine, the particular circumstances generally furnish best direction regarding the means to be pursued.

The dread prevailing in France and Germany as to the use of calomel, and the reprobation of English practice on this score, are well known. Unless partial cases of abuse be admitted as argument, such as may occur in the case of any other medicine, it cannot be allowed that there is much justification for these harsh views. It may indeed be affirmed, (and I state this on my own observation,) that the judgment is formed mainly on hearsay, and has gained weight by mere repetition. The actual knowledge from experience of the medicinal qualities of calomel is, on the continent, exceedingly limited; yet this is the only evidence which can fairly be brought to the question. Who, for instance, that has not seen the effects of the medicine, duly given in severe cases of croup,—or in certain affections of the brain,—or in cases of great congestion about the liver and abdominal viscera,—can rightly estimate the benefits procured from it? and procured, we are often able to say, without any injury to countervail the good. It is needless to multiply examples to this effect. The experience of every medical man in this country will supply them; but without such experience no censure, like that alluded to, can justly be applied.

It is of course not to be inferred that these results are derived from the use of calomel alone. Where the peculiar action of mercury is the main object, other mercurial preparations may be equally capable of fulfilling these intentions; and some of them are perhaps even better attained by the form of which I am about to speak. But the more explicit knowledge we have of calomel, and its undoubted sufficiency for many of the most important ends in practice, must ever sustain its repute, whatever equivalents may hereafter be acquired for the effects we now obtain through its agency.

The error of many continental physicians on this subject arises, I believe, from their connecting the large use of purgatives in English practice with the idea that calomel is the medicine chiefly employed for this object. I have spoken in another place of what I think to be the real excess in this part of our practice; and, as respects calomel, have allowed that it is often needlessly,—sometimes, and in particular temperaments, injuriously employed. But the admissions ought not to go further than this; and there remains to all who rightly estimate its use, a large balance in favour of the medicine, fully sanctioning the place it holds with English physicians in the treatment of disease.

Among the different mercurial preparations, the oxymuriate, or bichloride of mercury, is not so generally used as it merits to be, though doubtless more extensively now than heretofore. Under discreet employment it is one of the most valuable remedies we possess. The power of giving it in solution is a material advantage in various parts of practice; rendering its action more certain, more equal, and probably, by readier absorption, more effectual as an alterative upon the whole system. I have seen its influence in augmenting the secretions, procuring the absorption of morbid growths, altering the state of the skin in many cutaneous disorders, and changing the character of morbid actions generally throughout the system, in cases where I believe no other medicine, or combination of medicines, would have had equal effect. Its conjunction with bark, steel, sarsaparilla, &c., afford resources of the greatest value in the treatment of disease. And, though otherwise held by common opinion, I think it on the whole as safe a medicine as calomel in the hands of the practitioner; inasmuch as its distribution can be made as equal and determinate ; and its effects, from being given in a state of solution, are less likely to be interrupted by mechanical hindrances in the stomach and bowels.

It is worthy of note, indeed, how long this medicine may be continued in uninterrupted use, without obvious injury or inconvenience. I have often given from four to six drachms daily of the liquor hydrarg. bichlorid. (*Pharm. Lond.* 1836) for six or eight weeks; without affection of the gums, irritation of the bowels, or any effect making it needful to intermit or modify its use. In other cases this is not equally possible; but the difficulties which occur from idiosyncrasy, or other causes, are quite as readily surmounted here as in the case of any other mercurial, and are rarely such as to prohibit the use of the medicine altogether.

Perseverance in the use of this preparation is, according to my experience, of singular avail in certain cerebral or spinal disorders; where there is presumption that some effusion may have taken place, or that the state of obscure inflammation exists, tending to this effect. I have seen great benefit from it, thus steadily employed, in several cases of paraplegia; the usual slow progress of this disorder giving scope for its effects, and the danger in prospect justifying the full trial of the remedy.* In other instances, where the object has been to procure absorption of a deposit or thickened texture, or to change the condition of action leading to this, as in particular cases of hypertrophy, I have found equal facility in sustaining its action for a long period, and this without obvious injury to the system.

I may repeat generally my persuasion that much advantage might be gained from the larger and more various employment of this mercurial remedy. But to obtain the full benefit, we must be patient as well as decided, in its use. In those cases where it is of greatest avail, the processes of change are often slowest; and not testified by those instant and obvious results, which are sometimes needed to fortify the mind even of the physician in the perseverance proper to the practice; still more to satisfy the patient and those around him; alarmed, it may be, by the name of the medicine, and by the precautions taken as to its dose and effects. As a result of these or other difficulties, I have repeatedly known a course to be abandoned in the middle, (sometimes at the very moment when becoming most effective,) which there was every reason to believe capable of relieving eventually a distressing or dangerous malady.

* Adverting to this disease, I may remark that in those cases of it which appear (more perhaps in the results of practice than from any assured diagnosis) to be unconnected with atrophy or other change of the nervous substance itself, I know no remedy which can compare with mercury *adequately* used. One of the most remarkable cases I have seen, attesting this efficacy, was that of a patient about forty-three years of age; where the symptoms, beginning with weakness of the lower limbs and loins, preternaturally slow pulse, and slight confusion of mind, proceeded gradually in the course of a few months to total inability in these limbs, loss of power in the sphincters, extreme difficulty of articulation, failure of memory and intellect, and general want of nervous power throughout the whole system. Under a treatment of full doses of calomel twice a day for about five weeks, and then once a day for an equal time, without intermission, yet never proceeding to actual salivation, the symptoms were all progressively removed; the restoration of the voluntary powers and intellect being best proved by the patient regaining his power of walking and riding, and by being able to preside again as Chairman of the Quarter Sessions. The mercury was used in this case almost to the exclusion of other internal remedies. The only means, which could render the result ambiguous as to cause, were two issues kept open over the cervical and lumbar vertebræ. But, though these had doubtless some effect, the relation of date between the remedies and the relief obtained gave proof that the mercury was of greatest avail.

I ought to mention, that life was terminated half a year after this recovery by a sudden apoplectic seizure, the effect of some over-exertion in country sports; an event not invalidating the inference as to treatment, though showing that the same tendency still existed in the habit. No post mortem examination took place.

Such difficulties are best obviated by a right anticipation of what is to be done, and what expected; and by a steady recurrence to the same principles throughout the whole progress of treatment.

In these few remarks on mercurial medicines, as on so many other subjects in this volume, I have referred to those points only which seem to deserve further consideration than they have hitherto received, on a more direct application to practice.

CHAPTER XVII.

ON THE EXERCISE OF RESPIRATION.

MIGHT not more be done in practice towards the prevention of pulmonary disease, as well as the improvement of general health, by expressly exercising the organs of respiration?—that is, by practising according to some method those actions of the body, through which the chest is alternately in part filled and emptied of air? Though suggestions to this effect occur in some of our best works on consumption, as well as in the writings of certain continental physicians, they have hitherto had less than their due influence; and the principle, as such, is little brought into general application. In truth, common usage takes for the most part an opposite course; and, under the notion or pretext of quiet, seeks to repress all direct exercise of this important function in those who are presumed to have tendency to pulmonary disorders.

Yet, on sound principle, and with reasonable care, it is certain that much may be done in this way to maintain and invigorate health, even in constitutions thus disposed. Omitting some points of controversy, particularly as to what regards the mechanical influence of respiration on the circulation through the heart and lungs, (points meriting, however, much attention from their importance,) the free and equable expansion of the latter by full inspiration is beneficial,—*first*, in maintaining their healthy structure, by keeping all the air passages duly open and pervious; *secondly*, in preventing congestion in the pulmonary circulation; *thirdly*, in providing more completely for the necessary chemical action on the blood, by changing at each act of respiration a sufficient proportion of the whole air contained in the lungs, and giving it more complete access to the vascular tissues;—all objects of great importance, and all capable of being promoted more or less by the means in question.*

* The ingenious suggestion of Dr. Carswell, as to the cause of more frequent tuberculous deposit in the superior lobes of the lungs, is well known, and applies to the subject of this chapter. In the excellent work of Sir James Clark on Consumption will be found some valuable remarks having more direct reference to it.

The phrase of exercise of respiration may indeed be used almost in the same sense, and with the same fitness, as that of muscular exercise. Each is capable in its respective way of increasing the power and facility of the function concerned. It is remarkable how speedily this is often attained in the instance of the former. A person in ordinary health may so exercise the lungs by repetition of a given exertion, that what produced breathlessness at first is soon performed without effort or fatigue ; a fact familiar to common observation, in examples which show not only the speed but the extent to which the effect may be produced. This of course is not equally true where the liability to disease exists ; but even then the express exertion of the organs, under observance and regulation, may often be made a means of augmenting their capacity and power.

We might take lesson on this subject from some of the provisions made by nature for relief to these organs, when oppressed in their functions. The acts of sighing and yawning are instances to this effect. Coughing, another mode of expiration (less indeed to be dreaded in itself than from the inference it conveys) is an instrument in keeping the air tubes free from obstruction ; and there are cases often occurring, where it might be partially superseded, or lessened in severity, by the gentler exercise of respiration ; so performed under the direct influence of the will, as somewhat to exceed, without passing into labour or fatigue, the ordinary course of the function. Trial is necessary in each case to give assurance of the effect, and often the irritability of parts of the membrane may be such as at once to negative any repetition. But the test is so easy and certain, that no undue risk can be incurred in making the experiment.

However it be in this particular example, we may still affirm the fact that good is occasionally to be gained from the regulated exercise of respiration, even when diseased actions are already going on within the lungs ; much more, where there is yet only threatening of these, from hereditary or accidental causes in the constitution. Here such exercise is beneficial, as well through its influence on the general health, as more directly by its effect on the lungs themselves, in the several ways mentioned above. There is even reason to affirm that, under discreet use of the remedy, a larger proportion of good may be obtained from it in these cases, than in any other where it can be employed. It is a good we are in nowise entitled to neglect ; seeing the paucity of the means we possess for dealing effectually with the most frequent and fatal form of pulmonary disease ;—that which has been so often cited as a reproach upon medicine ; though perhaps unjustly, when the nature and difficulties of the object are fully taken into account.*

* In adverting to this disease of pulmonary consumption (tubercular phthisis), it must fairly be admitted that the progress of medical science has hitherto effected nothing towards a valid cure, whatever may have been done by methods for protecting the constitution against its earlier inroads, or in certain degree

It is scarcely needful to say that the same regard which is paid to the quality of air in ordinary respiration, and especially under tendency to pulmonary disorder, must be extended even more carefully to cases where the quantity inspired is thus by effort augmented. Where experience has clearly shown that air below a certain temperature produces irritation in the air passages, it is certain that this cannot be fitted for the exercise of respiration as here recommended. And the same with respect to a humid atmosphere, under which any given degree of cold produces much more effect on an irritable membrane, from the medium through which it is applied. These points, indeed, though adverted to as maxims in the treatment of phthisis and other pulmonary diseases, are not sufficiently made the subject of trial in particular cases. Two or three experiments, readily devised for each case and unattended with risk, might suffice to decide a question which applies alike to the preventive and curative practice in these disorders, and throughout every part of their progress.

As respects the modes of exercising the respiration, they should be various, to suit the varying powers and exigencies of the patient. The " clara lectio" is one recommended from antiquity, the good effects of which are not limited to this object alone. It might be well, indeed, were the practice of distinct recitation, such as implies a certain effort of the organs beyond that of ordinary speech, more generally used in early life, and continued as a habit and exercise, by those especially whose chests are weak, and who cannot sustain stronger exertions. Under judicious observation as to posture, articulation, and the avoidance of all excess, such exercises may be

abating the symptoms in their progress. This, however, as remarked above, is less an opprobrium upon medicine than on first view it might appear. The more distinct knowledge that has been acquired of the tubercular diathesis,—of the tendency in certain habits and in particular textures to the growth or deposit of a peculiar morbid matter,—and of that more especial direction to the lungs, warranting M. Louis's assertion, that after the age of fifteen tubercles are never found in any part without appearing also in this organ,—points directly to a specific constitutional disease, for which none other than a specific antidote is likely to be of complete or certain avail. Whether such will ever be found (either general for the tubercular disease in the habit, or more especially preventive of its deposits in the lungs), is still very doubtful; though the research is amply justified, both by analogy and by the urgency of the cause requiring it. This analogy, however, does not extend to the nature of the morbid matter itself, or its relation to other specific remedies. We have nothing yet which can be considered even a plausible clue; and the discovery, if made, is more likely perhaps to be the effect of accident than of any concerted plan of inquiry.

These difficulties, which can be rightly understood by medical men only, become a vindication for that which the science has not yet attained, though sedulously sought for. Meanwhile, and in conjunction with these efforts, attention has justly been directed towards the means best calculated to guard constitutions so disposed against the active ingress of the disease. This is obviously the only alternative as a principle of treatment; and it has been successfully pursued in many ways, so as undoubtedly to place the preventive practice in phthisis on a better footing than at any former period. More, however, is probably still attainable; and the subject of the present chapter is one which furnishes evidence to this effect.

rendered as salutary to the organs of respiration, as they are agreeable in their influence on the ordinary voice. Even singing may for the same reasons be allowed in many of these cases ; but within narrower limits, and under more cautious notice of the effects.

Of actual muscular excesses with this object, that of full and repeated inspration in the free air is perhaps one of the best. The exercises which open the chest, as it is termed, are salutary, provided they are not such in amount as to hurry the circulation, oppress the breathing, or occasion too large and sudden expenditure of muscular power. These precautions do not always receive the notice they deserve in relation to exercise of the chest, and especially in the case of those of feeble habits and disposed to pulmonary disease. If the exertion be such a kind or degree as to quicken materially the action of the heart, and hurry the respiration, no good is obtained, and much evil may be incurred. These are the best as well as most ready tests we can apply, to regulate what may expediently be done. Altered they are in degree even on the slightest exertion; but they ought not to be so to such extent as to prove distressing to the sensations of the patient at the time, or to leave the feeling of langour behind.*

The breathing, therefore, may be best exercised in these cases by full inspiration when the body is otherwise at rest, or in slight and easy movement. The lungs will thus be more completely filled than by hurried respiration, and without any evil to countervail the good. It is from this cause, chiefly, that exercises on horseback are frequently more beneficial to persons having weak chests than those on foot, in which greater muscular exertion is required, and where the diaphragm particularly is brought into more hurried action. But there are cases where neither mode of exercise is practicable, yet where the gentle exercise of inspiration by voluntary effort, so as to bring more air into the lungs than is done by the common act of breathing, is advantageous even to those who are deeply under the influence of pulmonary disease.†

It is worthy of remark that rapid motion through the air, on horseback or in an open carriage, is often felt as more beneficial to those in ordinary health than a slower rate of movement. It may be that the air thereby gets more thoroughly into all the bronchial

* This is particularly to be guarded against in those gymnastic exercises which have had their periods of fashion as well as other less commendable remedies. and have often been carried to injurious excess, both in this point, and in the over-strain given to the several parts concerned in motion. Rightly applied and limited, they have great value in various ways for the maintenance of health. and the restoration of parts enfeebled or altered by disease.

† A caution regarding exercise in such habits may be given here, which I do not recollect to have seen mentioned, though founded on a remarkable fact. This is, the increased difficulty of breathing for a time on stopping suddenly from any exercise by which the respiration has been much hurried. Without entering into the causes, it is enough to mention this circumstance as suggesting the precaution of making the change more gradual, when a state of breathing has been incurred which in these cases ought especially to be avoided.

cells, removes what has been stagnant there, and produces more rapid and complete arterialization of the blood. This is obviously the same case as that of moving against a wind, which is generally felt to be invigorating in its effects where the wind is not so strong as to produce much muscular toil in facing it. Other animals evidently share with man in the bodily feeling thus produced.* There is a distinct difference of sensation in the opposite case of moving together with the wind, and at the same or quicker rate than its motion; and I have even known instances where a certain degree of faintness appeared to be thus produced.

It is not improbable that these effects depend in great part on the different amount of change effected by the air upon the blood. Experiment and observation show us how very rapidly such changes often take place, and how sudden as well as singular is their influence upon all parts of the frame. Everything which tends to give full ingress of air into the lungs contributes to an effect, which may best be described by saying that the power of vitality is augmented throughout the whole being.

The remark just made as to the effect of rate of movement through the air without muscular exertion, might be usefully applied to many cases in practice, beyond those in which the chest solely is concerned. In dyspepsia, for instance, where the circulation is for the most part feeble, and both body and mind inapt to exercise, much good is attainable in this way; and those fitting changes in the blood, which are interfered with by the whole manner of life of the dyspeptic, may be procured without efforts to which it is difficult habitually or sufficiently to rouse him. The frequent conjunction of dyspepsia with the earlier stage of pulmonary disease affords suggestions here which merit much attention in practice.

In cases of this kind, and still more in chlorosis, it is worthy of note how very inertly the acts of respiration are often performed, and how little change is made in the air within the lungs. The chest is hardly seen to rise during common inspiration; the patient seems scarcely capable of aiding it by voluntary effort; and short spasmodic breathing comes on upon the slightest exertion. Here it is manifest that the proper changes in the blood do not take place, and that all the functions of the body suffer in effect of this privation. Many of the symptoms in the singular class of disorders to which we refer, are certainly derived from this source, whatever be the original causes in the state of the uterus, of the brain, or other parts of the nervous system. And it must be kept in mind, that the deficient change of the blood (testified in chlorosis by a want of the right proportion of fibrin and red particles; and by lessened power of coagulation) has effect not only upon the secretions to

* A coachman will say that his horses do not breathe so well, that they sooner become faint, with the wind blowing behind them, though the positive draught be less. Something is due here to the heat from exercise not being so freely carried away; but this will not explain the whole of the effect observed.

which this fluid directly subserves, but also, as we have every reason to suppose, upon the vigour and equality of the circulation itself. The action of the heart, the state of the capillaries, and the altered production of animal heat, may be received as the more obvious proofs of a fact, than which there are few of greater importance in the animal economy.*

I doubt indeed whether this point of the due arterialization of the blood, familiar as a physiological doctrine, has been enough considered by physicians in relation to the prevention or treatment of disease. Venous blood circulating in the arteries is a cause of speedy death to the functions of the brain, and thence indirectly (to say nothing of its simultaneous effect on other organs) to the whole body. Between this state of venous blood, and that perfectly arterial, there may be every possible grade of change. Such intermediate variations we know to exist in many cases, and most distinctly in some forms of disease. It is certain that each proportion between the two extremes must have its definite effect for good or ill upon every part of the system ; partly by altering the power and rate of the circulation itself; partly by ministering a fluid of different chemical composition for the nutriment, secretions, and other functions of the several organs ; principally perhaps by the more direct influence on the nervous system just referred to. The great agent in determining these changes in the blood is the respiration ; and commanding this function as we do to a great extent, both in the quality and amount of what is inspired, we are bound to take every advantage which this important power can afford us for the relief of disease.†

* Some interesting experiments by Dr. Alison (*Reports of the Fifth Meeting of the British Association*, 1835) lead to the presumption that the oxygen of the air has effect in exciting the flow of blood through the capillaries, independently of any action on the vessels themselves; confirming in this the curious notices of Haller as to the *drawing* of blood towards any part where an opening is made in a vessel, so as to admit the contact of air with the fluid within.

Though we have no proof that the physical peculiarities of chlorotic blood are owing to deficient respiration alone, yet there is reason to suppose this cause materially concerned ; more so, perhaps, than is usually adverted to in histories of the disorder.

† Though the experiments as to this point are the subject of controversy, yet, as they render it nearly certain that the forty or forty-five cubic inches of a single ordinary inspiration is less than a sixth part of the air constantly present within the lungs, it is manifest that there is great scope for change in the amount of that respired, without interfering too much with the natural course of the function.

The disappointment of earlier and more sanguine expectation as to the medicinal value of the protoxide of nitrogen (*nitrous oxide gas*) has had the effect of withdrawing attention too much from this remarkable agent. The inequality of influence upon different persons, and the disagreeable influence upon some, are circumstances common to all powerful remedies we possess, and not fairly to be admitted in argument against its eventual use. Looking to the functions of respiration in all its parts, it can scarcely be doubted that cases must occur where it may be important to add to the proportion of oxygen inspired ; and the evidence of effects from this particular compound is sufficient to suggest it, under modification, as the most expedient method of attaining the object.

CHAPTER XVIII.

METHOD OF INQUIRY AS TO CONTAGION.

AFTER all that has been written upon contagion, in angry controversy or sober reasoning, I cannot but think that the question still admits of greater precision in the methods of inquiry; whereby to reconcile the contradictions, and remove in some part the difficulties, which still perplex it in so many particular cases.

I take the subject in its most general form; and the term contagion in its broadest application; as implying the communication of disorder in any way from one person to another, without reference to time, or medium of communication. The term *infection*, being less limited in its derivation than contagion, may be preferred by some; but using the latter word in the wide and popular sense just stated, it cannot well be misunderstood. The particular proofs by which the contagious nature of certain diseases is established, and the enumeration of these diseases, important though the topics are, do not enter into my object.

I believe it may be assumed, that in every instance of communicated disorder of the same kind (except the ambiguous case of certain nervous complaints, where other principles are concerned) there is a *materies morbi*, a material cause, whatsoever and however subtle its nature and mode of transmission, which is directly concerned in the propagation. This assumption, though large, is justified by observation as far as it goes,—by strict analogy and probability, where observation cannot be had. It is likely that future research will rather augment than lessen the number of instances where such miasma or material cause of contagion may be presumed to exist. And it is further probable that we shall hereafter acquire more intimate knowledge of the nature of these morbid matters, of their relations to each other, and of the manner in which they are transmitted so as to propogate disease. The cause of modern inquiry directs through many channels to these results.

Looking, however, to the principle just stated, and admitting its truth, we shall find basis in it for all reasoning on the laws of contagion; that is to say, for all the conditions which determine and modify the communication of disease from one person to another. A disease is communicated by some morbid matter, thrown off from the first, and capable of producing like symptoms in the second; when conveyed either by inoculation, by simple contact, or indirectly through some medium of transference. Here then three main conditions present themselves, each open to many variations; and, in their combination, capable of producing the numberless varieties and apparent anomalies in the laws of contagion. These are,—first, the condition of the person giving the infection;

—secondly, the state of the person receiving it;—and, thirdly, the condition of the medium through which the transference is made. I believe that reflection will show the whole subject to be comprised under these three heads, and that we are bound to refer to them severally in all particular questions or instances which come before us.

The first is very important; inasmuch as it includes all that relates to the varying quantity and intensity of the virus itself. This forms a part of the condition of the patient giving the infection, and the most essential part,—one, however, by no means duly appreciated in the ordinary methods of viewing the subject. Though we have no present means of estimating the absolute quantity or activity of the material cause, or the relation which they bear to one another, this does in nowise lessen the certainty that such variations exist, and have effect, directly or indirectly, in every instance of infection. The modifications arising from the particular period of the disorder; from idiosyncrasies of constitution in those affected; and especially from the variety of the parts or textures through which communication takes place, are all concerned in this view; and have severally their influence in determining the power of the virus, and the course of propagation of the disease.

Under the second head, viz., the state of the person receiving the infection, we have modifications derived from the previous condition of temperament and general health,—from the actual health at the time, and particularly from the presence or absence of other specific disorder, counteracting or modifying the virus received,—and from the state of the organ or tissue first or most intimately affected by it. The latter is an important point, and, like another just mentioned, not sufficiently estimated as a part of the inquiry.

Under the third head, of medium of transmission, still more numerous variations may be presumed to exist. Putting aside the obvious cases of inoculation and contact of surfaces, and looking to the atmosphere as the medium in the great majority of instances, we have here the endless variety arising from changes of weight, temperature, humidity, electrical state, and direction of currents— circumstances capable of modifying indefinitely the action of any virus thus conveyed, even without regard to the chemical changes which it may possibly undergo during such transmission. And further under this head, we have the case of fomites or virus thrown off from diseased surfaces, imbibed by porous bodies, and again emitted;—occasionally, as some assert, in a more concentrated form.

Duly considering these several points, they will be found, I think, to show adequate cause for all the strange and perplexing appearances of contagious disease. So far from being difficult to explain, why a given disorder should occasionally appear infectious, at other times not;—why it should spread rapidly in some localities, and not at all in others;—why it should affect some persons, and leave others free;—why the cases should be violent at one period, mild in another,—it is rather perhaps matter of wonder that the circumstances are not still more varied and irregular. Where there are such numerous elements of difference, the combination of these may well give scope to every assignable variety of result.

It is clear that very many of the contradictions of opinion and statement, as to the contagious nature of certain diseases, may be solved by a reference to these considerations. In all common reasoning on the subject, infection is too much regarded as a simple and uniform act; and the virus transmitted as the same in quantity and intensity. Such views, however, carry error into every part of the discussion. If we can dilute the matter of small-pox, so that it is no longer capable of giving the disease by inoculation, equally may the effluvia of certain fevers, capable of communicating the disorder in one degree of concentration, be so diluted in other cases, either in their original emission from the sick body, or by distance, or by the state of the atmosphere, that they lose the power of reproducing the disease in its complete and specific form. Accordingly we find that in these fevers, as well as in diseases more undoubtedly and actively contagious, the proofs of infection multiply, in proportion as the causes exist which are likely to concentrate infectious matter; as proximity, stagnant air, want of cleanliness and fresh clothing, &c. And what is true as to these disorders, will equally apply to many other doubtful or anomalous cases in the history of disease.

In erysipelas, for example, though its occasional contagious nature is sufficiently proved, the instances of this are comparatively so rare, that it occurs in the light of an anomaly to common observation. Nor can I doubt (having seen cases which go far to prove it) that a patient labouring under genuine measles may be present to another, perfectly susceptible of the infection, without the latter receiving the disorder; in default of the quantity or other peculiar state of the virus, needful for its passage through the intervening air. And this point receives further illustration from those singular cases, where an imperfect and irregular evolutions seems to occur of an infectious disorder, the actual nature and presence of which cannot be doubted. These various conditions can in no way be so well explained as by looking to the difference in quantity or concentration of a given virus; a diversity which must be of constant occurrence, and can never occur without some change of effect.

It is another and frequent mistake, in reasoning upon contagion, to consider that the infectious nature of a disease may be disproved, by showing that it has been spread without any obvious communication through man or human means. The two cases in fact are perfectly compatible. If a virus can be transmitted from the body through a few feet of air, we are not entitled from the partial experiments hitherto made to set any limit to the extent to which, under favourable circumstances, it may be conveyed through the same or other medium. Common reason here concurs with our actual experience of the transmission of the virus of certain diseases, in various ways, and to remote distances.

Notwithstanding all the labours of the time past, the subject of contagious diseases still offers a spacious field for discovery. In the remarks just made I have sought merely to put into a precise form those considerations or methods which must, I think, be the groundwork of all inquiry on the subject; purposely abstaining from the many illustrations which might be drawn from all parts of pathology. These methods have application to every view of the nature of the virus of particular diseases; and, under the scanty amount of our actual knowledge, this general application is, perhaps, the best test we can have of their value. Neither the laws of contagion, nor the many collateral questions which have perplexed and angered medical authors, can be rightly settled without some common principles to which to refer for classification of facts, and guidance amidst the seeming anomalies they present.*

CHAPTER XIX.

ON THE MEDICAL TREATMENT OF OLD AGE.

THERE are some points belonging to the disorders and treatment of old age, which, though familiar to the experienced physician, are scarcely enough regarded in general practice. It is understood that the rules which apply to other periods of life require alteration here, but the causes and extent of this are not always considered. True it is that old age is not to be reckoned merely by number of years. Family temperament, individual constitution, and the incidents of life, all concur to modify the time at which those changes begin which warrant the term in a physiological sense; and to affect no less the rate at which they proceed. Old age, moreover, may be said to be unequal in different individuals, as respects the different parts and functions of the body;—this diversity arising out of the same general causes which have just been assigned. Hereditary malady, or incidental disorders, often bring on premature decay in one organ, while others are comparatively untouched by time. These are points of importance to the practitioner; but withal so complicated, as scarcely to admit of being classed or described. Experience alone can adequately teach them.

Taking the term of old age, however, in its familiar sense, there is no difficulty in recognising certain changes that have taken place, or are proceeding, in all parts of the animal economy; nor doubt as to the fitness of modifying medical treatment, whether preventive or curative, with reference to these.

* A valuable paper on the laws of contagion, by my lamented friend Dr. Henry, is contained in the Fourth Report of the British Association, in which will be found the notice of nearly all that forms our present knowledge on the subject.

Bichat has defined life, " l'ensemble des fonctions qui résistent à
la mort ;" and the description, however quaint (and perhaps not
strictly logical,) is true in one important sense ; viz., that living
organization is that which is withdrawn for a time from what we
understand as the ordinary laws and conditions of matter, and
seems in many points even placed in opposition to them.* I use
general terms here, because I believe that our knowledge does not
justify our drawing any distinct line between what have been severally named physical and vital laws. Such line may exist; but
the attempt to define it at present rather marks our own ignorance,
than any natural boundary between the laws which govern organic
and inorganic creation. All great discoveries in physical science
(and especially some of recent date) have had the effect of altering
this presumed boundary, and, for the most part, of extending the
domain of physical into that of vital phenomena.†

But the power of vitality, much better defined by what it does
than by what it is, cannot be regarded as one definite quantity. It
fluctuates much even during the vigour of life: it declines in amount
in old age ; and its decay gives scope in the same ratio to those impressions upon the body of common physical agents, to which life in
its entireness seems to stand in a sort of opposition. There are
few more curious subjects of research than the condition of the
human body, when, from the weakening of the vital power, agencies
and changes, purely physical according to our understanding of the
term, produce new and peculiar effects upon it ; the progress of
these showing the degree of decline in the power which we thus
name.

Gravitation, for instance, which has manifest influence on the
circulation in all parts of life, and against which many provisions
are made in the structure and arrangement of blood-vessels, acts
with augmented effect as the vital moving forces are enfeebled.
These changes, depending on mechanical causes, and including the
various depositions and obliterations which take place in the vascular or other parts of structure, have been so fully described by

---

* A grosser definition of life, though in the same sense, is given by another
author,—"Illud putredini contrarium." It is obviously easy to multiply definitions founded on this principle of description.

† Chemistry in its largest sense, connected on one side with the great mechanical laws which govern the universe ; on the other, with those imponderable
agents, light, heat, and electricity, which science is now fast submitting to the
same laws, is apparently the source whence we may expect the greatest and
most certain results.

It is needful here, however, (and especially for the student or general reader
on such subjects,) to understand the true bearing of these, even if carried far
beyond their present limits. They do in nowise alter or impair the evidence of
Natural Theology, but even enforce and enlarge it. If an agency, wholly
unknown to us before but in a certain series of effects, is proved to be identical
with one producing, under other circumstances, a different series, we extend in
our comprehension the scope of that power which can govern and direct the same
agents to such vast and various ends ; and we establish yet further the unity of
that design which pervades, associates, and sustains the whole.

different authors that it is needless even to enumerate them.* The further question as to changes in the blood, or the admission of chemical on the diminution of vital affinities, is a more obscure matter of research, and one upon which few certain results have been obtained. The increased proportion of venous blood in old age is one of these facts; and it is probable that some of the deposits and alterations in different textures are the result of the lessened power of life of resisting common chemical changes, especially in the minute vessels, where it is likely that such loss of power would first be felt. Whether we are to look to the same source, or more directly to the functions of the lungs, or to those of the nervous system, for the diminished faculty of producing animal heat, is a point not yet wholly determined; though belonging to one of the most interesting questions in physiology. However this be, the importance of the fact is obvious, as relates to the medical treatment and general management of old age.

I may notice in the same cursory way the other changes, less obvious in their origin, though equally familiar to observation, which belong to this period of the life of man. The senses, even without apparent structural disease, lose their power of being excited,—become less keen and discriminative. The energy of volition is enfeebled; and its influence over the muscular actions in all ways impaired, often to the extent of partial paralysis, independently of the changes in the muscular tissues themselves. The diminution of irritability in all textures of the body, from whatever parts of the nervous system this be respectively derived, seems to occur in some ratio to the decline of sensibility and voluntary power. And hence morbid changes in all the functions of absorption and secretion, on the skin without and the membranes within; and the incapacity of adequately repairing the injuries sustained from accident or disease.

The intellectual functions, and particularly the faculties of recollection and association, undergo change; but not in any obvious proportion of time or degree to the decline of those powers, which give us more direct connexion with the external world. Where there has been no express disorder of the sensorium, some of the higher faculties of thought, as well as of moral feeling, are occasionally preserved to a very late period of existence, and amidst much of general decay. Ultimately, however, they give way, under that provision of our nature by which the living mind has been attached in its present existence to a certain definite organization;— growing with this from infancy upwards;—independent in some of its faculties, as far as consciousness can inform us;—in others so related to the physical conditions of structure, as to be intimately affected by all changes in these;—the whole a deep mystery to

* What has been successively written on this subject by Boerhaave, Haller, and Bichat, may especially be referred to. Recent inquiries have chiefly added to our knowledge of the changes going on in the capillary vessels in old age. The observations of Dr. Carswell on the *Gangræna Senilis* are a very valuable example of these researches.

which human reason in its present state can seemingly make no nearer approach.*

It is well worthy of note to how small a sphere of action life is often reduced, either from old age or disease, before its utter extinction; and how long in fact it may continue, thus narrowed and girt in on every side, with little excitement, and as small expenditure of those powers upon which it depends. The vital organs tardily carry forward the processes essential to existence; respiration may be limited to a small fraction of the lungs; the blood, feebly projected by the heart, moves languidly through vessels obstructed in all their minute branches; and the mental faculties, so far as they can be estimated, appear under the condition of a vague dream,—an analogy capable of being extended in many ways, and of great and peculiar interest to our views of the nature of mind; but which it is not my business to pursue further here.

One observation I would yet further make on the general view of the subject; viz., that no previous reason or feeling can afford a

* The growth of the intellectual powers through infancy and childhood has been the subject of careful notice and inference. Not equally so the progressive steps of mental decay in old age; a more difficult study, from the inequalities introduced by state of health, and the habits physical and intellectual of previous life; yet still capable of yielding many curious results to the science of the human mind.

It is one opinion on this subject that the sensorial functions, later perhaps than others we possess in reaching their respective completeness in each individual, are the first which begin to decline. The assumption is a very doubtful one: but however this may be, the enfeeblement is certainly not in the same ratio as to time for all the faculties; the losses not equal of the ideas and knowledge of different classes, and different periods of acquisition. Does not the faculty of receiving and associating fresh impressions for the most part decline earlier, than the power of combining and using those formerly received? Is not the faculty of directing and fixing combinations or successions of ideas one of those earliest impaired? In a lady of 91, whom I am now attending, the decay of the mind shows itself especially in the dependance of the course of ideas on the sound of words. A word, or even part of a word, of double application, will suddenly, and without the consciousness of change, carry off the mind to a new and wholly foreign subject. In another elderly patient, whose memory is singularly tenacious as to persons and detached events of past life, there is a singular incapacity of associating them together by any reasonable link; and the slightest relations of time or place suffice to carry the mind wholly astray from its subject. Such instances, by no means uncommon, have close kindred to the state of dreaming; the power of combining and directing the course of thought being similarly impaired in both cases.

It would seem, as respects the decay of memory more especially, that the power of recollecting words and names is lost earlier and more readily than that of events, both in effect of old age, and of accident or disease. This fact is strikingly attested in paralysis and other cerebral disorders; where, the ideas still remaining distinct, words are partially or wholly wanting for their expression; or others, by a strange and inexplicable perversion, are substituted, having no relation to the intended sense.

In another chapter I have noticed (what perhaps is more hypothetical) the absolute tardiness of mental operations in old age, whether of perception, volition, memory, or thought. It seems impossible to exclude the direct notion of time from these cases, as compared with others where the functions are in full vigour of power and exercise.

right estimate of the relation the mind assumes to death in the latter hours of life, even where no impairment of its faculties has occurred. This is especially true when long and painful sickness has been the prelude to the event. But the exhaustion also from acute pain of short continuance alters this relation; and even without sickness or suffering of any kind, the mere diminution of vital power by the decay of age produces the same effect. The earnestness to live abates, as the possession of life is gradually withdrawn. Every physician is witness to these things, as he watches occasionally over existence slowly ebbing away, without toil, suffering, or alarm.

> Gathered, not harshly pluck'd, for death mature.*

Familiarity with all the circumstances which thus designate the natural progress of old age, and with the modifications they produce in disease, is obviously of much value in practice. I shall refer in what follows to a few of these points, which seem especially to deserve attention.

The first practical conclusion which the prudent physician will draw from his knowledge here is, in some sort, a negative one; viz., not to interfere,—or, if at all, with care and limitation,—in those cases where changes, irretrievable in their nature, have occurred in any organ or function of the body. To urge medical treatment, in face of distinct proof to this effect, is to sacrifice at once the good faith and usefulness of the profession. This is a point the more needful to be kept in mind, as the patient himself, and those around him, are rarely able or willing to recognise it. It is often an exceedingly nice question of conscience, as well as of opinion, to define the extent to which practice may rightly proceed in such instances; always admitting, as must be done, that something is due to the feelings of the patient; something also to the uncertainty of our own judgments, antecedently to actual experience. This question in medical morals, like so many others, cannot be treated as a general principle only. The integrity and discretion of the practitioner must ever be appealed to for guidance in the endless variety of particular cases. In some, concession to a certain extent is safe, or even justified by indirect advantage to the patient. In others, mischief alone can arise from this meddling with the course of nature; and bad faith or bad judgment are involved in every such act of practice.

Illustrations of the latter kind may be drawn from a class of cases meriting much attention; those, namely, where discharges occur from some part of the body; the fitness of checking or suppressing which is the main question of treatment. The discredit injuriously cast upon the humoral pathology, had the effect during a long period of withdrawing the attention due to this class of disorders; and which, with inferior means of research, the ancient physicians had more sedulously bestowed upon them. Modern inquiry has again

* Paradise Lost, xi. 536.

reverted to the subject; and with the assurance, already sanctioned by results, of finding in it a wide field of discovery. Whether these discharges be habitual, or critical, or vicarious (for they may be understood as occurring in each of these senses), equally do they express functions of life, which cannot too sedulously be kept before us in practice.

This important consideration applies to cases occurring at every period of life, and not least to certain symptoms common in old age. In the *catarrhus senilis*, for instance, and the various bronchial affections of old persons, we have to consider whether it is expedient to put an active check upon them (therein complying with the demand almost always made from the physician), or whether the mucous or other discharges they involve are not really a safeguard to the constitution; an outlet provided for that which, retained in the blood, would create disorders of more critical kind? Without affirming it to be so in every case, my experience assures me that, in many, the practice of restraining such discharges is injurious in the attempt, hazardous if it be really effected. I entertain no doubt, from proofs furnished at every period of life, and particularly from the evidence by metastasis (of which I have noted many curious instances) that these large mucous secretions are often as essential to health as the secretions from other organs, which we assiduously seek to sustain. The necessity for them, having doubtless some relation yet unknown to the healthy properties of the blood, varies exceedingly in different habits, and at different ages; and this variation we can often distinctly connect with the state of other secretions; sanctioning the term vicarious, though not perhaps in the absolute sense in which it is sometimes used. We may seek to moderate occasional excess; to facilitate expectoration; and to regulate the cough so that it shall interfere as little as possible with rest. But to urge practice beyond this, in control of habitual symptoms, is more frequently a mischievous interference than a right direction of medical treatment.

The latter symptom, of cough, is that for which the physician's aid is most generally invoked, and where concession is too often and indiscriminately made. For, whether the secretions from these membranes be necessary or not, the act of coughing is at all events needful for their extrication or removal; and cases must have occurred to every practitioner where it is difficult to avoid the conviction that the sudden arrest of this, by opiates or otherwise, has accelerated a fatal event. This point is always to be kept in view in treating the disorders of advanced age; as well from the frequency of the symptom, as from the mistaken views regarding it, which are constantly pressing upon the better judgment of the physician.

A similar caution may be given as to interference with the secretion of lithic acid from the kidneys, generally increased in amount in old age. Alarm is often excited by the large quantity of this coming away, and alkalies are as largely given to obviate it. When there is tendency to concretion or occasional lodgment in the kidneys, this may be proper; but where the discharge is free and without distress, and there is no obvious disorder of internal organs attending it, the wisest practice is, generally, that which most refrains.   This discharge indeed is often the most effectual outlet for that which, retained and accumulated, becomes a source of active disease, particularly to the brain, in those of advanced life.   I have known many patients never well, unless when such removal of animal matters through the urine was largely going on.

I may further allude, under similar view, to habitual discharges from the bowels; resembling often those of active disease, yet attended with no distress, and indicating only the need of separation of these matters from the body.   A meddling or rude practice in these cases is rarely effectual for good; and may do serious harm if it alters or suspends actions salutary to the system.*

Though less frequent occurrences than some of the preceding, the same remark applies to certain passive hemorrhages incidental to advancing age; epistaxis; hæmaturia; hemorrhages from the bowels, uterus, &c.   In conformity with the oldest opinions in physic, these may often be regarded as salutary evacuations, critically occurring to the relief of particular organs, or of the general circulation.   On the approach of old age, as indeed at other marked periods of life (without getting too far into the mystery of epochs), various new balances are struck in the allotment of the blood to different parts; and in the course of such changes, congestions and discharges are prone to occur; the latter relieving or preventing the former.   The tests by which this is to be determined are generally simple and well marked, requiring only care to note them. And all experience teaches how frequently these discharges, even when most profuse, proceed safely to a termination: their continuance being defined by the relief they afford to the exciting causes. But here also the physician is occasionally drawn out of the temperate observation which is his best practice, by the alarm and anxiety of those who surround the patient.   Without evidence of inflammation or organic disease, the lancet is taken up to control, as it is presumed, the internal hemorrhage; or lead and other astringents given, with vague relation to the cause or seat of disorder, and often with mischievous effect in other ways.

Taking into fair view the average of such cases, and without any undue favour to the doctrine of critical evacuations or vicarious discharges, I believe more evil to be inflicted by eagerness to check or alter the course of hemorrhages of this kind, that can be incurred by a cautious forbearance and observation of their progress; with due care to sustain the system under any exhaustion which may attend them.   Even in common cases of hemorrhage from diseased structure, this consideration is to be kept in view; but particularly where there is presumption of its taking place from mucous sur-

* See Chapter XIII. (On some Points in the Pathology of the Colon.)

faces, or in the parenchymatous structure of organs, without actual disease.

Though noting this point here, as one which demands especial attention when life borders on old age, the remark might be made much more general as respects the treatment of hemorrhage. Instances there doubtless are in which speedy restraint is the only safety ; and many more in which prevention, or change of direction, are sedulously to be sought for. But there remain numerous cases, at all periods of life, where present hemorrhage, even of active kind, is best treated by simply withdrawing all that may excite or protract it; and where the causes of the bleeding are most relieved by its occurrence. Hæmoptysis even is not so much to be dreaded in itself, being often a partial relief to the pulmonary circulation, as in the indications it gives of future evil. Hæmatemesis, however large in amount, rarely needs any active control. It expresses more distinctly, perhaps, than any other hemorrhage, the need of the relief which it actually affords to a part of the circulation ; and I believe more injury than good to be done by the means often used to check it. The same remark will apply to hæmaturia ; with some qualification for cases where it originates in calculi, or disease of the kidney. On these points, as on so many others, the experience of the physician must be brought to judgment on particular cases. Where precepts, to be applicable at all, need to allow for such numerous and important contingencies, they lose much of their value in practice.

Connected with this subject is the question as to the relative fitness and extent of bleeding, as a remedy, in advanced life; a matter of frequent doubt to the practitioner ; and, like the preceding, best to be solved by sound experience applied to each case. The general rule, doubtless, is that of comparative limitation, and a still more cautious observation of the tests by which this limit is marked in actual practice. For the various disorders of inflammation or congestion occur in the same organs, and of the same kind, as in earlier life ; but with diminished means in the system itself of resisting the disease, or repairing any losses sustained in its treatment.* Under the latter consideration, it becomes especially needful in old age (though the rule applies to all ages) that the remedy, when required, should be promptly used; before the disease gains stronger hold, before parts are disorganized, or the nervous powers exhausted by long illness.

The latter point is one to which attention is singularly due at this time of life ; lest by continued active treatment of symptoms, which might have subsided after the first remedies, we bring on others more injurious in result. Here, too, there is need of a particular caution as to the pulse of old age. The artery brought nearer to tho surface by the absorption of other parts, with its own texture

---

* The observations of M. Louis, on inflammations occurring under debility of the system at large, well merit every attention here.

and elasticity also changed, gives a pulse to which common interpretation will not apply, and which deceives the inexperienced or
careless by the impression of more vigour of circulation than actually exists. A like deception often arises from ossification of some
part of the heart or vascular system, so common at this time of
life. An irritable jarring stroke is thereby produced, mistaken
sometimes for one of power; and leading to a mischievous activity
of depletion, the effects of which are not readily repaired.*

One of the best tests here is the equality, or otherwise, of the
heart's action; and the more needful to be observed, seeing the frequency of structural changes in this organ in advanced age. If
intermitting, and unequal either in strength or frequency of beat,
caution as to bleeding must be doubled; and this caution is no less
to be maintained, where there is presumption of the irregularity depending on sensorial disorder. In this case it expresses more frequently deficiency of nervous power, than a state of brain requiring
depletion: while if originating in the vascular system, it is oftener
the result of mechanical difficulty from structural causes, or of unequal supply of blood to the heart, or of change in the quality of the
blood itself, than of actual excess in the quantity of this fluid.
Where, nevertheless, the symptoms are deemed to require bleeding,
its influence upon the regularity of the heart's action must be carefully looked to as a test; and this not merely at the moment of depletion, but even yet more when the circulation has recovered from
the sudden change of balance thus produced.

The effect upon the sensorium and nervous power is, undoubtedly,
the most important part of the question as to bleeding in old age.
In another place I have made some remarks which bear especially
on this subject.† It is certain that there are states of brain, with
which its general condition in old age is closely connected, where
sudden or considerable loss of blood brings on various morbid effects,
paralytic or convulsive in kind, the occurrence of which is too exclusively attributed in common practice to fulness of blood in the
vascular system. Errors in treatment, founded on this view, may
be repaired at other periods of life, when such state of brain is
brought on by casual causes: but in old age, where it is more or
less permanent, and depending on organic changes, the mischief
done is sometimes irreparable in kind. And the greater care and
discrimination are needed here, from the singular similarity, as far
as general aspect is concerned, of symptoms really arising from
different causes, and requiring opposite treatment.

* In the application of the valuable means we now possess for discovering
organic changes about the heart and great vessels through the parietes of the chest,
the separate indications to the same effect through the pulse are too much neglected.
It is probable that there is no structural disease of the heart, certainly none of
consequence, which is not represented in some manner in the pulse, beating
along a vessel of the size of the radial artery. The difficulty, of course, is in
estimating the slighter modifications, and in separating them from the analogous
or identical effects of other disorders; the latter difficulty, indeed, one that is common in part even to the more delicate methods just referred to.

† Chapter III. (On Bleeding in Affections of the Brain.)

Further, it may be remarked that bleeding in advanced life, when manifestly required by the symptoms, does not of necessity preclude the use at the same time of means to support the nervous power.   On this point, indeed, as respects all periods of life, common practice is too straitened and exclusive.   A disorder which requires depletion by bleeding, as the chief and earliest remedy, is presumed to admit none other than antiphlogistic means while this state continues: and, as a general rule, this is so ; but there are cases of exception, and old age includes many such.   The nervous and circulating systems, though so closely connected in every function of life, have yet their separate powers.   Even taking the whole of each system, these powers are not always, it would seem, in exact relation to each other ; and this is more particularly true where the vascular changes, whether of inflammation or simple congestion, are limited in extent. We may need for relief the change in circulation which bleeding affords ; yet may require at the same time that support or stimulus to the nervous power, which is essential to the equal distribution of the blood, and without which disorders of a new kind may supervene, or the one for which the remedy was applied be kept up under an altered form.   We cannot rightly refuse the name of inflammation to certain cases which occur, not simply during debility, but even consequently upon it ; and the just application of remedies of the two classes, concurrently or consecutively, to these cases, forms one of the most delicate points in medical practice.   It is sufficient to mention it here, in its application to the treatment of the diseases of advanced age.

Several of these observations as to bleeding apply equally to the use of purgatives.   The frequent employment of drastic medicines .. of this kind is injurious to the general powers of life, as well as to the particular organs on which their impression is first made.   The necessity of many cases, even in extreme age, does of course supersede this rule ; but it is one fitly to be kept in mind in every part of practice.   In applying it we must advert to the fact, that the feebler circulation, and deficient sensibility and secretion of the mucous surfaces in old age, often render medicines and doses ineffective which have acted readily at other times of life: so that here, even more than in other cases, we are to measure our means not by common table of doses, but by observation of effects on the body.

Many of the foregoing remarks are applicable to general practice ; but I specify them here as comprising the principles which may best regulate the use of depleting remedies in old age.   Another question regards the employment of opiates at the same period of life : nor is this without its peculiar perplexities.   Besides the modifications which are required from the different relation of years to bodily powers, and those further made necessary by the various idiosyncrasies as to opium, we have another specialty in this part of treatment from the changes which the functions of the brain, and often even its obvious texture, undergo in advanced age.   Some of these changes are of kind to render the action of opiates ambiguous at least, if not in many cases distinctly hurtful. The vague dozing state, which steals gradually upon the aged, and without any acute disease, seems in the end to turn life into a mere dream,—this express an altered condition of the brain and nervous system, in which narcotics probably quicken the change and render it more complete. Happily these are the cases in which they are generally least required. The state in question is a benign dispensation to the extreme term of life, rarely coming within the proper scope of medical treatment, unless there be some sudden passage into what is obviously a condition of coma. And even where other organs are more actively diseased, the sensibility in such cases is often so far lessened, as to supersede the remedies which are necessary at other periods of life to relieve irritation alone.

All questions of practice in these instances are manifestly those of degree ; nor can any rule be given general enough to preclude attention to the individualities of each case. We have often, too, in old age other symptoms which seem more directly to require the aid of opiates ; such as a habitual restlessness at night, under the influence of vague images and sounds, harassing the mind by a sense of reality beyond that of dreams. The effect of the remedy, however, even in these instances, is by no means an assured one ; and benefit can only be attested upon trial. For progressive or permanent changes in the brain are generally concerned in such cases, and of a nature often to render injurious the stupor produced by narcotics, as well as to make uncertain their effect in procuring repose. There are doubtless cases where it is otherwise ; but it is difficult to find other criterion than that of experience for determining these.

In the eneuresis of old age, especially when not depending on any disease of the prostate gland, I have often found more benefit from moderate opiates than from any other remedy. And in that harassing complaint, the *prurigo senilis*, which is ever so difficult of relief, this treatment is probably the best. Where the internal use of opium is objectionable on any account, the irritation may be greatly abated by lotions or ointments in which this is the main ingredient. Its combination with some mild mercurial, under the same form of use, frequently adds to the benefit obtained.

The principles as to diet in old age do not differ essentially from those applicable to every period of life. The questions are chiefly those of degree, and to be answered under the same modifications and exceptions as in other cases. Regularity in the times of food seems, indeed, as in infancy, more essential to the well-being of the system than when the body is in the full vigour of life. It has now fewer resources, whether animal or vital, for righting itself: the functions are all less prompt to repair any partial injury or deficiency. Stimulants also, which either in kind or quantity might be injurious in midlde age, are often fitting or needful at a more advanced period. The questions as to particular articles of diet may for the most part be settled on the same principles for both these periods ; making due allowance for the difficulties of mastication in old age, and for the want of those active exercises of body which tend to obviate obstruction, and to assist all the powers, mechanical as well as vital, upon which digestion depends.

All that relates to the preservation of warmth in old age, and, through this, of equable circulation, is too familiar to need being dwelt upon. The functions upon which animal heat depends have lost their vigour; and its production is in the same ratio diminished. We are bound with the greater care to save from loss by diffusion that which remains. This is important, not alone as sustaining the functions of the skin, the action of the limbs, and the general comfort, but also as lessening that tendency to congestion in internal organs which is one source of particular maladies, as well as a cause of general decay. We cannot restore the balance between absorption and deposition, in the loss of which some define old age to consist; but if these changes admit of retardation, as it is likely they do, this is probably best effected by whatever tends to maintain animal heat, and a free circulation throughout the vascular system.

Connected in some sort with this latter topic is the common question respecting old age (but one of deep interest, though common), to what extent the bodily powers may be preserved by maintaining their assiduous exercise :—whether, to take a single instance, the muscular organs may be longer kept in vigour by exertion to the full extent of ability at each successive period of life? or whether the powers, whatever they be, which minister to these actions, are longer and better maintained by comparative repose?

Though the question may seem easily solved by ordinary observation, yet is this not so. It involves some of the most subtle and obscure points in physiology; those, to wit, which regard the nature and origin of vitality, its mode of distribution and manner of decay; —questions which, under different forms and various phraseology, have perplexed reasoning men of every age, and begotten theories and controversies without end. Taking life, however, not as a definite exhaustible quantity of an unknown influence, but as expressing a common result of the actions of many parts differently constructed and endowed, we are furnished with what comes nearest to a satisfactory reply. Whatever habits of living sustain the greatest number of organs or functions in healthy state (having regard also to the relative importance of these functions) may be considered as most conducive to length of life. The positive fatigue of any organ from its exercise must always be deemed an excess; —of little import, it may be, in single instances; certainly injurious by frequent or habitual repetition. All exercise of a natural function of the body within this limit may be viewed, without material risk or error, as salutary in itself, and maintaining the integrity of the organ concerned longer than the opposite habit of inertness and disuse.

This practical distinction is simple and probably just. It is applicable, moreover, to every period of life, and very appropriately to old age in all its stages. The limit of action without exhaustion becomes more and more contracted, and in the same ratio must action be abated in degree. Exercise, short of this exhaustion, and with due allowance for casual fluctuations of power, may be admitted as maintaining the functions in their healthiest state, and thereby tending to lengthen the term of duration to each.

The same principle and rule may be applied without error to the mental functions also. Here, equally, there is a power, naturally diminished in old age, susceptible of exhaustion from excess of use, and liable to be permanently impaired where this excess is frequent and severe in degree. On the other hand, disuse is not preservation; and we have every cause to believe that the integrity of these faculties is best and longest sustained by habitual exercise, within those bounds which are reached without fatigue at each successive period of life.

With all the desire that has existed to discover rules conducive to length of life and preservation of its powers, it is doubtful whether any can be found which are not directly subordinate to the principle just stated. We have no simple element, cognisable by our means of research, to deal with here. Organs and their functions are the sole interpreters of life to our present reason ; and the maintenance of these in healthy action is all that can be done to solve the problem, and satisfy the desires, which have been entertained by mankind of every age on this subject.

CHAPTER XX.

ON THE USE OF EMETICS.

AMONG the changes which time and fashion impose upon the treatment of disease, emetics as a remedy have fallen into comparative disuse in English practice. It is no longer now, as heretofore, one of the first questions before the mind of the practitioner, when called to prescribe for a disorder, whether the stomach should not be thus immediately relieved. The suggestion of the patient himself is for the most part needed, or some other equally express indication, to lead to their use. I am speaking here only of a general alteration that has occurred. The exceptions to it are of course numerous; but the truth of the fact so stated will probably not be denied.

The cause of this change may chiefly be found in that larger and more various employment of purgatives which forms the character of our modern practice. To what extent is the alteration of method a beneficial one? I believe a fair consideration will justify the opinion that in many points it has been carried too far. Vomiting, especially when brought on at the outset of fevers and many other diseases, produces effects of a kind, and with a speed, which no purgatives alone can equally obtain. Beneficial as is the action of emetics in unloading the stomach and upper part of the alimentary canal, it is certain that their influence goes far beyond this; and that other parts of the body, even the most remote and different in structure, are powerfully acted upon. The emetic, moreover, if rightly used, is beneficial not merely in the effect of morbid matters removed from the body, but often even by the nausea attending its operation, and by the mechanical effort of vomiting; a combination of advantages scarcely belonging to any other remedy.

The experiments of Magendie seem to have proved that the stomach itself is passive in vomiting; and that the action is due to convulsive movements of the diaphragm or abdominal muscles, brought on, not solely by emetic or other irritating substances in the stomach, but by similar agents introduced directly into the blood, as well as by certain states of the brain and nervous system. As I have in view only the practical application of the remedy, I need not advert to these points in physiology, further than to remark, that they illustrate much more satisfactorily the various causes of sickness, and the effects of emetics, than the old notion that the stomach alone was concerned in this action. There are still points of question as to the proximate causes of vomiting; even such as relate to the state of the diaphragm in the act, and in what particular way it is connected with the function of respiration. Something also may be learned of the manner in which particular irritations produce sickness, by reference to reflex nervous actions through the spinal cord. But, for the reason just given, I merely allude to these topics of inquiry.

It is unnecessary to say much of the effects of vomiting as a remedy upon the stomach itself. The relief got by rejecting undigested food, or morbid ingesta of other kinds, is not, however, to be regarded as the only benefit thus obtained. The secretions from the mucous membrane lining this organ are frequently such in kind and quantity, that their removal becomes necessary to all further treatment; and accordingly we find that instant good is often derived from emetics, where these matters alone are discharged. While still left on the stomach, all other treatment by internal remedies is injurious or unavailing; a point not sufficiently regarded in ordinary practice, where the failure of one medicine is too often made the prelude to another of similar kind. It may be that emetics have influence also in changing the nature of the secretions from this organ, either by inducing the state of nausea, or the act of vomiting; each, as it would seem, capable of this effect, though perhaps in different manner.

Much caution, however, is necessary as to the use of emetics in another state of the stomach and alimentary canal, where the secretions from the lining membranes are almost wholly suspended; and where there is general gastric irritation, tending to inflammatory action, indicated by redness and dryness of the tongue, fauces, and throat, and often by tenderness over the region of the stomach itself. These, indeed, are cases where the effort to vomit is often a symptom, and a very distressing one, of the disorder; and where emetics of course are interdicted by the most obvious circumstances present.

The value of emetics in the treatment of *cynanche tonsillaris,* though understood as matter of medical precept, is not equally regarded in practice. Nor, indeed, as a general fact, do we sufficiently keep in view the close relation between the several parts of the internal fauces, and the membranes of the œsophagus and stomach ; and the frequent and singular translation of morbid action which takes place along this continuity of surface. Many more exact interpretations of disease might be derived from looking to this connexion through the medium of contiguous structure and function, than from that minute nomenclature which is formed upon the mere locality of symptoms: and the indications of treatment would in the same proportion become more exact, as in the use of emetics under the circumstances to which I am now referring.

The liver, and the whole system of the portal circulation are singularly under the beneficial influence of this remedy. Congestion, so prone to occur in this part of the body at the commencement of most fevers, as well as in other diseases, is lessened or removed by vomiting,—the passage of bile into the bowels rendered more free,—other secretions promoted or restored,—purging often obtained without further aid,—and a general state of all these viscera induced, peculiarly tending to lessen febrile action, and especially in those cases where it arises directly from gastric disorder.

In most of the slighter cases of jaundice with which we have to deal, emetics will be found much more capable of speedily restoring the passage of bile into the bowel than any other means ; and the instances are numerous (including particularly those fevers of warm climates, which, however variously designated, have all such close relation to the functions of the liver and the circulation through the chylopoietic viscera) where the direct combination of an active emetic and purgative medicine in the outset of disease, with repetition of the same means when needful, has effect in subduing the violence of disorder beyond any other remedy. This combination is not sufficiently employed in ordinary practice, in the many cases where speedy disgorgement is required of the part of the system just referred to.

The effect of emetics upon the circulation is a complicated one, including, as it does, both nausea and the mechanical effect of vomiting ; each capable of influencing greatly the heart's action, and the general movements of the blood. From both, however, may much benefit be obtained ; though with different application according to the nature of the case. When the circulation is morbidly excited, nausea may be longer sustained ;—where there is congestion about the heart and great vessels, vomiting is speedily to be brought on. Nor is there cause for the degree of apprehension which exists as to the rupture of blood-vessels, or pressure upon the head, from this effort. Though cases of such kind have doubtless occurred, they are comparatively very rare, and generally depend upon causes peculiar to the individual. It is singular indeed to what extent, and with what violence, vomiting may take place, without producing any injury of this nature. Sea-sickness, and that attending every stage of pregnancy, are evidence of the fact; and it is important the inference should be kept in mind, that there may not be undue discouragement to the use of the remedy in many cases where it is of singular value.*

The influence of emetics upon the nervous system is also complicated, and one in which it is not easy to separate the direct from the indirect effects. It is unquestionably powerful, and capable of being very beneficially applied. The circumstances, not yet wholly understood, which give such peculiar sensibility to the region of the stomach, and so closely associate it, not only with all others of the vital organs, but also with the functions of animal life, render the several conditions of this part very important to the well-being of the whole system. No illustration of this is needful to those who have felt the influence, both upon mind and body, of the sensations arising from disorders having this seat, even such as are casual and temporary in kind.† Here the action of emetics is well marked, and often of singular avail; and from hence their effects are largely diffused over other parts of the nervous system. Some part of the good they produce, when given at the outset of fevers, may depend on this circumstance, in concurrence with the others already mentioned.

In illustration of the benefit to be obtained from emetics in this stage of disease, I would refer again to the epidemic influenzas, which have so repeatedly prevailed of late years. I have already stated my conviction that no remedy is equally safe and expedient, at the commencement of the disorder, in diminishing the severity of the attack; or apparently, when slight, in suspending it altogether. In the progress of the malady, too, there is often benefit from the repetition of the same means; and especially in the case of children,

---

* I may mention in further proof the common use of emetics among the workmen in coal-mines, for the relief of the state brought on by breathing fixed air in excess, as well as after being subjected to fire-damp. I have had recent occasion of learning this fact in visiting the mines at Whitehaven. It might be supposed in these cases, if in any, that congestion in the vessels of the brain was to be avoided. Yet if injury be thus produced, it is seemingly of much less import than the good gained by renewing the action of the diaphragm and restoring respiration.

† The fitness of the term of *foyer epigastrique*, as expressing a fact respecting this particular part of the body, has been made the subject of some controversy. Bichat denies its propriety as applied to any one spot; but, in connexion with his hypothesis that the vital organs are the proper and sole seat of the passions (an hypothesis which has foundation in language alone), he makes a sort of admission of the phrase in question as expressing a central influence of these organs.

where the want of due relief by expectoration is best thus supplied. I may name this as an instance where the comparative disuse of emetics has certainly interfered with the general success of our practice.

The mention of emetics as aiding expectoration brings us to one of the most important uses of this remedy. Though yet insufficiently employed for the express object, their effect in relieving the chest, when the bronchial cells and tubes are gorged with mucus, is scarcely less beneficial than their action in unloading the biliary system. They may justly be reckoned the most powerful expectorants we possess; speedy in effect, and often complete in relief. In bronchitis and other cases, where, from accumulation of mucus in the air passages, the breathing and pulmonary circulation are greatly oppressed, and the patient under much suffering, the change thus produced is sometimes surprising in degree, and such as we can obtain in no other way. Their value in croup is well attested by the concurrence of all modern experience with that of the excellent physician who first enforced this treatment.

I have already commented on the apprehension of hemorrhage, or pressure on the head, which checks one important application of emetics. In the case now before us, their use is often abandoned from the like fear of making undue pressure on the vessels or producing suffocation; an apprehension unwarranted by fact, and which the most common experience might correct. The converse of this is nearer the truth, and forms, indeed, the especial value of the remedy in the instances alluded to. Even in cases of actual inflammation of the lungs I believe the risk of their use to be exaggerated, though undoubtedly more watchfulness is here required.

There is greater cause for referring to this application of emetics, from our vague and imperfect views as to the whole class of expectorant remedies. Scarcely indeed is the term defined in its ordinary use in practice. It is left doubtful whether the expectorant is a medicine which promotes the secretion of mucus from the bronchial surfaces,—or facilitates, after being formed, its removal from the chest,—or combines both these effects in its single power. The natural result is that of rendering practice almost equally vague on these points. And, though there is less liability to dangerous error here than in many other classes of remedies, yet it is obviously important to gain more distinct views than those currently received.

The emetic is probably the only agent which both promotes secretion and discharges it; the latter action being chiefly, if not altogether, a mechanical effect of the effort of vomiting induced. There is reason to believe that no one of the medicines termed expectorants can act in freeing the chest from mucus in the air passages, unless they be so given as to produce vomiting, or to bring on cough by irritating the membranes; or unless they increase or attenuate the actual secretion, so as in this manner to excite cough, and render it more effectual for expectoration. Their influence upon secretion is indeed the circumstance we must chiefly regard among me-

dicines of this class; and here, again, their effects and relative value are very ill defined.   It is probable that the expectorants, so
termed, which act as emetics when given in larger doses, are principally of avail in augmenting the secretion when used so as to
keep up a certain degree of nausea.   This state has manifestly
much influence in relaxing the exhalant and secreting vessels; and
though I do not venture to affirm it, where proof is so difficult, I
believe that it is chiefly in this way that the medicines in question
come to be of any avail in practice.*

The question as to the proximate cause or seat of the sensation
which we term nausea, and its relation to the act of vomiting, is
indeed a curious and difficult one.   If anything like explanation is
to be found, it will probably be through the results obtained by Magendie and others, to which I have already alluded.

Connected with this subject is the alleged effect of emetics as a
remedy in the early stages of pulmonary consumption; an opinion
held by many eminent physicians from an early period down to the
present day; and which has gained rather than lost weight by recent inquiries on the subject.   The researches of Dr. Carswell into
the origin and seat of tuberculous deposits afford a more explicit
notion how emetics may act, by removing or preventing the growth
of tubercle on the membrane of the bronchial cells.   It is easy to
understand that any means which can promote the natural secretion into these cells, render their contents more liquid and easy of
removal, and aid in actually procuring it, may be of singular advantage;—especially in that earlier part of the disease, where the
presumption exists that tuberculous deposits are only beginning to
take place.   The action of emetics reaches further towards these
several objects than that of any other remedy;—it is compatible
with every other part of treatment—and under regulation of their use,
and with due regard to any acute inflammatory states which may
occur in the progress of the disease, I believe them to be the safest
and most effectual means yet suggested for the relief of incipient
phthisis.

Unfortunately this must still be stated more on speculation than
on certain experience.   A few continental physicians have made
systematic use of the remedy; but in England its employment with
this object seems to have been very partial, though enforced by
medical authorities which claim every respect.   The difficulties, indeed, which oppose themselves to the treatment, especially among
the higher classes, are not easily overcome.   The remedy, from various associations, is regarded as more formidable than is really the
case;—the present habit of practice is adverse to it;—and, further,
the suggestion of the treatment comes at a time when fears may

* The whole class of expectorants, however divided and defined, needs revision, as do so many other parts of the Materia Medica.   The progress of
medicine, as a science, requires that we should not bind ourselves too implicitly
to old tables and formulæ, which have their origin in doubtful sources, and gain
authority chiefly by long transmission from one book or lecture to another.

hardly yet be awakened, or when there is repugnance on the part of the patient and those around, to admit what argues a dangerous disease at hand. The influence of these causes is well known to every physician.

The use of emetics in producing absorption of effused fluids, or of parts morbidly enlarged, seems sufficiently attested. But we have no reason to suppose that they have any effect on tubercles actually formed; and their employment therefore in phthisis, when we can obtain trial for them at all, is probably to be limited to the earliest stage of the disorder.

I need advert but slightly to the benefit derived from emetics in asthma; though here again it must be admitted that there is an insufficient use of the remedy, seeing the great good gained in many such cases by unloading the stomach and liver; and the equal advantage, though less obvious in explanation, from its influence on the actions of the circulation and nervous system. A single emetic may cut short a paroxysm for which opiates and antispasmodics have long been employed in vain.

The use of this remedy in the disorders of children is at present much less general than it ought to be. In very many cases emetics would beneficially supersede that employment of purgatives which often adds to the irritation it professes to remove. In the infantile fever, for example, which is a type of various disorders, an occasional dose of ipecacuanha, so as to excite vomiting, (especially where there is much of the cough which attends this complaint, and large secretion from the mucous membranes,) will be found more effectual than any other means. It is to be noted, further, that the action of vomiting is for the most part singularly easy in children; more immediate, and generally less distressing than that of purgative medicines.

In these remarks I have attended rather to the general effects of emetics, than to the several qualities and manner of action of the medicines so termed; it being my object only to draw attention to the fitness of their larger and more defined use in ordinary practice. The question of preference among different emetic substances is indeed of less moment, from their action in emptying the stomach of its contents. In the majority of cases, that may be deemed best which fulfils its purpose without actual pain, and with greatest certainty and speed. It ipecacuanha were invariably of good quality, which unfortunately it is not, it might be sufficient in almost every instance. Antimonials, from sustaining nausea longer, and producing more distinct sedative effect on the nervous and vascular systems, may be preferred where excitement of these exists. The emetic of simple mustard ought never to be lost sight of as an immediate resource, and one producing its effect with less previous distress than any other.

In considering, however, the effects of emetics, we must separate such as belong to the direct action of the medicine on the coats of the stomach, from those produced by the act of vomiting. The former may be more or less hurtful, as depending upon a peculiar irritation of the part; and here the action of emetic medicines must be assimilated to that of acrid or poisonous matters received into the stomach or generated there. But the mere effort of vomiting itself is much less injurious to this organ than might on first view appear likely. Without referring in proof to the " *vomitus luxuriæ causâ*"* of the Roman dinner tables, I may again mention sea-sickness, the sickness of pregnancy, the frequent vomiting of infants, and the habit some individuals have of rejecting constantly in this way a portion of all food taken, as evidence that little mischief comparatively can be derived from this source.† The point is one which must always be kept in view in judging of the effect of emetics in practice, and of the frequency and particular methods in which they may best be employed.

CHAPTER XXI.

ON THE USES OF DILUENTS.

THOUGH there may seem little reason for considering these as a separate class of remedies, yet I doubt whether the principle of treatment implied in the name is sufficiently regarded in modern practice. On the continent, indeed, the use of diluents is much more extensive than in England; and, under the form of mineral waters especially, makes up in some countries a considerable part of general practice. But putting aside all question as to mineral ingredients in water, the consideration more expressly occurs, to what extent and with what effects this great diluent, the only one which really concerns the animal economy, may be introduced into the system as a remedy? Looking at the definite proportion which in healthy state exists in all parts of the body between the aqueous, saline, and animal ingredients,—at the various organs destined directly or indirectly to regulate the proportion,—and at the morbid results occurring whenever it is materially altered,—we must admit

* Celsus, lib. i. cap. 3.
† I have known a patient, a young lady of delicate and irritable habit, who, during fourteen months, rejected invariably some portion of every meal; the quantity rejected, and the interval before vomiting occurred, depending much on the quality of the food. In this case (in which the malady depended not on organic disease of the stomach or pylorus, but seemingly on irritation translated from another part), the patient suffered chiefly from an uneasy distension preceding vomiting, little from nausea or the vomiting itself; and she even gained considerably in flesh while the disorder was going on.
In another instance I have known the habit of vomiting continue for many years, after every meal of which animal food was the principal part; without any apparent injury to the constitution or increasing mischief to the stomach. In cases of this kind, the act of raising the rejected food is generally attended with very little nausea or distressing effort.

the question as one important in the animal economy, and having various relation to the causes and treatment of disease.

Keeping in mind then this reference to the use of water as an internal remedy, diluents may be viewed under three conditions of probable usefulness;—first, the mere mechanical effect of quantity of liquid in diluting and washing away matters, excrementitious or noxious, from the alimentary canal;—secondly, their influence in modifying certain morbid conditions of the blood;—and thirdly, their effect upon various functions of secretion and excretion, and especially upon those of the kidneys and skin. Other more specific effects there may be; but these are presumably the most important, and each may be made to contribute respectively to valuable ends in practice.

The first is an obvious benefit in many cases, and not to be disdained from any notion of its vulgar simplicity. It is certain that there are many states of the alimentary canal, in which the free use of water at stated times.produces good which cannot be attained by other or stronger remedies. I have often known the action of the bowels to be maintained with regularity for a long period, simply by a tumbler of water, warm or cold, on an empty stomach, in cases where medicine had almost lost its effect, or become a source only of distressing irritation. The advantage of such treatment is still more strongly attested, where the secretions taking place into the intestines, or the products formed there during digestion, becomes vitiated in kind. Here dilution lessens that irritation to the membranes, which we cannot so readily obviate by other means, and aids in removing the cause from the body with less distress than any other remedy. In some instances, where often and largely used, its effect goes farther in actually altering the state of the secreting surfaces, by direct application to them. But it is difficult for the most part to distinguish this result from the effect taking place through the circuit of the blood.

I mention these circumstances upon experience, having often obtained much good from resorting to them in practice, when stronger medicines and ordinary methods had proved of little avail. Dilution thus used, for example, so as to act on the contents of the bowels, is beneficial in many dyspeptic cases, where it is especially an object to avoid needless irritation to the system. Half a pint or more of water taken when fasting, at the temperature most agreeable to the patient, will often be found to give singular relief to his morbid sensations; and, where such is the effect, may even become a valuable aid to the other treatment pursued. Or in cases where there is habitual excess of acid in the lower bowels (a source of frequent distress, though not so easily recognised as acid on the stomach), the solution of half a drachm or more of carbonate of soda in the quantity of water taken, will add greatly to the good gained. It is often more beneficial in this way than given in smaller proportion of liquid; a point connected with the action of mineral waters, which clearly influence by quantity and dilution the me-

dicinal effect of their contents, while having at the same time the
mechanical operation due to water alone.

In reference to the foregoing uses of diluents, it is to be kept in
mind that the lining of the alimentary canal is to all intents a surface, as well as the skin ; pretty nearly equal in extent ; exercising
some similar functions, with others more appropriate to itself ; and
capable in many respects of being acted upon in similar manner.
Medical men themselves, and still more those with whom they have
to deal, are prone to attach undue importance to the mere fact of
a substance being taken into the stomach, as if this were equivalent
to its being received into the system.   As respects the subject before us, it is both expedient and correct in many cases to regard
diluents as acting on this internal surface analogously to liquids on
the skin.   And I would apply this remark, not only to the mechanical effects of the remedy, but also to their use as the medium for
conveying cold to internal parts,—a point of practice which
either the simplicity of the means, or the false alarms besetting it,
have hitherto prevented from being duly regarded.

The abstraction of heat from an inflamed or irritable membrane
within, is often indeed quite as salutary as the cold directly applied
to a hot and dry skin without.   The extent of use is from obvious
causes much more limited ; but I have seen enough of the benefit
from cold liquids freely given in the acute stage of gastric disorders,
inflammatory and febrile, with express reference to this point of
temperature, to justify the recommendation of more frequent recourse to it in practice.   This is a point where the feelings and
desire of the patient may fairly be taken in guidance, and we can
rarely go wrong in following them.   The test, in fact, is simple and
immediate ; depending on sensations which cannot readily be mistaken, and the changes in which indicate the extent as well as
suggest the use of the remedy.

The second condition under which diluents may be viewed, as
altering certain morbid states of the blood, is one of more difficulty,
and connected with questions in physiology and pathology still under
active research.   Independently of those recent observations of
physiologists, which show the natural difference of proportion between the fibrin and serum of the blood in the two sexes, and under
different ages and temperaments, we know as matter of fact that
there are such morbid states, in which the proportion of water to
the solid animal contents of the blood is below the healthy standard.
Slight variations of this nature, as well as those of opposite kind, may
be presumed to be perpetually occurring ; delicate and beautiful
though the adjustments of function are, through which the balance
is maintained, and all inordinate deviations arrested in their progress.

But passing over lesser instances, the singular facts observed as
to the blood in the Asiatic cholera, show the extent to which such
change may take place under the influence of disease ; and give
wide scope to the existence of gradations between this and the state

of perfect health.* The importance of these changes of proportion, however produced, is best inferred from the experiments which prove how essential are the fibrin and colouring particles, not merely to the right constitution of the blood, but to all the phenomena of life; how many functions concur and are needful to their elaboration; and how speedily distress or death ensue in many cases, where they are exposed to the agency of foreign substances introduced into the circulation.

The question with which we have now concern is, how far the actual use of diluents may be capable of repairing such altered proportion of the serous part of the blood, whether the result of chronic causes, or of more acute malady? The tendency of modern inquiry regarding absorption has been to show that it takes place much more rapidly than was supposed; and through textures and by means which were once believed to have no concern in this function. The conception that the processes of absorption, as well as those of secretion, must be carried on through the open mouths of the vessels, and that communication of fluids can only take place by means of tubular structure, has given way to the distinct experimental proof of imbibition and exudation through the coats of vessels or other parts of animal texture. In the phenomena of endosmosis, more particularly, we find curious and satisfactory explanation of facts as to the transmission of substances by the animal fluids, which formerly perplexed all our views of the economy of structure and function.†

These points, however, are only important here as proofs of the facility and speed with which liquids taken into the stomach, especially when fasting, may be absorbed into the circulation. It still remains a question, how far the blood can appropriate to itself, in alteration of its quality, fluids thus received? There can be little doubt that it does so in those cases where the proportion of its watery parts is from any cause materially lessened.‡ Perhaps in

---

* Andral, in his " Anatomie Pathologique " (vol. i.), has given a summary of most of the facts in this interesting part of pathology; and Lecanu, in his " Etudes Chemiques sur le Sang," makes this specification more distinct by the results of very exact analysis. It is part of our knowledge likely to be extended hereafter.

† These discoveries of Parrot and Dutrochet, remarkable as the exposition of a new physical law, have great interest in their application to physiology, and show especially how much may be added to our knowledge of the vital functions by every such step in physical science. The views as to respiration, suggested by Dr. Stevens's valuable observation on the affinity of carbonic acid and oxygen, are another instance of similar kind, having various relations indeed to the former.

‡ The experiments of Orfila and other physiologists have shown the connexion between thirst and the proportion of water present in the blood, by the relief given to this sensation from the injection of different fluids into the veins. In that intense thirst passing into febrile state, which follows the long privation of liquids, and appears to be the most vehement of all appetites, there is every reason to suppose that these feelings are the result of changes in the blood itself; depending on the altered ratio of its fluid and solid parts, and affecting the vascular system to its most minute extremities.

all instances the tendency to absorption bears some ratio to the state of the blood in this respect; unless there be counteraction from causes of disease in active progress at the time. But it is equally probable, and for the same reasons, that little alteration is made in its state or proportions by any excess of liquid beyond this natural demand. The processes for separating water become more active in the same ratio as the increased imbibition; and even admitting, what is now rendered very doubtful, that the whole or greater part passes through the blood, there is every reason to believe that the extrication thence through different channels is so speedy as never to allow any material change in the proportion of its several parts. There is manifestly a constant and mutual relation between the blood and the kidneys, the organ most especially destined to this function of balance. Whether change of condition begin in the former or the latter, equally is it followed by reciprocal change in the other; tending always, it may be presumed, to adjust or restore those proportions in the blood which belong to the natural state.*

We cannot indeed prove, when there is habitual excess in the quantity of fluid taken, that there may be not some effect of this kind; producing thereby a sort of chronic disorder of the blood, and affecting more or less every part of the system. A difference existing by natural temperament may be induced by habit also, but probably to no greater extent, unless the change be aided by the operation of actual disease. And, in the latter case, the altered proportion probably depends rather on the insufficient power of supplying the fibrin and albuminous part of the blood, than on any change tending directly to increase the ratio of water contained in the circulation.

Applying these considerations to the medicinal use of diluents, it may be inferred that we have little justification for giving them, with direct intent to alter the qualities or proportions of the blood, independently of actual experience. Our knowledge on these points is still too limited to admit of any practice founded on theory alone. But on the other hand, we have reason from the same considerations to believe that liquids may freely and without fear be given, wherever there is demand for them from the sensations of the patient. There is, in truth, no motive or rule of treatment upon which better to depend than these natural feelings; and even when partially vitiated in their nature, we have the assurance that it is a case in which the system is well provided with means for remedying any excess. This conclusion, fairly attained, is one of great practical value.

Viewing the subject, indeed, in relation to actual disease, where the appetites are in part removed from the dominion of habit, there

---

* Many extraordinary cases are recorded of the enormous quantity of water habitually taken, and urine voided, even without actual disease. In most of these instances it is difficult to determine where the excess of action begins, or by what causes it is produced.

are few rules in practice which may be admitted with such slight limitation as the one just given. Even in diabetes, I have never found any continued good from opposing the inordinate thirst of the patient, nor aggravation of what are the essential symptoms of the disorder by assenting in full to this desire. The restraint as to liquids to satisfy the thirst in malignant cholera is still less justified by any reasonable principle or experience in practice. Without admitting, what some have affirmed, that cold water is an actual remedy here, we may at least presume that it is beneficial, if finding access to the circulation, in modifying that state of blood which is so characteristic of the disease. The eager demand for liquid is in some sort an evidence of this; nor is it disproved by the occasional rejection from the stomach of what is so taken. The thirst occurring as an ordinary symptom of all fever, is for the most part to be viewed as authority for its gratification. In the greater number of cases, more harm will arise from opposing it, than from any excess in the use of liquids to which it can lead.

The remaining point of view under which we have to consider simple diluents, as remedies, is in their effect upon various functions of secretion and excretion. This subject is closely connected with the preceding, inasmuch as the effects must take place chiefly, if not altogether, through the circulation; and some change be produced in the blood itself by every alteration occurring in these functions. The kidneys and the skin are the organs most concerned here, though it is probable that the lungs also have part in the effect, and that no secreting organ is wholly independent of it. Any large and rapid addition of water to the mass of blood brings into activity that part of the vascular system, whether glandular or otherwise, through which separation of the superfluous fluid may take place. The pressure of volume upon the extreme vessels, or upon the membranes through which exudation takes place, must have influence on the functions of these parts: and the same might be inferred, if we regard as vital phenomena exclusively, the actions by which superfluous fluid is thus separated from the system. Under either supposition the secreting vessels or exuding membranes certainly undergo alteration for a time; and this of nature to affect the qualities of the blood, by altering the amount or kind of matter which such secretions carry away. In the kidneys, for instance, the proportion of the lithates or other saline ingredients, removed through these organs, may be augmented by a large and rapid passage of water through them; and the functions of the skin, as an excreting organ, may equally be rendered more active by the same means. It is probably in this indirect way that diluents have greatest influence upon the blood; and here we find best explanation of their utility in certain cachectic cases, in which there is general disorder or deficiency of the secretions.

It seems certain further, in the medicinal use of diluents, that something is gained by mechanical effect on the secreting tissues. These may become in any part less permeable than in the healthy state ; a condition apparently capable of being removed by the more copious passage of fluid through them. The remark applies to many states of the skin, both in fevers and other disorders, where simple diluents, freely given, form the safest and most effectual sudorifics we can employ. And the same remark applies to various cutaneous disorders, where the use of this remedy, even in its simplest form of pure water, might be very beneficially extended, to the exclusion of many diaphoretics and alteratives of much more doubtful character and effect.

This is, according to my experience, a point singularly meriting attention in practice ; and the simplicity and safety of the trial warrant every recommendation of it. In exanthematous fevers, though the treatment by such means is more ambiguous, yet I believe that a freer employment of diluents might be beneficial than is commonly adopted ; certainly to the fullest extent in which they are called for by the feelings of the patient.

On the same principle, there is good reason for their use even in certain cases of dropsical effusion, where the object is to restore a due action to the kidneys. Popular feeling, and indeed medical opinion, inclines to the opposite treatment ; and with some reason, as respects the habit of drinking largely in such cases. But I have experience of the good often obtained by the sudden and copious use of diluents in recovering these organs from a dormant state ; an object which may most readily be effected after the bowels have been freely relieved. The latter fact is important in regard to the action of almost all diuretics. They have little effect as such, while there is need of alvine evacuation ; and in ascites and anasarcous swellings, particularly, it is commonly desirable to preface all other treatment in this way. The ignorance or neglect of these precautions in practice often produces a hurtful activity where nothing can be gained, and a delay no less injurious in the actual relief of disease.

As I have been treating of this remedy only in its simplest form, I do not advert to the use of the different mineral waters further than to state that they confirm these general views ; separating, as far as can be done, their effect as diluents from that of the ingredients they contain. The copious employment of some of them in continental practice gives room for observation, which is wanting under our more limited use. I have often seen five or six pints taken daily for some weeks together, a great part of it in the morning while fasting, with singular benefit in many cases to the general health, and most obviously to the state of the secretions. The functions of the kidneys and skin were maintained in great activity during the whole of this period ; but without assuming any disordered character, and passing readily again into their natural state when the cause of increased action was removed. These courses, however, were always conjoined with ample exercise and regular habits of life ; doubtless influencing much the action of the waters, and aiding their salutary effect. In cases where such aids are omitted, or only partially employed, a much smaller quantity generally disturbs the stomach, and the treatment altogether is of little avail for the amendment of health.

Without reference, however, to these extreme cases, it must be repeated, that the use of water, simply as a diluent, scarcely receives attention and discrimination enough in our English practice. This is a point wholly distinct from the question regarding the fit proportion of liquids as a part of diet. The process of digestion suffers more or less from any excess in quantity of these; and, though the natural appetite may be unduly controlled, yet some rule is often required, in dyspeptic cases especially, to obviate such excess, even where the simplest and most innocuous liquids alone are concerned. For in these cases a morbid craving for them is often created, partly by the vitiated sensations of the patient, partly from the actual state of the membrane lining the palate, œsophagus, and stomach, and from the disordered secretions and products of digestion acting on this surface.

It is obviously another question, how far and in what way diluents may be employed, expressly as such, for medical purposes? including under this question what relates to thirst as a symptom of disease, to the use of liquids in disordered states of the alimentary canal, and to their employment in cases of general cachexia and vitiated secretion. These are the points to which the preceding remarks apply; less, however, as furnishing explicit rules, than as suggesting the views upon which this part of treatment may best be founded, and rendered more generally useful.

CHAPTER XXII.

ON MORBID ACTIONS OF INTERMITTENT KIND.

HAS sufficient weight been assigned in our pathological reasonings to that principle, which associates together so many facts in the history of disease, viz., the tendency in various morbid actions to distinct intermission, of longer or shorter duration, and more or less perfect in kind? Few objects of inquiry are more interesting than this, either to the physician or the physiologist. The subjection of so many diseased actions to this common law establishes relations which could not have been learnt from other sources, and which have much value even in the details of practice. To the physiologist the facts are of great interest, as being effect and part of that more general principle in the animal economy by which various natural and healthy functions of the system are subject to like intermission.

This principle, though in some of its workings it must ever have been obvious to all who observed the phenomena of life, has in later times only been distinctly recognised as such. And to modern inquiry also we owe the remark, that this intermittent or periodical character belongs especially to the animal functions; and that those of organic life show it in a much more obscure and indeterminate form. The most dubious cases are those in which both functions seem concerned in supporting one action, as in the instance of respiration; but the general distinction may be admitted as well-marked and striking.*

This tendency to intermission in the animal functions may justly be termed a law; inasmuch as it is natural, general, and manifestly designed. All the phenomena of mind, and all those of body which have direct relation to mind, are more or less submitted to it. The alternation of sleep and waking,—a phenomenon in which so many separate functions have part—is the instance at once most familiar and remarkable. The organs of sense are all more or less connected with this one important condition of existence; while they have besides various shorter and more irregular intermissions, depending on changes in the action upon them from without, and the proportion of this action to the excitability they possess. A closer view may lead us to associate these also with the phenomena of sleep; admitting the view as to this function, that though for the most part simultaneously extending to many different organs and actions, these are not necessarily affected in the same degree, nor always at the same time. Thus considering it, one sense may be said to be partially asleep, when all the others, as well as the mental functions, are in state of perfect wakefulness. This general principle, stated at length in another chapter, is one which not only associates more distinctly all intermittent actions with the great common function of sleep, but is also important in illustrating many varieties of intermittent disorder, and indicating methods for their treatment.

It may be that, in the case of the senses, the principle of intermission exists even in those elementary actions through the nerves, upon which sensation as a function depends. We have no direct evidence here, and from the nature of the subject it would not be easy to obtain such. But there are some reasons for supposing alternate action and remission even in these subtle movements, which seem scarcely to be submitted to the laws of time and space; and it is possible that analogies drawn from other agents, now under active examination, may hereafter give more weight to the slight presumptions we possess.

* Bichat was one of the earliest to call attention to this principle under the name of the " Loi d'Intermittence," in its application to the function of muscular action, sleep, &c. (Anatomie Générale, tom. i.) It cannot be doubted, however, that he has limited the law too exclusively to the animal organs, as opposed to those of organic life; in conformity with his other views of the relation of these parts in the animal economy. And the same is the case with respect to the kindred law of habit, which he has been led, by attachment to this principle of distinction, to confine too especially to the parts of animal life.

The several actions and conditions of the voluntary organs furnish examples to the same effect as the senses; and interesting, more-over, from the other questions to which they lead us. Of these, one of the most remarkable is that which regards the nature of the exhaustion following muscular action; in what way, and in what proportion, the diminution of nervous power, and the diminished irritability of the muscular fibre, respectively contribute to this effect? Here, too, more distinctly than in the case of sensation, we have proof of different grades or periods of intermission; from those instantaneous changes of action and relaxation which we know to exist in certain actions of the muscular fibres, to various longer periods, determined by causes of which we have little cog-nisance, but which are doubtless connected with the two conditions just noted. It seems not impossible (and there are some phenomena of morbid action which best admit the solution) that both are con-cerned in producing these variations of interval. The irritability of the fibre may be exhausted, or the nervous power which acts upon it; and the concurrence or separation of these effects may alter variously the periods at which intermission takes place. The inquiries now suggested appertain to the general theory of muscular action; a subject on which so much research has been bestowed from the time of Haller downwards; yet scarcely perhaps with proportionate attention to that part of it in which the principle of intermission, and its many variations, are concerned.

Though all evidence is more obscure as to the involuntary muscles, yet can we not wholly omit here the question regarding the ryth-mical contractions and relaxations of the muscular substance of the heart, as well as of other organs of the same class. This has been explained in certain cases as depending on the stimulus given by the fluids or other matters they convey. But the hypothesis is doubtful; and in the case of the heart it is still uncertain, after all the experiments and reasoning directed to this point, how far, and in what way, its action depends for continuance and uniformity on nervous power supplied to it? from what particular part of the nervous system this power is derived? or how it is sustained for a certain time even when the heart is removed from the body?* The

* In regard to this important question, less attention has been given than they merit to those curious cases where great irregularity of the heart's action, con-tinued sometimes for a period of years, (and attributed, as I have more than once known, to assured disease of the organ,) has wholly or in great part disappeared, in sequel to a paralytic seizure. I have the notes of two cases now before me; in one of which, the patient, a gentleman who had suffered much during ten or twelve years from intermission and other disorder in the action of the heart, un-derwent an attack of hemiplegia three years ago; since which this irregularity has wholly ceased. The other instance is that of a patient, who during a period of fourteen years, possibly longer, had a pulse rarely below 120; the action of the heart so feeble as scarcely to be felt; cold extremities; and much tendency to œdema. Here a very slight paralytic attack altered the whole character of the heart's action, reducing it in frequency to seventy or eighty, with much more vigour or even irritability of pulse, and greater warmth and freedom of circulation throughout the body; but giving at the same time an acute sensi-

source of action and intermission in the muscular part of respiration is open to the same doubt ; augmented, indeed, by the mixed automatic and voluntary character which belongs to this function.

Passing over these and other questions, which have been so much discussed by physiologists, one general inference may be drawn, which it is difficult indeed to avoid ; viz., that nervous power, or the agency upon which sensation and voluntary action in their material part depend, has the element of quantity in it in the most express sense ;—that it is literally capable of being exhausted by action, and renewed by repose. The fact is familiar in common statement and application ; but not duly appreciated in all the deductions to which it leads. In every intermittent action more especially, whether of long or short interval, the notions of quantity, of expenditure, and reaccumulation, appear needfully to be involved ; and most distinctly where the intervals approach to uniformity in time. It is difficult, if in any sense possible, to conceive a principle of intermission which does not virtually include these conceptions; and all our views regarding the phenomena become more clear in proportion as we keep them before us. It is less indeed an hypothesis with which we are here engaged, than a necessary exposition of undeniable facts. And connecting with them the circumstance already noticed, of the variety of intervals of action even in the same function, as testified particularly in disease, we obtain a general view, widely applicable to pathology, and founded on a principle which extends to the whole economy of life.

This argument is more obvious, and apparently stronger, as applied to the voluntary-functions than to those of sensation, though complicated in the former case by the *vis insita* of the muscles themselves, already mentioned as modifying all these actions. Nor have we indeed any authority for referring the two functions to a single nervous agent. Conception fails us in seeking to assimilate effects so widely different in their nature. All we know is that they depend in each case on certain nervous structures (alike, as far as the most minute observation goes, for the sentient and motor nerves), the lesion of which impairs respectively all the functions to which they subserve.

Observation must further lead us to admit that the mind and body have some common relation to the principle just stated. Exhaustion of the one by over-action produces in most cases a like state of the other also. They are not simultaneously capable of strong and continuous efforts, such as imply at once intent thinking, acute attention to sensations, or powerful voluntary action ; but one set of functions must give way to enable the other to remain in full exercise. The mind cannot safely or successfully be exerted while

bility, not previously existing, to the least irregularity of the organ, which made the change a very equivocal benefit to the patient.

These cases have relation to the recognised effect of many cerebral disorders upon the heart, but they are more remarkable in the peculiarity of the circumstances, and in their rarer occurrence.

the body is under actual toil, or the fatigue consequent upon it; and for any great and continued effort of voluntary power it is needful that the intellect be in state of comparative rest.* Circumstances which force both into strong action at the same time do so at the expense of great exhaustion of the living power.

I allude to these topics, however, merely as they give basis to every view of intermittent actions of morbid kind. These admit of being classed in several different ways; but here, as in many other instances, no arrangement is so clear, or practically so useful, as one which connects the morbid actions with the natural and healthy functions of the same parts. The former grow gradually out of the latter; and though presenting in this morbid state many peculiar modifications, yet are there none which may not be referred, directly or indirectly, to some equivalent phenomenon of healthy action. For an outline, therefore, of the subject, the best division may be into intermittent disorders of sensation; those of voluntary organs; and those again of more mixed and indefinite kind:—each of these forming particular cases of disorder in the system, of which intermission is a marked and often a leading symptom; though the latter are so far distinct from the two preceding that it is. not easy to connect them by any common theory.

The phenomena of simple pain may be taken as an explicit instance under the first of these classes. Though often obscured, or rendered very unequal by the complexity of particular cases, yet the tendency to intermission, more or less distinct, will probably be found in all; and most obviously in those instances where the pain is acute, and limited chiefly to one nerve, as in the tic douloureux, toothache, and other neuralgic affections. Some varieties of headache also will occur as examples, in which the pain seems to occur by pulses or fits, with intervals between. Where, on the other hand, extensive and complicated parts give origin to pain, and different nerves convey the sensations thence derived, the proofs become less distinct, possibly because the intermissions are separate, and do not necessarily coincide in time with each other. This consideration, however, leads us into abstruse questions regarding the functions of the nerves of sense, and their relation to the sensorium, which do not strictly pertain to the subject.

It is easy for any one to make observations on the intermission of simple pain, with the precaution of allowing for this complexity of parts; and with care also to distinguish between intermission, as a condition of nervous action, and the rapid alternations of more or less pain, which depend on the pulses of an inflamed part, and cor-

* A remarkable instance of this, though it may escape attention as such, is the difficulty or impossibility of carrying on any earnest train of thought, when running quickly, or otherwise strongly exercising the body. We approach here again (as through so many different channels of inquiry) to that view which contemplates existence as a series of states inseparably blended in their sequence, but strictly speaking never in activity, or really present to the consciousness, at the same absolute moment of time.

respond in fact with the action of the heart.   These throbbings may generally by a little attention be distinguished from the former.

The degree of intensity of pain seems also to modify the tendency to intermission, and the rate of its occurrence.   This might perhaps be inferred, when admitting the notion of physical quantity into that agency, whatever it be, which ministers to sensation.   Pain is in fact among the causes which tend directly to exhaust nervous power; and, when violent, often very suddenly and remarkably.   The collapse which follows any acute bodily suffering, even though of short duration, is well known both to physicians and surgeons.   The instances are familiar of sleep ensuing instantly upon the remission of such suffering; as in sequel to a severe operation, or in the intervals between labour-pains, or on the remission of acute inflammation or spasms.

The principle thus illustrated by an action of one of the senses, derives similar illustration, and not less distinctly, from the functions of the others also.   However natural the mode of excitement of any one of these, yet if it be excessive in degree, or unduly protracted, it becomes a source of morbid action; creating intermissions of sensibility, more or less complete, and which vary in uniformity or duration according to the nature or intensity of the cause. The instances of this deficient or disordered action of the different senses, testified by intermission, are equally numerous and familiar, and especially as might be presumed, in those of sight and feeling; taking the latter term (however vague its general use) to express all sensations throughout the body, which are not included under the attributes of the other senses.*   The function of hearing affords many similar examples; as do more obscurely those of smell and taste.   All these cases may be said to graduate from the slightest . variations incidental to the healthy state, to others where for a time the sensibility is wholly destroyed,   Yet all depend, I would again remark, upon a common principle, which in its healthy action is natural or even neccessary to the animal frame.

Though the treatment of the disorders forming the subject of this chapter is not now in question, it is proper to advert to the many ways in which these considerations apply to practice; particularly in what relates to the prevention of injury or premature decay in the organs of sense.   A due regard to the principle of intermission, both in health and disease, will furnish many general rules as well as particular admonitions, in aid of this important object; and more likely to be stable from having their foundation in a natural law.

* Physiology, and pathology no less, may be said to labour in every part under the difficulties of language as applied to the subject of internal sensations, derived from the different organs and actions of the body itself.   The inquiry speedily merges in metaphysics, and is ever tending to be lost there.   One portion of it, however, has been rescued from this obscurity, owing principally to the acuteness of Dr. Thomas Brown and of Magendie;—that, namely, which indicates the relation between the simple sense of touch, and the muscular sensations invariably connected with this function.

The difficult questions to which I have already alluded, again occur here, respecting the nature and source of the changes which constitute these intermittent actions. That they are material, and affecting the material instruments of sensation, cannot be doubted. That one modification of the agency, which circulates through the nervous system, and ministers power and action to all parts of the frame, is principally concerned in them, may with reason be presumed. It is probable, however, that some condition of structure in the organs themselves has part in the effect, in the same manner in which the proper contractility of the muscular fibre modifies the action of the nervous power upon it. Beyond this general view we are not called upon to proceed at present; the question before us regarding only the morbid changes to which the principle of inter·mission is subject.

Morbid intermittent actions of spasmodic kind, in which the voluntary muscles are concerned, are more distinct and remarkable than those of sensation, and form a larger page in the history of disease. They possess great interest, moreover, from their peculiar and compound relation to the functions of mind and of organic life; the voluntary muscles being those especially subject to this morbid condition; but subject to it independently of volition; and in many cases from causes of excitement with which the sensorium is in no way directly concerned. Epilepsy, catalepsy, chorea, hysteria, hooping-cough, and hydrophobia, furnish the most curious and characteristic instances of this class of morbid intermittent actions; very irregular in kind and interval, and depending on a great diversity of indirect causes; but all having it in common that the voluntary muscles are affected by other agency than that of the will; and for the most part with clonic spasms, or those of alternate contraction and relaxation.

The common hiccup, familiar though the instance is, becomes for this reason one of the best illustrations of the simple intermittent spasm; occurring with regular intermission from causes and nervous actions independent of the will, but capable to a certain extent of being controlled by voluntary effort. Another example may be given in the *tremor tendinum*, or shaking palsy, where the separate spasms are slighter, and the intervals less distinct; but where the morbid actions sometimes continues more or less constantly present through a series of years. And we have another remarkable instance in that quivering of the substance of muscles which is seen under certain circumstances of injury or disease, and may be occasionally noticed in the muscles of a palsied limb;—a phenomenon the more interesting, as it seems in some degree to interpret the natural action of the muscles under the will, which we have reason to believe performed by an infinitely rapid series of movements in their minute fibres.

This double capacity of the voluntary muscles, of being excited respectively by the will and by the actions of organic life, is one of those remarkable facts, or rather laws, in physiology, which link

together functions seemingly the most remote; and a full understanding of which would solve some of the greatest difficulties in
this branch of knowledge.   While thus strikingly exemplified in the
effects of certain diseases, it must be regarded in itself as strictly
a natural part of the economy of life ;—the subjection of the same
muscular structure to two different kinds of nervous agency, to
voluntary and involuntary excitement, being manifestly an important condition of health, though becoming in its excess or irregularity a symptom of disease.*

Many singular anomalies indeed of the latter state are solved, by
looking to the concurrence or opposition of these two agencies directed to the same point.   The more definite character of voluntary
movements, and the consciousness of the will creating them, may
give the belief that these are the most natural and first in order.
But the fact is certainly otherwise.   We may even venture to
affirm, that while organic or involuntary muscular actions occur at
the earliest period, of the same kind and perhaps of greater relative
intensity than in adult life, voluntary power is a function of slow
growth,—a nullity in infancy,—unequal in its progress as applied to
different muscular parts,—capable of cultivation,—governed by
habit, sometimes almost to the suppression of the will,—lessened or
lost by disease.   This manner of viewing it is most accordant with
known facts, and will best obviate the many difficulties of the subject ;—as, for example, the complex actions of respiration; the
double relation of which to the will and involuntary power has furnished material for so much controversy to physiologists.

The spasmodic diseases already mentioned, not only exemplify
these singular relations, but furnish instances of another fact, very
important ·in general pathology, viz., the great length which the ·
periods of intermission occasionally reach, while the series and

---

.* Modern research has done much for the illustration of this interesting subject.
It is now more distinctly recognised that the cerebral nerves, and those belonging appropriately to the spinal system, are separately and respectively instruments
in the effects by which volition and other states of mind are related to the involuntary actions of the body.   The researches of Dr. Marshall Hall, and other
physiologists, into the reflex actions of the spinal marrow, by attaching to definite
portions of this nervous structure the relations of excitement and reflected motion
which pervade every part of the system, have given much clearer insight into
these singular connexions of function : and it must be allowed that no other view
explains with such precision and consistency the symptoms of the remarkable
class of spasmodic diseases alluded to above.   I might cite from my own recollections in practice many curious examples illustrating these topics.   At this
time I am attending a patient who is scarcely able to raise his right arm to his chin,
in effect of an hemiplegic attack three years ago ; but in whom the dressing of a
seton, near the lumbar vertebræ on the same side, often twitches the arm forcibly
to a much higher level.   In the same patient, when yawning, the fingers of the
right hand become suddenly extended ; though at other times bent closely and
tightly inwards, without any power of opening them by voluntary effort.
The valuable Memoir of Stromeyer (*Gottingsche gelehrte Anzeigen*, 1836), on
the production of sensations by certain motions and contractions operating through
the intermedium of the brain or spinal marrow, furnishes, if the principle should
be established, a remarkable appendix and proof to this doctrine of reflex actions.

character of morbid actions at each occurrence remain the same. Epilepsy may be taken as a remarkable example to this effect; in which disorder the principle of intermission and repetition is often distinctly maintained, with intervals exceedingly protracted between,—tending sometimes to a regular period; though more frequently irregular, and liable to variation from causes of temporary excitement. Here, though in a new form, we must again recur to the element of quantity, to aid our conception of nervous power thus brought into action. In some forms of epilepsy particularly, it seems essential to any just theory of the symptoms to suppose accumulation, or irregular supply, of this or other agent; with the further presumption that, if it be the nervous power, it is for a longer or shorter time taken out of the dominion of the will, and expended in producing spasmodic muscular movements.

Expenditure is here the fit expression, because in no other way can we adequately explain the progressive increase of irritability up to the moment of a fit, which so often occurs in the epileptic patient; and the almost entire absence of this which afterwards ensues. Such effect is more especially observed where the intervals are long, and the fits succeeding to them repeated and violent; the irritation subsiding more completely, as it would seem, in proportion to their severity. There is clearly, in these cases of lengthened periodicity, some direct relation between the time of exemption and the violence of the succeeding attacks, equally in conformity with the same general view of the cause.

I have recently seen a case of epileptic seizures, supervening upon apoplexy, in which there was singular proof of the accumulation of the cause of spasm at regular intervals of time. Six attacks occurred, with intervals of sixteen or eighteen minutes between; so exactly recurring, as noted by the watch, that it was impossible to suppose it a mere casualty. The convulsions appear afterwards to have been less frequent, and in a few hours they ceased altogether. I have notes of another case, where a spasmodic seizure, more of tetanic than epileptic character, occurred twice a day for many weeks successively, and almost exactly at the same hours each day. In another instance, which happened to me lately, where the remarkable symptom at the time was that singular shock or jar which patients themselves often compare to an electric shock, and which in this case occurred with frequency and violence in the lower limbs, the attacks, when most severe in degree, came on almost exactly at equal intervals of somewhat more than two minutes; the muscles of the legs, during the intermission, being in a state of constant tremor, felt by the patient and visible to those around.*

* The patient in this case described the sensation as "a sudden shot into the limbs, seeming as suddenly to disperse itself into innumerable sparks, which penetrated into every corner of them." Most persons will probably recognise in this description a frequent occurrence of ordinary health, where a sudden shock or jar is felt to spread in an instant through the whole body; happening generally without obvious cause, yet most frequently during the approaches of sleep.

The hooping-cough, however different in its nature and causes from epilepsy, furnishes also a curious example of intermittent spasmodic actions, tending to like intervals, and these often of considerable length. When no casual irritation is present to provoke the fit, and more especially perhaps when the disorder is declining, it is remarkable how regular the times of seizure occasionally become, retaining the periodical character even to the last.

It must still be admitted, that there are many difficulties in the theory of these spasmodic disorders; depending in great part, as is probable, on their mixed relation to the animal and organic functions. Two distinct causes seem to be concerned, operating through different channels, upon the same organs; separately sometimes, sometimes concurrently; and with every possible variety of combination in different cases. In these numerous conditions, we have large scope for explaining the actual diversities which occur to our notice, both in health and disease. In some convulsive disorders for instance, as hydrophobia and hooping-cough, it would seem that any direct influence of the sensorium is almost, if not altogether, absent. In chorea more of this influence is perceived, modifying in various ways the aspect of symptoms, which yet belong chiefly to the class of automatic actions. In hysteria, the interference is still more marked, and the circumstances become complex in proportion. Epilepsy presents altogether great difficulties, from its complication with apoplexy, paralysis, and other states of cerebral disease; and from its relation at the same time to so many other organs and functions of the body as exciting causes of its attacks. I can find no better general expression for the facts regarding this disease than that already given, viz., some anormal distribution and action of nervous power, in which the brain and its nerves are chiefly concerned, and of which the accumulation and expenditure of this power seem to be a frequent or principal part. The effects on the circulation and respiration, as well as the convulsive motions, may all be received as subordinate effects. And even the singular phenomenon of the *aura epileptica*, in which the action seemingly begins from the extremities of nerves, is not more difficult of explanation under this view than by any other theory.*

In these considerations on spasmodic diseases, I have not thought it necessary to dwell on the distinction usually made between the two kinds of spasm, seeing that in fact they graduate into each

* In that common but curious state, called *fidgets*, we find certain analogous circumstances, though of minor importance. Here there appears to be (whether depending on a state of the circulation, or more directly of the nerves themselves) an accumulation of some cause of irritation which requires muscular action for its relief. The effect so produced is, however, taken partially out of the power of the will; and testified by sudden, uncertain, or almost spasmodic movements, preceded by a sort of uneasy thrill through the limbs, which this action seems to remove for a time; but which returns with a regularity of interval often very distinctly marked. Illustration from these familiar sources is frequently of more value than that furnished by rare and anomalous cases.

other. The clonic spasms best illustrate the principle of intermission; but it is frequently well marked in those of tonic kind also.

It is an important question regarding these intermittent spasmodic actions, whether there is not in certain cases mischief, or even danger, in forcibly arresting them? It would seem, as I have before mentioned, that there are some conditions of body (or we may more explicitly say of the nervous system) where the amount of the exciting cause present at the time renders this expenditure in the form of convulsive action necessary for relief. The involuntary movements are a sort of outlet or discharge for that agent which, either by excess in quantity or intensity, or by other manner of change inaccessible to research, has become a cause of undue excitement to the system, and requires to be removed from it.

These phrases may seem too mechanical, but illustrations of the reality of the fact will be found in many cases; particularly in the instance of the *vis epileptica*, already mentioned. I have never seen, but have heard on good authority, of the serious mischief produced from suddenly arresting by mechanical force the convulsive motions of chorea. One instance has been related to me of fatal event, apparently from this cause, in a young child strongly affected with the disorder. In a singular case, which I have lately seen, of spasmodic twitching of the muscles on one side the neck, (very incessant, and of such violence that the head was forcibly drawn backwards and downwards, so as to touch the point of the left shoulder,) the patient had apprehension from his feelings of any strong restraint put upon these motions, and considerable distress when it was attempted.*

This fact, if sufficiently attested, is a curious one in the animal economy; and well deserving inquiry in relation to the healthy as well as morbid actions of the nervous system. In connexion with the law of intermission in these actions, it involves the notion of quantity more explicitly and irresistibly than any other, concurring therein with all the conditions before stated as belonging to them.

* In this case, which I attended with Sir B. Brodie, the patient was about fifty-two years of age, and had been subject for some years to irregular action of the heart, partially relieved by a first fit of gout, but more completely when this spasmodic disorder came on. There was nothing to explain its original occurrence, and no other affection of the head or spine, except an occasional headache on the left side. The convulsive twitching continued for nearly a year with much severity; so great in degree for some time as to make it impossible even to read from the incessant motion of the head. At the expiration of about twelve months from the greatest severity of the complaint, its symptoms had almost wholly disappeared; the treatment pursued being that of periodical small cuppings on the nape of the neck, bichloride of mercury and morphia; and, at a later time, the sulphate of copper, persisted in for a long period. The same affection recurred, however, about six months after; equally without obvious cause as at first, and scarcely less severe in its degree. In this instance it was seemingly mitigated by cupping, calomel, and a perseverance for some time in the use of colchicum, though never wholly removed. I do not dwell, however, on the effect of the remedies in this case, believing these. with the exception of the cupping and the calomel, to have been very ambiguous in result; and at all events subordinate to other causes of change in the body.

It is somewhat difficult to class the several forms of intermittent headache with other affections of this kind; but those having lengthened periods of intermission may best perhaps be noted here. The equality of time often observed, even where the intervals extend to two or three weeks, or yet longer, is a very remarkable feature in these cases; and denotes a cause specific in its nature and uniform in its operation. I know instances where such intermittent headaches have occurred during the greater part of a protracted life. More frequently, however, it happens that they affect especially certain periods of life;—in this, as in many other circumstances, showing singular relation to various disordered actions of the gouty constitution. In conformity with the same relation, there is reason to believe that the kidneys are the excretory organ most concerned in giving relief in these cases, and principally by an increased separation of the lithic acid or its salts. Such action may readily escape notice, where the attention is directed by the presence of pain to another part; but I infer it from close observation of many intermittent headaches, and think the remark likely to be confirmed by others.

I have thus far spoken of morbid intermittent actions, chiefly as they occur in the functions of sensation and muscular motion. There exist besides some remarkable forms of intermittent disorder, which I have noticed as a third class; having no direct or certain connexion with either of the others; though not impossibly related by some common principle of morbid action to the headaches just described. The best type of these diseases, which chiefly belong to the order of fevers, is the regular intermittent fever; whether quotidian, tertian, quartan, or other variety. The cause of periodicity here has hitherto baffled all inquiry. We have no longer before us the fact of distinct intermission of nervous action; which, under the notion of exhaustion and reparation of a definite power, seems at least to afford some explanation of the cases before cited. If admitting anything like the principle of nervous intermission in fevers, or the reaccumulation of a power capable of exciting anew certain trains of action after stated intervals of time, it must, to meet the phenomena in question, be under different and much more obscure conditions than those hitherto known to us. Still, on whatsoever side we approach the subject, we can scarcely avoid the admission of some morbid matter, generated in equal or definite periods of time within the system; the phenomena of the paroxysm, as in exanthematous fevers, not coming on till the accumulation or maturation has reached a certain point; carrying away in their progress this active cause of disorder, whatever it be; and thereby producing the interval which ensues. The present state of our knowledge does not entitle us to go beyond these vague expressions of probability.

Though referring here to intermittent fevers, expressly so termed, yet must any general views on this subject include those also of remittent kind. The principle of remission is analogous, if not actually identical, with that of intermission; the regularity of period is often as well marked; and the two conditions not unfrequently pass into each other without obvious change of other kind between.

This is not the place for entering upon the theory of fever, even had I any new views to offer on this difficult topic, our imperfect knowledge of which carries difficulty and incertitude into every part of the history of disease. But, in connexion with the subject of intermittent actions, I must refer to one of the most remarkable facts in pathology; viz., the great variety of forms which simple intermittent fever assumes; not merely by changes of type, as they are termed, but still more singularly by affecting particular and limited parts of the body, with equal regularity of interval. A few of these neuralgic affections, from their greater frequency and distinctness, have been recognised by name; of which the *brow-ague* is a familiar instance. But I believe the cases to be much more numerous than is generally supposed, in which a determinate connexion exists with this common principle of morbid action in the system. The fact is capable of being proved in several ways;—first, by the regularity of the intermissions in these local affections, and by their following the various types of common ague;—again, by their succession to, or alternation with, intermittent fever in its ordinary form;—and further, by the influence of the same specific remedy in removing or relieving all such varieties of disorder. The application of these proofs to particular cases might be largely made, but it is enough to mention a few in illustration of the fact.*

Of the unequivocal transition from regular forms of ague to these local neuralgic affections with like periods of intermissions, I have seen a singular instance in a gentleman, who, within the space of a few months, underwent tertian fever of the ordinary kind, brow-ague, and a similar affection of intermittent pain in one knee; each state manifestly suspending the other, and all relieved eventually by the free use of bark.

Among the more recent cases in my note-book, I find several to this effect, connected with the constitution left behind by the influenzas, so frequent of late years. In one family, a brother and sister, who had both undergone scarlatina and influenza in the early part of 1837, were severally affected in the course of the autumn with a severe pain in the upper jaw on one side, coming on every day precisely at the same hour, with complete intermissions, and continuing in this regular course, until removed by the sulphate of quina.† In another case lately, I have observed a large and painful

---

* This long duration of the tendency to recurrence of intermittent fevers is a fact so familiar, as almost to conceal the singular conclusions it involves. I have seen numerous and remarkable examples of it in the Peninsula, in soldiers who joined the army there, after having been previously in the hospital at Walcheren. At this time I have two patients, residing in London, in whom variations of weather often reproduce distinct ague of quotidian or tertian type, the result of original seizures of this disorder when travelling in the south of Europe three years ago.

† In one of these cases the attack, precisely similar both as to seat and regula

swelling of the tonsils to appear at a stated hour every day; and so continuing until relieved by bark. Several instances occurred to me at the same time of inflammation of the tunica conjunctiva and eyelids, coming on at a given hour each afternoon for nearly a fortnight together; similarly relieved, but showing distinct tendency to return for many weeks afterwards. The recurrence of fits of coughing at one or more stated times every day was a very frequent symptom succeeding to these singular epidemics.

Another instance is known to me, on good authority, in which the patient was affected by urgent thirst at a regular hour on alternate days, without other obvious symptom of disorder. Here also the character of the case was attested, not only by the periods of intermission, but by speedy cure under the use of the quina, when other means had failed. It is known that epistaxis sometimes occurs with the same regularity of interval, and is obviated chiefly by the employment of the same means.*

Examples of this kind, not always noted in their right connexion, though familiar to the observant practitioner, make it certain that there is a common principle pervading these intermittent disorders of regular type; the development of which forms an important object of future research. The translation of one form and seat of malady into another, and the subjection of all to well defined laws of time and order of occurrence (admitting, however, of certain familiar exceptions and anomalies) render this question one of the most interesting in pathology. Whether we may ever surmount the difficulties encumbering it is yet uncertain; though the prospect is better perhaps now than at any former period in medical history.†

intermission, occurred in the following autumn, and a third time late in the autumn of the succeeding year; in each instance again removed by the same means.

* Dr. Leonhard, of Muhlheim, relates a singular case of a woman in whom an attack of influenza (the severe epidemic of February and March, 1837) passed into a local quotidian intermittent, affecting first the left, afterwards the right arm, with every successive symptom of regular ague; the rigour, heat, and stage of perspiration all distinctly marked in each fit;—other parts of the body wholly unaffected;—the disorder cured by quinine. The most remarkable statement connected with the case is, that the pulse in the affected arm gave 90 beats, that of the other arm only 80, at the same moment of time.

We still indeed only partially recognise the many varieties which occur in intermittent fevers. Mr. Oldfield, who went up the Quorra in a steam-vessel with Lander, describes with much exactness a quotidian which affected him in this river voyage; the paroxysm coming on at first about noon; then half an hour later every day, till it reached six o'clock; at this time an entire intermission of two or three days, recommencing afterwards at noon. This order was so often repeated that he could anticipate the daily time within a minute or two.

† The late Dr. Maculloch, in his work on remittent and intermittent diseases, has dealt with this subject more explicitly than any other writer; and in assuming a single generic disease, the product of malaria as a specific virus, has associated with it many neuralgic and other affections, sciatica, headache, tic douloureux, toothache, ophthalmia, palsy, &c. Though the generalization is obviously far too extensive, yet it marks throughout the acuteness of this author; and in connecting neuralgia generically with intermittent fever, offers something of more plausible arrangement for the curious facts noted above.

One path of inquiry is that which directs towards the diurnal changes in the bodily functions, as well in the healthy state as under disease. The tendency in various disorders to exacerbation or remission at stated hours comes in evidence of such natural changes within the daily period, distinct from the more obvious changes produced by sleep. It is not easy to obtain unequivocal evidence on this subject, from the disturbing influence of digestion in its several stages, and from other contingent habits of life equally affecting these phenomena. Nevertheless averages have been obtained, sufficiently free from error, to show that the functions of respiration and circulation do undergo certain determinate changes within the day; such as can scarcely exist without influencing the period and source of morbid actions, when these are in existence in the system.* Such natural diurnal changes, inexplicable on any known principle, may depend on periodical alterations in the nervous power, of which sleep is the chief index and example. But whether so or not, the main question is, if they are sufficient to explain the tendency in certain diseases to definite periods of one or more days, and the fluctuations from one type and time to another ? It must be admitted in the present state of our knowledge that they are not so. No adequate explanation has yet been drawn from this source; and the suggestion is merely one which seemingly leads us further than any other in an inquiry where hitherto so little has been attained.†

* Dr. Prout has found that more carbonic acid is formed in respiration from daybreak to noon, less during the remainder of the twenty-four hours. Something of periodical change in other functions must needfully be produced by this difference, on whatsoever cause it depend.

Observations on the pulse seem to show that there is an average acceleration of the motions of the heart in the morning, and retardation in the evening, independently of all causes of external influence; and greater excitability of the heart by stimulus, whether of exercise or food, at the former period than the latter. The recent researches of Dr. Knox upon this subject (*Edinburgh Med. Journal, April,* 1837) are very valuable. These changes in the action of the heart, depending, it may be, on prior changes in the nervous system from sleep or other cause, have probably some effect on all functions of the body; but whether they are adequate to explain any periods of morbid action is very doubtful.

The electricity of the atmosphere appears to undergo diurnal changes; the positive electricity being stronger during the day than in the night, with subordinate increments and decrements also during the day. The influence of these may not be great, but some effect they must have, and we have no means to appreciate its amount.

† If venturing to name any particular periods in the twenty-four hours at which changes most obviously take place, both in health and disease, I should be led, on experience, to refer to the hours of two or three in the afternoon, and the corresponding time in the night. Such statement, however, has little value, seeing its vagueness, and the numerous exceptions to it which arise on every side. The individualities of each disease produce perplexity here; and, equally so, all peculiarities of temperament and habit of life. Every variation of diet, and each particular stage of digestion, have their appropriate effect on the other functions, even on those apparently the most remote.

In adverting to the causes, whatever they be, which give an aspect of daily periodicity to some of the bodily functions, the proofs may be admitted that they

The influence of certain medicines, and particularly of bark, in curing even the most anomalous varieties of these intermittent disorders, is a fact of great interest. Like the use of mercury in obscure syphilitic affections, or of colchicum in the most irregular forms of gout, it enables us to denote and class together symptoms apparently the most remote in kind; but which presumably could not be thus relieved unless depending on some common morbid cause. We have therefore, in the specific nature of the remedy, a sort of practical test of the character of the disease; often of great importance to the consistency and success of our treatment; and related, through the principle of inquiry, to some of the most interesting questions in all pathology. This it is, as was noticed when speaking of colchicum, which gives peculiar value to all that illustrates the action of these remedies. They are the interpreters of facts far beyond their momentary effect; and of connexions between morbid states which are in no other way so definitely made known to us.

In closing these remarks on morbid intermittent actions, I may observe, that they form a bare outline of a wide subject of inquiry, which well merits a much more complete investigation of all its parts.* The principle of intermission is one so marked and characteristic of some of the most important functions of life, and affords such curious results in the variations of interval even in the same function, that we may well rank it among other bases of classification for disease. And though some of the morbid actions, thus designated, are seemingly remote from others, as respects both periods and causes of intermission, it is probable that the tendency of further inquiry will be to give them closer association, by the discovery whence these modifications arise. Every relation to general principles is of so much practical as well as theoretical value in medicine, that there is often advantage in viewing diseases under new connexions, even though less intimate than those previously adopted into use.

have influence on the mind also; chiefly as respects the aptitude for exertion of its intellectual faculties, but partly even in relation to the character and intensity of the feelings. The physician, as well as common observer, have frequent opportunities of noticing this. The best evidence, however, is that which the cautious and candid observation of each person may furnish to himself.

* If the subject of intermittent disorders were pursued in the more extended manner I have ventured to suggest above, numerous illustrations, to which I have scarcely alluded, would occur from every part of the healthy economy of life. Menstruation is, doubtless, the most remarkable example in point, but many others might readily be cited.

CHAPTER XXIII.

ON DIET, AND DISORDERS OF DIGESTION.

Looking over the notes I have made on this subject in the course of practice, I find them almost wholly superseded by the many and valuable treatises which have been published of late years. These works, founded upon an improved physiology of the organs of digestion, have done much to give dietetics the character of a branch of science, which it certainly in nowise possessed before.* Even now it may be doubted whether our materials are ample or exact enough for methodical arrangement; and whether many of the rules founded on them are not calculated to foster, rather than repress, the vague and changeful fancies which prevail on this subject. It is certain on experience that no proportionate benefit has yet been obtained from all hitherto written upon it. For this there may be many causes. One doubtless is, the difficulty of establishing or applying positive rules for conditions so infinitely varied, that the evasion of these rules becomes easy, or is even apparently sanctioned, by the peculiarities of each case. Nor can it be affirmed that the precepts of medical authors themselves are concurrent on the principles of diet, and the management of dyspeptic disorders. Many points are still disputed; and on few perhaps are the criteria of truth so complete as to possess the influence that is required for their successful application to practice.

These circumstances, and still more the habits of society among the higher classes, and the influence of dyspeptic complaints on the minds of those affected, render the treatment of such disorders a matter of great interest, even in a moral point of view. They unhappily furnish an arena on which all the worst parts of medical practice find their readiest display. Fraud, intrepid in its ignorance, here wins an easy triumph. Seconded on every side by prejudices, fashions, and foibles, and taking advantage of the mind and body in their weakest mood, it deals out precepts and drugs with a pernicious facility;—sometimes altogether at random;—sometimes, and even more injuriously, with one common scheme of treatment applied to the most variable and incongruous symptoms.

These abuses indeed, in their worst form, exist only on the

---

* I may mention particularly the works of Dr. Combe, Dr. J. Johnson, Dr. Southward Smith, Dr. Paris, Dr. Wilson Philip, and the article on Indigestion, by Dr. Todd, in the Cyclopædia of Practical Medicine. The physicians of the United States, who now contribute so eminently to medical science in all its branches, have added to our knowledge on this subject. And their writings have the greater interest, as stating the result of manners of life differing in several respects from the ordinary habits of our own country, and of other parts of Europe.

outskirts of the profession. But it will be admitted by all who have candour and experience, that there is no part of medical practice where knowledge and good faith are put to equal trial as in the management of dyspeptic complaints. Even the effect of the disorder in obscuring the judgment, and rendering impotent the will of the patient, becomes an embarrassment to the physician. If his own judgment be slow and wavering, he is deprived of aid;—if hasty and rash, of that control from the opinion of his patient which is frequently needful. The mind of the dyspeptic is uncertain and fickle. He interprets falsely his own sensations, and the effects of the treatment employed;—is unduly confident at one moment and under a new remedy;—at another time as irrationally desponding;—prone, moreover, to change his medical adviser, and to resort to any person or remedy where there is largest profession of relief.

All these things, familiar in practice in this country, make the situation and conduct of the physician in cases of dyspepsia hardly less difficult than in acute and dangerous diseases. Though the symptoms before him are not so critical in kind, they need sound moral management as well as discreet methods of medical treatment.* Forbearance and firmness are both required; and, together with these, integrity and good faith. The admirable precepts as to uprightness in practice, which came down to us under the great name of Hippocrates, obtain here their closest application; and may well be impressed upon all who are entering on a medical life. The mind must be fashioned early and strongly in these professional principles; as they are rarely attained afterwards, and even with difficulty preserved, amidst the many difficulties which beset the conduct of the physician.

For the reasons already named, I shall not seek to give any method to the few remarks which follow respecting diet and dyspeptic disorders. They are drawn from my experience, on no other principle of selection than that of appearing to be least regarded in proportion to their practical importance. If desultory, it may be truly affirmed that the subject to which they relate is so likewise.

It is needful to say in the outset, that rules of diet may be pressed too closely, as well as too vaguely, in the treatment of dyspeptic cases. They may come to exercise a morbid influence over the mind of the patient, countervailing all the good obtained. Attention to his sensations is already too much awakened in the habitual dyspeptic; and often the greatest benefit which can be conferred is that of weaning it away from them. In another chapter I have alluded to the singular influence of the mind, simply directed to the digestive organs, in altering or disordering their natural functions; and this even where no solicitude exists on the subject.† Every

---

* What Aretæus says regarding the treatment of chronic diseases in general, applies singularly to dyspepsia, as one of the most frequent of them. Ενθα δη αρετη διαιδεται ανδρος ιητρου, και μακροθυμινς, και ποικιλινς, και χαριτος αβλαβους των ηδεων, και παραφασιος.

† Chapter V. (On the Effects of the Attention of Mind on the bodily Organs.)

such effect is greatly aggravated in the case of the dyspeptic. His minute and anxious watch over his sensations generates the very evils which it is the object to remove. A system of rules for diet and other management of the digestive organs may be necessary in such cases; but their effect on the mind must be observed, to see that they do not usurp too much upon it, and sanction injuriously those morbid habits which, arising out of the malady, augment the symptoms and retard their cure. A strict rule, good in itself, may often expediently be relaxed or dispensed with, if found thus to influence the temper of the patient. Austerity must bend before the variable conditions with which we have to deal in the treatment of disease.

Many points of practice connect themselves with this state of mind in dyspeptic disorders. It may be well, for instance, (though the rule is by no means an invariable one,) that the bowels should act each day in such cases. But if the patient becomes morbidly intent on this object, as often happens, all value of the habit is lost in the anxiety it creates, and mischief is generally incurred in the means employed to promote it. Here every effort must be made to disengage his mind from the presumed need. It is often even expedient for this purpose to advise expressly that there should be action only on alternate days; gaining thereby the chance of some interruption to these habits of morbid feeling. The disorder they produce in the various parts and stages of digestion does generally, itself, indeed, prevent that regularity which is sought for.

So also it may be very desirable that the dyspeptic should dine at regular and reasonable hours, and from a simple and discreet table; but if this rule brings him to a solitary meal, set apart for his express condition, more of ill than of good is the result. It is rarely expedient that he should feed alone. His mind needs to be solicited away fom attention to the functions and feelings of he stomach; and this can only effectively be done by society at the time of eating. The apprehension of indigestion creates it;—sometimes almost as an instant effect. When the stomach is full, the less the mind has to do with it the better. We are often then obliged to strike a balance between these evils, and to sacrifice something of principle for a practical expediency of greater importance.

Upon the same principle it is obvious that rules of diet lose much of their value in practice, if too various and minute. This applies alike to the treatment of actual dyspepsia, and to general methods for preserving a healthy digestion. Multiplicity of rules may become as ineffectual as no rules at all. We are bound to take human nature and society as we find them; amending where we can, but not by aiming at too much, forfeiting that which may be gained by simple and more compendious means. The dyspeptic patient feeds his disordered fancy on minute maxims, adopting and dismissing them with equal facility and forgetfulness. The patient who seeks only a rule by which to preserve health, disregards a series of small observances, which he feels as burdensome; and which in reality, if strictly observed, often become an unwholesome restraint.

It may be difficult indeed to say how far rules should go, to attain the greatest amount of practical good. The physician must be furnished with full knowledge of all that are sanctioned by reason or experience, in order to give them direction to particular cases. For the guidance of patients themselves, those of course are best which are most promptly and safely applied; neither harassing the mind by anxieties of choice, nor the body by encouraging wayward fancies as to methods of prevention or cure. If, for example, I were to specify any general maxims as to food, preferable to others from distinctness and easy application, and serving as a foundation for lesser injunctions, they would be the following :—

First, that the stomach should never be filled to a sense of uneasy repletion. Secondly, that the rate of eating should always be slow enough to allow thorough mastication, and to obviate that uneasiness which follows food hastily swallowed. Thirdly, that there should be no urgent exercise, either of body or mind, immediately after a full meal.

The simplicity and familiarity of these rules may lessen their seeming value; but in practice they will be found to include, directly or indirectly, a great proportion of the cases and questions which come before us. And many such questions, as for example those which relate to different qualities of food, would lose great part of their difficulty, were these maxims successfully enforced. When the quantity taken does not exceed the just limit; where it comes to the stomach rightly prepared by mastication, and by admixture with the secretions of the glands which aid the first stage of digestion; and when no extraneous interruption exists to the proper functions of the stomach in this stage; the capacity of digestion is really extended as respects varieties of food, and tables of relative digestibility lose much of their value.

It is certain that different temperaments require, whatever be the causes of this diversity, different proportions of aliment; and the same constitution alters its demand at different times both in health and sickness. No rules of diet, therefore, can be made positive as to quantity; and the attempt at such is now generally abandoned. The criteria to be taken for particular cases are those furnished by the state of the several organs concerned in digestion, both immediately, and at various intervals after food ; and also by the effect of digestion, while in progress, upon other functions of the body. This is for the most part too intricate an observation for the patient himself. It is enough for him (and much indeed of positive good), if his adherence on conviction can be obtained to the simple rule stated above; viz., habitually to stop eating at a point short of uneasy repletion. In effect, this maxim is nearly identical with the more familiar one of not eating beyond the appetite. But it is to be preferred for practical purposes, as being less liable to ambiguity and self-deception. Though with apparent relation only to the first stage of 'digestion, it is in truth more or less a provision for every succeeding part of the process, and for the well-being of all the organs concerned in it. A meal, which sits lightly on the stomach in the outset, giving during the first hour no oppression, drowsiness, heat, acidity, or other uncomfortable feeling, will probably pass healthily through all succeeding stages of digestion. If otherwise, the evil arises from some accidental or especial cause, against which no ordinary rule can provide.

That there is a general excess in quantity of solid food among the higher classes in this country, perhaps in all highly civilized countries, may be admitted as certain. In its effects, direct or indirect, it is one of the, circumstances which tend to equalize the actual condition of different classes. No reasoning or quotation of cases is needful to the proof of the mischiefs hence derived. Daily experience is the argument here; both as to the effects of single excesses, and of that smaller habitual excess, which, little felt at the time, does nevertheless accumulate a store of ills for the whole of life, affecting in various degrees all the functions both of body and mind. The observations of Dr. Beaumont, under the singular facilities afforded in the case of St. Martin, add more direct proof to this ordinary experience. In showing to the eye the immediate effect of excess of food, as well as wine, in producing an erythematous state of the mucous coat of the stomach, they render more explicit the influence of such excesses long continued; and the passage from slight and transient disorder to permanent disease of texture. These living observations have a value tenfold that of any attainable in other ways, and especially as applied to an organ of such complex condition as the stomach, so variously acted upon by mental as well as physical causes.

The proper regulation of diet under actual disease is not, if rightly viewed, so difficult a matter as it might seem from the infinite variety of conditions with which we have to deal. The great law of the living economy comes in here for our guidance,—that the appetite for food is lost or diminished, in exact relation to the impairment of the powers by which it is digested and converted to the uses of the system. The exceptions to this law (many of them such only in appearance), are too inconsiderable to require enumeration. Its truth is singularly denoted in all cases where there is febrile action present in the body; and its 'generality gives it value as an index of disorder, as well as of the right methods of dietetic treatment.

I have mentioned elsewhere the aids we are entitled to draw from the patient himself in this point of practice, where disease has retored nature for a while to its dominion over the appetites. It is rare that any mischief can arise from following this guidance, if care be taken to ascertain its reality. Nevertheless, the physician is liable here to various difficulties, created chiefly by the mistaken importunity of those around the patient. No conviction is harder to be removed than that which regards loss of appetite as itself the disorder,—food as the proper and certain remedy. Even the concurrence of the patient's feelings with the judgment of the physician is scarcely of avail against this persuasion. And when the former are altered in part by returning health, and old appetites and habits begin to recur, the risk of excess becomes greater, by the enfeeblement of that natural control which is the best security against it.

The adult patient, however, is better able than the child or infant to protect himself against such hurtful importunities. In the case of the infant, more especially, a facility is often afforded to the commission of this mischief by the thirst of fever, which allows liquid food to be largely given, and under the deception of appearing to be taken eagerly, when most unfit for the disorder that exists. These evils are familiar in practice, and not easily obviated altogether. They may best be diminished by consistency and firmness in the medical man, whose unwilling concessions in a few instances weaken his influence in all.

As to what regards the manner of taking food, little can be added to the maxims which are familiar on this subject. The recent experiments of some German physiologists on the properties of acidified mucus and other products from mucous membrane, as agents in digestion, give new proof of the necessity that the food should be well mixed with the saliva and secretions of the mucous glands in the early stages of this process.* And the observations of Dr. Beaumont, aided by the facilities just mentioned, on the secretion of the gastric juice as an effect of the stimulus of food received into the stomach, and on the peculiar manner in which its inner coats contract on each fresh morsel, show the necessity of allowing due time to these operations, and not disturbing them by matters hastily swallowed and imperfectly prepared. In youth, the activity of the system, seeking fresh materials for growth and other remarkable bodily changes then in progress, readily overcomes all difficulties. But at more advanced times of life, and when these demands are diminished or have ceased, the stomach needs to be dealt with more leisurely and gently. Common experience will tell every one of the uneasiness and sort of convulsive reaction, produced by hasty swallowing and hurried meals. This, in fact, is one of the many causes of dyspepsia to those of sedentary habits who feed alone; and not less to those who eat, as they live, in a tumult of business, measuring their meals by minutes stolen from the labours of the day.†

---

* I allude to the researches of Eberle, Schwann, and Muller, which have been repeated and extended by Dr. Todd in this country.

† In Thomas Paynell's *Regimen of Health*, 1557, (a translation of the Regimen Sanitatis Salernitanum,) this matter is quaintly but well expressed.—" Prolongynge of tyme in eatynge moderately (as an hour's space), to chawe and swalowe our meate well, is aloweable, and helpeth moche to the conservation of health. For good chawinge and swalowynge downe is as halfe a digestion. And

With the latter case is connected the further rule, that there should be no sudden or urgent exertion soon after a full meal, nor indeed immediately before it; for the same general reason applies to both cases.   The stomach requires (as does every organ for its appropriate function) a sufficient supply of nervous power whencesoever derived, and a proportionate increase of blood in its circulation, to minister to the actions of which digestion is the result.   It may be a physiological fact that these two conditions are identical; or that one involves the other.   But whether so or not, it is equally certain that both the nervous power, and the blood needful to digestion, are diminished and disturbed by strong exercise immediately before or after a meal.   And this independently of the effects of mechanical agitation in the latter case, which is no doubt often concerned in disturbing the process.

The proofs of these facts are furnished by constant experience, and are familiar to us amongst other animals; yet is attention not sufficiently given to them, either in the habitual directions of physicians, or in the rules which men apply themselves to the management of their diet.   Hard exercise and fatigue are often understood as a sanction for immediate and ample food, without regard to the expenditure of power that has taken place, or to the direction which the circulation has got towards the muscles and capillaries of the skin.   Those who are exposed to the necessity of long and fatiguing journeys speedily learn the error of this.   But experience of such kind is generally needed to teach it; nor is this always sufficient against the force of early impressions, and the faulty habits of society.*

What is true as to bodily exercise after food is equally so as to mental emotion, or intellectual labour.   Neither with sound nor unsound digestion ought there to be any intent exertion of mind at this time.   Strong or sudden emotion will instantly disturb or even stop the whole function; and short of this there is every degree in which the moral feelings habitually derange it.   To this cause we may in part attribute the frequent occurrence of dyspepsia in middle life; when the excitements are more active and various, and the passions inflict greater disturbance on the body.   Their influence is familiar to observation in the sensations of the moment; and not less in the symptoms which arise from repetition of the disturbance.   Two or three days of continued anxiety will bring dis-

ill chawinge doth eyther let dygestion, or else doth gretly hyndre it. But prolonginge of tyme in rallying and tellying of tales two or three houres is ryght hurtful."   And the reason for the latter clause is just, though that of probable excess of quantity in such cases might also be added. " For when the last meate is received the first is well neare dygested. Therefore the said meates in divers of their parties, as touching dygestion, be not like."

* I know from my own observation how well Government messengers, and the Tartar couriers of Turkey, have generally learnt this lesson, derived from the necessities of their manner of life, which are far more effectual for teaching than any other maxims. We apply the rule carefully and extensively in the management of our horses and dogs, without rightly heeding it for ourselves.

order and debility into all parts of the digestive organs, however healthy their previous state.

But even urgent intellectual exertion, unattended by any emotion (unless a laborious effort of the attention be so termed) interferes for the most part with easy and perfect digestion. The ancient precept, "*sin lucubrandum est, non post cibum id faciendum, sed post concoctionem,*" will ever remain good. We have in this an example of that remarkable law, which stands at the threshold of every theory of life, that one function in vigorous or excessive exercise diminishes more or less the power of simultaneous exertion of any other. One must give way, or both be imperfectly performed.

We may, as before, seek explanation of this, by estimating the common nervous power as a given quantity at each moment; capable therefore only of a certain amount of effect, and requiring replenishment. Or we may look otherwise to the quantity of blood required by every organ for the complete performance of its functions; and its distribution according to this demand expressly interfered with in the case before us. But whatever the manner of viewing the subject, it is certain that this is a point of importance to good digestion, and that it ought to enter into every rule of treatment for disorders of the stomach. And the rather so, as the dyspeptic is often by temperament prone to what may be termed intellectual excesses, as well as to earnest and easily excited moral feelings.

The relation of digestion to sleep is one of the most important in the economy of life. These two functions severally aid or disturb each other, in proportion as they are perfect or imperfect in their course; and no rules are more important than such as apply to this relation. It must be admitted, however, that they are exceedingly scanty and incomplete, notwithstanding the perpetual experiment which life affords on the subject. It is difficult to extricate clear results from so great a variety of conditions; and unhappily the current fashions and phrases tend rather to perplex than inform our judgments on the subject.

Setting aside the effects of particular articles of diet, which it would be impossible to specify, the practical questions chiefly regard the relation of time and quantity of food to sleep; and these are the fitter objects of study, as some averages are attainable and convertible to use. It is clear, for example, from observation both of man and other animals, that a certain quantity of food in the stomach, concurring especially with the habitual time of rest, tends to produce sound and healthy sleep;—that an excess in quantity brings on such as is broken, uneasy, and oppressed;—while sleeplessness is usually the effect of the stomach being empty and needing support. To these general facts, without inquiring into their physiological cause, may be referred most of the particular relations between sleep and food, and the precepts founded upon them. The fashions of society infringe largely upon the principles thus established; and though the powers of habit and accommodation in the system do much to lessen the evils that result, yet it is certain that some methods are greatly preferable to others, and that observation cannot better be employed than in ascertaining these.

In another chapter, on Sleep, mention will be made of the relation between the principal meal of the day and the time of rest. This is a question of constant occurrence in practice; and, without going into details, it is enough to say that much may be done for the restoration of sleep, where this is at fault, by altering the time of dinner to an earlier hour; so as not only to admit some bodily exercise in the interval, but also a light supper before going to bed. The benefit of such change from the ordinary usage is often immediate; depending partly on the avoidance of the recumbent posture, and of efforts to sleep at a period of digestion unfit for this state; and further, and not less, on the direct effect of moderate repletion in disposing to rest. The latter circumstance, again, may depend in part on the mechanical influence of such repletion; principally, perhaps, on its furnishing material for the secretions of the stomach to act upon, which otherwise would fret with uneasy sensations the nerves of the organ itself Various suggestions will occur in practice, founded more or less directly on the facts just stated. When well substantiated, they are of great value in every part of the treatment of disease.*

The reciprocal importance of sound and sufficient sleep to a healthy state of the digestive organs, is familar to all. This influence is probably in great degree of indirect kind; in some respects certainly so. There is a circle of relations here, which, even if it were expedient, could scarcely be viewed separately. The connexions are those upon which all right practice is founded, and the knowledge of their causes is that which gives medicine its character as a science.

Treating the subject thus cursorily, I may omit all those details as to particular articles of food which are to be found in the works on diet and digestion. The number of such facts has been materially increased of late, and more certainty and value given to them both by direct experiment, and by their association with organic chemistry. Notwithstanding this, fashion still too largely tampers with the whole subject of dietetics; and injuriously, as regards the stability of its principles, and their application to practice. Of late years, for example, this fashion has directed itself against vegetable food;—an erroneous prejudice in many, perhaps in the majority of cases. Allowing, what is partly proved, that vegetable matters are carried indigested to a lower part of the alimentary canal than animal food, and admitting that more flatulence is usually produced from them, it still is the fact that a feeble digestion suffers no less, though it may be in different ways, from an exclusively animal diet.

* It is a somewhat curious contrast to modern habits, that the early dinner, in the time of Augustus, appears to have been a mark of luxury and fashion.

Morbid products are alike evolved; and some of these affecting not only the alimentary canal, but disturbing other organs and functions through changes produced in the blood.

I know the case of a gentleman, having the calculous diathesis strongly marked, in whom animal food, taken for three or four days, even in moderate quantity, invariably brings on discharge of lithic acid, as sand or gravel; suspended upon return to vegetable diet. This is a particular instance; but experience in gouty cases furnishes frequent and striking notices of the same general fact; thus indicating a large class of disorders, having much kindred with dyspepsia, in which excess in animal food rapidly becomes a source of mischief not merely by overloading the alimentary canal, but by introducing morbid matters into the system at large. A persevering abstinence from any such excess may be reckoned among the most effectual preventives of gout in all its forms.

The rule of health being obviously that of blending the two kinds of food, I believe the exception more frequently required to be that of limiting the animal part in proportion to the other. The fashion of the day sets it down otherwise; and this is one of the subjects where loose or partial opinions easily get the force of precepts with the world at large.

The singular and seemingly wayward appetites which are common in illness or during convalescence, and the gratification of which is sometimes even a means of cure, give proof how much we have yet to learn as to the various states of the stomach, and their relation to different kinds of food. However difficult to apprehend, it is clear that this organ, together with the parts associated in the function, is often an exponent for the rest of the system of other wants beyond those of mere quantity of aliment. And upon this remarkable instinct in the animal economy (for it is difficult otherwise to express it) depends, doubtless, the preservation of that balance among the constituents of the blood which is essential to the healthy state. In all diseases it is probable that this balance is in certain degree altered or impaired; in some certainly much more than in others. The anomalous appetites of illness or convalescence are often, it may be presumed, natural efforts to restore it. There is enough of authority for this view from observed facts, to justify the physician in keeping constant watch upon such suggestions, hower fanciful in kind. Separated by due caution from certain obvious sources of error, they become frequent and valuable aids in the treatment of disease.

Another fashion, as it may be termed, among rules for diet, has been that of limiting the more solid part of the food to one or two articles, under the idea that digestion is better performed upon simples than on food variously compounded. In dyspeptic complaints, or with any active disorder present, there is general truth in the maxim. But even here limitation of quantity is more important than that of quality; and care is ever needful not to oppose our partial knowledge to the natural appetites just mentioned, when well attested to be really such.   In ordinary health, the habits of life rarely allow the rule to be persisted in, and the conditional objections to it are on this account of little moment: otherwise it might be urged that extreme simplicity in the kind of food is not required by any proof we have of its effects on health; and is even contradicted to a certain extent by the best experiments we possess on the subject.   The researches of Dr. Prout, founded on a simple and just principle, have rendered more exact than heretofore our knowledge of the elements of nutritious matter; and in referring them to three separate classes, with different chemical properties of each, have enabled us to understand the fitness of combinations of food, and even of some of the more artificial refinements which luxury has devised.   It is obvious that there may be excess from a disproportion of these several elements; but it is equally true in principle, that there may be fault on the side of limitation and simplicity; and this inference is justified by various experiments on animals, attended with very remarkable results.*

The various questions regarding wine as a part of diet have always had much interest; and reasonably so, from their importance to the welfare both of individuals and communities.   Here also much has been written, and many maxims and fashions are current; but without inferences precise enough to afford a rule for those who seriously seek it.   It is difficult indeed to obtain this rule, where the results are so far complicated by individual temperament, by the kinds and qualities of wine, and by the manner of its use.   That it is powerful as a medicinal agent is certain; that its habitual use, within fixed limits, is beneficial to some constitutions is equally so. But we have not less assurance that in numerous other cases it is habitually injurious, in relation both to the digestive organs and to the functions of the brain.   And it may be affirmed generally (as a point wholly apart from the enormous abuse of spirits among the lower orders) that the use of wine is far too large for any real necessity or utility in the classes which consume it in this country. Modern custom has abridged the excess: but much remains to be done before the habit is brought down to a salutary level; and medical practice is in general greatly too indulgent on this point to the weakness of those with whom it deals.

It has been a maxim anciently, as now, that habitual excess in liquors is less injurious than that of food.†   And, with regard to wine, this may perchance be true.   But we are hardly entitled thus to let off one evil by comparison with another, where each is in itself so great, and where they so often concur in fostering one common usage, injurious to all the functions of life.

* The most striking of these experiments are derived from M. Magendie, to whom we owe much in this as in other parts of physiology.

† Sæpe, si qua intemperantia subest, tutior est in potione quàm in escâ.— *Celsus.*   Many other remarks on this subject might be quoted from the ancient physicians, remarkable for the truth of their present application, notwithstanding the great diversity both as to the materials and preparation of food, and the habits of life most pertaining to digestion.

As respects quantity, kind, and admixture of wine or other liquors, general rules of ready practical application are the best which can be given. Those which aim at being more precise involve such various conditions, that evasion on the part of the patient is easy and sure to follow. Here, indeed, it is essential to engage his good faith and understanding in concurrence with the precept imposed, as the only protection against the facility of indulgence every where at hand. Even under the eye of the physician, appeal must be made more or less to his own observation of effects; and this observation, therefore, it should be an object of all rules to cultivate and direct with as little ambiguity as possible.

Much may be done in this way. As regards quantity of wine, for instance, the tests of what is to be deemed excess lie within the scope of ready remark, provided attention be fairly directed to the repetition of similar effects under circumstances reasonably alike. If the excitement of the spirits exceeds that of simple comfort (a condition not difficult to note), then is it certain that there is a state of brain, the frequent recurrence of which becomes a source of serious mischief both to body and mind. Or if, as happens in other constitutions, heaviness and drowsiness ensue speedily on the wine taken, equally is it certain that the quantity is in excess, and will be injurious in proportion to the frequency of repetition.* Or if a hot, dry skin, and increasing thirst, the inference is the same, and the result no less assured. Or, again, if the early hours of the morning are languid and oppressed, with headache of one kind or another, foul mouth, and weak or disordered stomach, the " *hesterna vitia*" may fairly be called to account, and wine probably as principal among these.

The familiarity of such tests makes them more valuable for practical enforcement; and there are few cases where the patient may not obtain from them, if fairly dealt with, a sufficient rule for his guidance. The same tests will apply to kind of wine as to quantity ; but more ambiguously, from the many new conditions brought in, which neither chemical examination, nor common experience, has yet been able to explain. The importance of the question is fortunately much less than in the other case. It is true here, as with regard to solid food, that, if the quantity be duly limited, the kind, though by no means to be disregarded, becomes of much less significance. It may even be doubted whether any practical good has hitherto been gained by our researches into and classification of wines. The comparison of qualities, of the influence of which upon the body we are very slightly informed, gives a specious license to the indulgence in certain kinds, often quite as hurtful as the more careless use of which the preference of the moment forms the only rule.

* As regards the two opposite effects here noted, I believe it will be found that the latter is more common where the kidneys act but little under the influence of wine : a result, if correctly stated, which it may not be difficult to explain.

We may admit, then, the simple tests just stated as the best that can be had, either for medical precept, or the self-direction of the patient. And, if strictly attended to, they would probably suffice for every purpose in practice. It may be added further that it is the part of every wise man, once at least in life, to make trial of the effects of leaving off wine altogether; and this even without the suggestion of actual malady. The point is one of interest enough in the economy of health to call for such experiment; and the results can seldom be so wholly negative as to render it a fruitless one. To obtain them fairly, however, the abandonment must be complete for a time; a measure of no risk even where the change is greatest; and illustrating, moreover, other points of temperament and particular function, which it is important to every man to know, for the right guidance of his habits of life.

In the common treatment of dyspeptic disorders in this country, it cannot be denied that injury is inflicted by the use of purgatives to excess. I have noticed this elsewhere; but the frequency and ill effects of the abuse warrant a recurrence to the subject. It may in truth be affirmed that the complaint is often brought on by the prevalence of such treatment in modern practice. The imagination of the dyspeptic solicits the momentary relief thus obtained, at the expense of his future health and comfort. Scarcely a symptom of the disorder which is not aggravated by the habit of frequent purging; either directly from irritation of the alimentary canal, and disturbance of the natural course of its functions; or indirectly, by morbid influence on the mind of the patient, an effect no less noxious than the former. The general course of English practice is doubtless open to much reform on this point.

A point of consequence, also, is the manner of using bitters in the treatment of stomach disorders. Experience leads me to think that this is generally too large and indiscriminate. Even were our knowledge of their relative qualities more exact than it is, and our adaption of them more just in consequence, we still might often render this action more beneficial in these complaints by lighter preparations than are usually employed. Bark, as having other and specific objects, may be expected in part from the question. But there are various states of stomach in which the ordinary doses and strength of bitter infusions are injurious; while obvious good is got from a more moderate employment of the same means.

Frequently the best mode of using bitters in these cases is in direct combination with the aperient which may be necessary. Thereby a smaller quantity of the latter is usually rendered effectual; and the noxious effects of repetition materially abated. The addition of creosote to laxative medicines is beneficial in similar way; and for this, as well as other reasons, it deserves more trial in dyspeptic cases than it has yet obtained.

The theory and uses of tonic medicines—exceedingly vague, it must be owned, in every part of practice—are not least so in their relation to disorders of digestion. Of those fitly thus termed, iron, in one or other of its preparations, is, according to my experience, the most generally beneficial. Comparing it with the whole class of bitters, I doubt whether there is any one among the latter capable of being made so variously useful. Regard of course must be had, in employing it, to the cause and particular character of the dyspeptic symptoms. But the circumstances which create apprehension, often most needlessly, as to its use, may be readily obviated by its conjunction with whatever laxatives are required; and this, as in the instance of bitters, is often better done by direct combination than by separate employment. The ammoniated iron with an aloetic medicine, or the sulphate of iron in solution with the sulphate of magnesia or soda, will be found among the most beneficial of these forms; and applicable in numerous cases, without other difficulty than what may arise from the patient himself. For the imagination of the dyspeptic, as before mentioned, is ever awake to discover sensations and draw inferences; the latter often as much diseased as the feelings which prompt them. His prejudices, easily excited against any remedies, obtain a sort of countenance, in the case of steel medicines, from the phrases vaguely applied to them by the ignorant; and it often needs discretion and firmness in the practitioner to insure that persistance in their use which alone can render them of avail.

Though not seeing cause for the apprehension as to alkaline medicines which some have entertained, I believe that they are often employed in needless, perhaps injurious, quantity, and indiscreetly as to the time of taking them. As they cannot fitly be termed a remedy for dyspepsia, but a relief merely to one symptom of the disorder, there is reason for closely conjoining their use with that part of digestion which it is the object to alter. Taken together with the food requiring this correction, the effect is generally more beneficial than when used after acid has been actually formed. It is a manner of prevention better according with the whole function of digestion, and avoiding that sudden extrication of fixed air, which, if the alkaline carbonates are employed, is sometimes injurious to it.*

Celsus mentions the "*clara lectio*," among remedies for dyspeptic complaints; and this merits more attention than it receives. As

---

* The suspicion that the alkalies, taken medicinally, may produce a morbid state of the blood, and thereby disease in different organs, though it cannot be affirmed impossible, under excess of use, yet is not warranted by any ordinary experience on the subject. The effects of sudden injection of carbonate of soda into the circulation cannot be received as sufficient evidence. At the same time, the singular importance of this great relation of acid and alkali in every part of the chemistry of animal life, and the unquestionable agency of alkalies on certain secretions, presumably through the blood, fully prove that the habitual use of this remedy is not negative in effect; and we have probably yet to learn some of its effects, only partially shown when taken to neutralise acid in the alimentary canal. The liquor potassæ, sufficiently diluted, (a point of some consequence to its successful employment,) is perhaps the most beneficial form when a constitutional effect is desired.

the condition of the abdominal viscera affects the organs of respiration and the voice, so reciprocally does the free exercise of the lungs and diaphragm influence beneficially the organs of digestion. This in part, perhaps chiefly indeed, is a mechanical effect. But, since in dyspepsia the arterialization of the blood by the lungs is generally deficient, it may readily be conceived that certain sustained and equable efforts of the voice are beneficial in exercising the respiration, and thereby remedying the default.

The influence of free air and sufficient respiration is, in fact, a point of singular importance in the treatment of this disorder, even independently of those exercises of the body which are usually and fitly recommended to dyspeptic patients. Good air is essential to perfect digestion: close and crowded rooms evidently disturb and impair it. The experience of every one may afford proof of this; yet is it certainly not enough regarded in common practice.* The dyspeptic, distempered in his feelings, languid in muscular power, and with feeble circulation, willingly indulges his indolence by making drugs the sole remedy for his ills; and this preference is too much sanctioned by the ordinary course of medical treatment in such cases.

The habits thus generated are the reverse of those which lead to cure. Neglecting or avoiding fresh air, the patient forfeits the safest and most effectual of all remedies; one which goes furthest towards the root of his disorder. For, in dyspepsia, no symptom is better marked than the languid circulation of the blood through the extreme vessels. This is especially obvious in the state of the skin and extremities of the body; and, looked to as a habit, forms one of the most essential characters of the disorder. If we might suppose, what is probable from the corresponding feebleness of the heart's action, that the same condition of faulty circulation extends to the capillaries of internal surfaces and secreting organs, we obtain a general expression of altered state and balance of blood throughout the system, which might well admit of being received as a proximate cause, and as rendering explanation of many of the multiform symptoms of the complaint. The absence or diminished quantity of blood in the capillary system, through which all the more important functions are performed, and its stagnation in the great vessels, and particularly within the venous system throughout the body, illustrate in special manner some of the more singular anomalies in the disorder.

Here the better arterialization of the blood is a main remedy; and without which none other can be of thorough avail. Open air and free respiration are to be sought for; under some condition of bodily exertion, if possible; but without it, if this be prevented. In

---

* A familiar illustration may be drawn from the singular difference of effect in travelling on the outside or inside of a carriage, immediately after a meal. Though the food be alike in both cases, digestion in the first goes on easily and healthily; in the second, often with much disturbance and difficulty, increased in proportion as the air is more confined,

another place I have mentioned the benefits to be derived from the express exercise of respiration ; and these are scarcely less obvious and assured in dyspeptic complaints than in others which seem more expressly adapted to them.   All that can give air free ingress to the lungs and to the blood, if not a primary remedy, is, at all events, so powerful an accessory to cure, that it behoves the physician to keep it ever before him in his treatment of the disorder.

These considerations involve in some part the theory of dyspepsia ; a topic, however, which I refrain from here, as implying a more exact definition and history of the complaint than is intended in these cursory remarks.   The ordinary states, bearing this name, are produced chiefly by circumstances in diet and mode of life acting topically upon the organs of digestion.   But that one remarkable form of it, connected with the hypochondriasis, and often inducing atrophy, depends on a state of the nervous power, is likely, or perhaps even certain.*   What this state actually is, whether of deficiency or deprivation, or what part of the nervous system is chiefly concerned in it, our present knowledge does not enable us to affirm ; and we are equally, and in the same way, at fault regarding hypochondriasis itself.   These are points involving many curious relations in pathology, and upon which we have much still to learn.†

An example illustrating the connexion between the states of dyspepsia and hypochondriasis, and not less remarkable in itself, is the effect of nursing in certain female habits, or of great excess of nursing in all.   The experience of most practitioners will furnish them with instances where this cause has brought on extreme disorder of the nervous system ; sometimes verging on maniacal state; more frequently shown in general debility and hypochondriacal depression ; and in the latter case generally connected with obstinate dyspeptic symptoms.   I have known cases where effects, manifestly having this origin, have continued in certain degree even for years.   The more rapid mischief occurring in some constitutions is familiar to all.

* In the writings of Dr. Whytt, so fertile throughout in sound and original views, will be found some excellent remarks on atrophy from morbid state of the nerves of the stomach and alimentary canal.

† The frequent occurrence of hypochondriasis among the people of the Western Islands of Scotland, is a fact for which we have the authority of Dr. Macculloch. It is curiously corroborated by an observation I made in Iceland (confirmed to me by the information of the priests and other intelligent natives) of the great frequency of the same disorder in that island.   There is reason to suppose that certain similar conditions of diet and manner of life are concerned in this effect. And the relation to scurvy is of some interest here ; a disease in which there is similar depression of the nervous powers ; and which depends chiefly, as far as we can see, on non-acescent or salted diet, confinement to one spot, &c. ; circumstances to which the almost entire deficiency of vegetable food, the long winters, and possibly the singular contrast between the physical condition and intellectual culture of the Icelanders, peculiarly expose this remarkable people. Accordingly, scorbutic complaints are common and severe in Iceland ; treated, when even these remedies can be had, by decoctions of trefoil, juniper, the sedum acre, and scurvy-grass.   In a Thesis I printed in 1811, on the Diseases of Iceland, may be found some more detailed notices on this subject.

Nor can we even assert the affection of the nerves to be itself a primary cause in these and other instances. It may be that the first condition is that of an altered state of blood, or in some cases a morbid matter, like that of gout, present in the circulation; and thence producing its effects, more or less directly, on other parts of the system. And there is some argument for the latter view in the undoubted connexion between dyspeptic disorders and the irregular forms of the gouty constitution; a connexion sufficiently close and familiar to observation to justify the belief of relation to some common cause; acting under different modifications from age, sex, and other temperament of body; as well as from variations, it may be, in the quality or proportion of the morbid matter itself. Though much here is still speculative, yet we know enough to see that future discovery lies before us in this direction.

Recurring to the feeble state of the capillary circulation in dyspepsia, whether this depend on altered state of the nervous power or not, equally is it important to obviate the evil of such tendency. For this object, exercises, friction, and bathing in different forms, together with change of air or scene, may rightly find place before most of the internal remedies which are usual in such cases. And our treatment of the disorder would be one of greater success, were these points more steadily insisted upon, and less concession made to the morbid preference for medicines: arising partly from the natural indolence of the complaint, partly from the fashions ever prevailing in respect to it. This is one of the instances where the general course of practice might be greatly altered and amended. Much is got, if the dyspeptic can be rescued from means, for the most part of doubtful or injurious effect; much also, if he can be led into habits which invigorate the circulation with safety to every part, and may be modified under more certain rule than any remedies of internal use.* Here, unhappily, as in so many other cases, the simplicity of the means forms a hindrance to their sufficient application. What is obvious can rarely be brought into

---

* The ancients, as is well known, employed friction under a more general conception of its use than we do; not merely as a remedy for feebleness or swelling of limbs, but as altering the condition of the whole body. And, without adopting all they have affirmed on this subject, it is certain that its employment, even in our climate, might be beneficially extended in a variety of cases; in none more than those of enfeebled or disordered digestion. So applied, it affords another example of the many important relations subsisting between the external and internal surfaces of the body.

Of the use of anointing, as practised by the ancients, we know from experience much less. Some explanation of its employment in tropical climates may be found in the protection it gives against the direct effects of solar heat on the skin. There is reason, as well as scope, for making larger trial of it as a curative means, even in disorders of the alimentary canal. The harsh dry skin of the dyspeptic patient might be improved in its texture and functions by rubbing with warm oils, &c., where wholly unaffected by internal remedies given for the same object. In one or two cases, I have had cause to infer that much benefit was obtained by this method; but, like most other external means, it would require more time and perseverance than the temper of the dyspeptic will often concede to such remedies.

successful competition with what is vague and obscure in the treatment of disease.

The recommendation of travel to dyspeptic patients is familiar and reasonable. Some caution, however, is needed as to details; nor ought these to be considered below the notice of the physician. The dyspeptic cannot wisely be sent to travel alone. His earlier way must be smoothed to him; and some concessions be made to his indolence and extravagant demands for comfort, for the better chance of surmounting them in the end. I have known many patients return from the experiment, jaded and dispirited, with whom a more judicious plan would have prevented all disappointment. It is well, in the outset, to keep their journey apart from the tumult of cities and spectacles. The dyspeptic cannot thus violently be removed from himself and his own sensations; and the failure of a first attempt renders others more difficult. Open or mountain air;—varied scenery, yet avoiding any such frequent change as may too greatly excite or fatigue the attention;—occasional pauses in travelling, to obviate any heat or excitement that may exist, or to prevent such;—the bodily exercise regular in amount, varied if possible in kind, and rarely passing into fatigue;—short passages by sea, if they can be managed with comfort;—early and regular meals and hours of rest;—and due attention to the state of the bowels, by the mildest means adequate to the effect;—all these points are worthy of attention in advising the remedy of travelling to the dyspeptic. Their importance, of course, varies in different instances; but I know, from a good deal of experience in such cases, that it is never wise to disregard them, as unimportant to the result. And this is the more true, as it is peculiarly the character of the dyspeptic patient to be incapable of determining these things for himself.

Among the minor conditions to be looked to in dyspeptic cases is that of habitual posture. The patient should be led, as much as possible, to keep the trunk of the body upright, and opened out freely in front. The compression of the stomach, pylorus, and duodenum, by the bending of the body upon itself, is exceedingly injurious to the functions of these parts; as is proved from the sensations produced by making this movement suddenly, and with some little effort, when the stomach is full. Disturbance to digestion is immediately felt; continued or increased as the act is repeated. The frequency of stomach disorders amongst those of sedentary pursuits, is doubtless owing in part to habits of posture unfavourable to digestion.

It may seem a trivial remark, yet is worth notice, that dyspeptics have frequently the habit of touching or pressing upon the epigastrium; a practice readily induced by uneasy sensation there, but bad in its effects on the complaint. Whatever the causes, no part of the body claims exemption so much as this from every interference. I have known the habit to such extent in one or two cases, as to form a principal cause of disorder; the symptoms ceasing when it was discontinued.

Another aid in the treatment of these complaints, deserving more notice than it receives, is the application of some uniform support, amounting to slight pressure, around the abdomen. The dyspeptic gains by this, not only in the avoidance of many uneasy sensations from distension, and in the better performance of the functions which distension impedes; but also by the uniform warmth and freer circulation in the superficial vessels of this part of the body; effects of no small import to the healthy state of the internal membranes, the relations of which to the functions of the skin are so numerous and unceasing. The chest, as matter of-custom amongst us, is carefully watched over with reference to these effects; though it may be doubted, looking to the structure and function of the respective parts, whether such care is really more beneficial here than in the case before us. Whether so or not, we cannot question the value of this aid in stomach complaints, and are bound to consider it enhanced by the simplicity of the means employed.

Among the external remedies insufficiently resorted to in dyspeptic cases, bathing may certainly be mentioned. The warm bath under certain conditions, attested chiefly by the state of the skin;—the shower-bath, cold or tepid, in other cases;—or occasionally the salt-water hip-bath, similarly varied as to temperature;—offer means both of prevention and relief which no discreet physician will neglect. Here, also, we must keep in view that important relation of external and internal surfaces, ever operating in all the phenomena of health and disease, and which serves as a basis to so many facts both in pathology and practice.

I may state again, what indeed will be seen on the face of the foregoing observations, that they are not to be viewed in the light of a dissertation on this copious subject; but merely as remarks drawn from my experience, on points which appear to have obtained less than their due share of attention, or which are especially recommended by their general and ready application in this part of practice.

CHAPTER XXIV.

ON DISEASES COMMONLY OCCURRING BUT ONCE IN LIFE.

THE title, thus including only a single character of these remarkable diseases, might be extended to other circumstances in their history; which, though not exclusively limited to this connexion, are still so closely associated, that it is impossible to view them asunder. Such are, the perfectly definite course of their symptoms in the ordinary form; the frequency of an external or eruptive stage in each; and the well-marked power of conveying infection by the reproduction or diffusion of the virus respectively peculiar to them;—all points of the highest interest in pathology; and which, under the relations just expressed, involve some of the most abstruse questions in the whole range of science. Controversy, as might be expected, has made itself busy with various parts of the subject; but has yet done little to remove the obscurity which hangs over it.

In pursuing the above connexions, even in their most general form, we seem ever on the verge of some discovery, giving new inlet to the more mysterious parts of the animal economy, whether in health or disease. Such discovery indeed, if hereafter made, is not unlikely to be derived from methods of inquiry in which these relations are directly involved. In their nature it is scarcely possible they should be unproductive to research, however great the difficulties attending it. The simple enunciation of the fact, that certain diseases of definite course, and communicable by some manner of specific infection, do generally occur but once in the term of human existence, abounds in the most curious suggestions, and carries us at once into the higher and more hidden parts of the philosophy of life.

The familiarity of the facts prevents indeed an immediate conception of the great wonder they involve. What in itself more strange, than that a minute speck of matter (if indeed what is actually the virus of disease be ever the object of sight)—in other instances, agents wholly imperceptible by any sense, and admitted into the body through unknown channels,—should be capable of exciting there certain trains of morbid actions, determinate in their character and duration; reproducing or perpetuating, if so it may be termed, that which is the principle of infection and element of disease; and, above all, giving exemption more or less complete to the remainder of life, from the action of this principle, or the recurrence of the symptoms depending upon it! What again is the nature of that definite change in the body which makes it inaccessible to a certain disease, yet apparently does not affect any other property or function of the animal economy? Though processes of diseased action are concerned in all this, yet is it a mystery of the same nature as that of generation and growth, and creating similar difficulties to our comprehension.

The consideration of these topics involves certain general views as to the course and changes of philosophical inquiry, at different periods in the history of science. It is impossible not to be struck with the fact, that modern research, armed with all its powers of experiment and exactness of induction, has carried and is yet carrying us back, to the realization of many ancient opinions, which have hitherto been viewed only as vague hypotheses, without other sanction than the hardihood or ingenuity of thought which first suggested them. The inquiries respecting the ultimate particles of bodies, their forms, relative weight, and manner of combination, —accredited though these now are by the most exact evidence which number or geometry can furnish, do yet represent in a more substantial form certain theories which may be termed the poetical dreams of antiquity, and were apparently so regarded by many of those who propounded them.*

Even on points, however, where no such stable foundation is yet secured, the tendency is strong at the present time to carry speculation forward beyond the bounds of actual knowledge. The very advance of science itself; the application of new methods of analysis; the discovery of new and subtle agents, universal as the more palpable forms of matter on which they act; the assignment of definite proportion, forms, and polarities, to matter in almost all its combinations; the successful research into conditions of the earth and of organized life anterior to those which now exist; and, further, the high perfection and power given to instruments wherewith to work in these deeper mines of knowledge;—all such attainments may be said to have forced philosophy upon bolder conceptions than heretofore, and nearer to what seem the ultimate bounds of human research. Still it is the wider generalization of facts which serves as starting-place to these speculations; and they are speedily lost, if not supported by extension of the evidence on which they depend. The fortunate but unproved and fruitless, anticipations of a former age curiously approach them on this still uncertain ground; gaining admission into the domain of science at the same time, and through the same channels only.

These remarks apply to medicine not less than to other sciences; and in singular manner as respects the relations of the blood to the production and progress of disease. Here modern research, by showing the very compound nature of this fluid; the frequent changes it undergoes in the proportion of its component parts; the generation of morbid matters within the circulating system; and the extraordinary influence of even the most minute quantity of certain substances introduced from without, has sanctioned to an unexpected extent doctrines which, after centuries of reputation and general adoption, had fallen almost wholly into disrepute. There is no more striking feature in the history of medicine than the rapid recurrence to these opinions;—in very different form and phraseology indeed, and now based upon the most minute analysis which modern chemistry can furnish; but still involving the same principle, and even conducting to many similar practical results.

It is difficult, in truth, to conceive how a doctrine, which, even

---

* There is much that might tempt one to enlarge further on this subject, and to fetch, from the incomparable poetry of Lucretius, passages (stript of their conclusions) which stand in singular relation to the most recent speculations of the present age. But this belongs rather to the history of the human mind, and of general philosophy, than to the subject before us. All indeed who read, as well as write, on medical topics, will find how difficult it is to attain any opinion or truth that has wholly escaped the genius or labours of those who have gone before. This is especially true on every point of theory and general doctrine. Little that is new can here be looked for, except what is expressly founded on further discoveries in anatomy and physiology; and on fresh relations, thereby disclosed, to what was already known.

in the infancy of physical science, forced itself into acceptance by its obvious nature, and by the very necessity of the principle it involves, should ever have been so far neglected, or supplanted by other views. When the circulation of the blood was unknown, and its uses in growth, reparation, and secretion—in the production of animal heat and of nervous power—scantily defined, still was there evidence enough to show that its alterations in quantity and quality formed a great part in all the phenomena of disease. What has been done by chemists and physiologists of late years, in the examination of its healthy and morbid states, renders this now, if not the richest department of medical science, at all events that which gives largest augury of future advancement. It would be impossible, and useless from their familiarity, to recite here all the facts which have connexion with the subject of this chapter. In the note below I have referred to a few of the number, which seem most necessary to be kept under consideration.*

* The main difficulty in this investigation, and bearing closely on all its relations to pathology, is that of interpreting the state of the blood within the living body, by its appearances and changes when withdrawn from the vessels. It is yet a question whether all the principles asserted to exist in this fluid (or even in the organized animal textures) do exist there in life ; or whether they are not produced, or their combinations wholly altered, when vital actions cease, and coagulation and the ordinary chemical affinities supervene. The state of the fibrin, of the globules, and of the iron or other colouring matter in circulating blood, are particular instances of this difficulty ; but it extends to other ingredients and conditions also, which the most exact observations have not been able to determine or explain.

The fact, however, is now well assured, that the blood does undergo great changes in the living vessels ;—that these changes may commence from within, or be excited by agency from without ;—and that they consist, not merely in fluctuations of quantity, or of proportion of the watery to the saline or coagulable parts, but also in alteration of these solid parts themselves ; and in the generation of new compounds, either by anormal combinations of the elements of animal matter within the circulation, or by direct absorption of substances not previously there.

In regarding those causes of morbid change which belong especially to the body itself, the points chiefly to be noted are, the absorption into the blood of animal products already found in the system ; and the retention there, by deficient or disordered action of the secreting organs, of materials that ought to be separated from the body. It is ever to be kept in mind, in relation to the functions and diseases of the blood, that it contains some parts to be assimilated ; others that have passed through assimilation, and are to be removed by excretion. And though the latter in the healthy state may be so incorporated as to lose all distinction in the uniform nature of the fluid (a point not indeed well ascertained), yet under morbid conditions it is manifestly otherwise ; and products are found in the blood representing those which ought to have been eliminated from the body ; or sometimes, though more doubtfully, such as may have been absorbed from parts under disease. The curious evidence, lately obtained, regarding the occasional presence of pus in the blood, may be named as an instance to this effect.

These and other analogous facts, now familiar to us, show some of the ways in which the blood may become the subject of disease ; and all have reference to, though they do not explain, the phenomena which form the subject of this chapter. This is a topic, moreover, on which, as I have mentioned above, speculation may be allowed to pass somewhat beyond the limits of actual proof. Looking,

To the views so reëstablished regarding the blood, we must mainly look for whatever partial solution may be given of the questions before us. It is impossible to seek from any other source, explanation of morbid changes, so diffused in their nature, so active yet defined in their progress; involving the phenomena of fever, metastasis, and reproduction of the same virus from which they had their own origin; and analogous in so many points to those natural functions in which we consider the blood to be the agent. Even were the inference to stop here in evidence, and to be ever unfruitful of further results, I know not how this general conclusion could be avoided, or any other reasonably substituted for it. But the methods of inquiry, just referred to, render it very unlikely that the proofs should remain limited as at present; and though it would seem that there are parts of the subject wholly beyond attainment yet the very narrowness of our actual knowledge gives reason for not drawing the line closely or arbitrarily around us.

The remarks which follow are merely an outline of some of the questions belonging to this remarkable inquiry; with such comments as may seem justified by what we have hitherto learnt upon it, or by analogies drawn from other parts of physical science.

There might be a preliminary question, what diseases are properly included under the title of the Chapter; and medical opinions

for instance, at the specific difference of form and size of the globules of blood in different animals, and the immediate fatal effect of mutual transfusion in such cases, it is impossible not to suppose that varieties in the number or state of these globules, whencesoever arising, may produce essential alteration in the blood, and through it in all the functions of the body. And again, with respect to the agents which affect coagulation, looking at the singular way in which electricity is found to operate through intervening tissues, we must admit the likelihood that certain definite effects from this cause may take place even in the living body. All the phenomena of coagulation, indeed, are of primary importance in the pathology of the blood; seeing the numerous causes which modify it; and that some of these (the alkalies and certain alkaline salts, for example) are of such simple kind as to give the liability to continual variations by their amount, and by the state in which they are present.

Many other questions apply to the curious subject of the influence upon the blood, of matters not duly separated from it, or reabsorbed into the circulation. As an instance, recognised by medical experience, may be noticed the effects of the semen, or the elements of it, retained in the habit; or possibly reabsorbed again after being actually separated:—and, on the other hand, the results when excreted in too large quantity, or at periods of life unfitted for the activity of this function. Of the existence of such effects on the nervous system, as well as upon the functions of particular organs, there can be no doubt. The manner of their production is wholly unknown to us, but we have every reason to infer that the blood is the medium through which they severally take place.

That there is, independently of what has been theoretically termed *innervation* of the blood, some constant influence of the nervous system upon the physical conditions of this fluid, seems highly probable, though the proofs are too vague to be admitted into any argument on the subject. This may take place indirectly, through changes in the capillary vessels; or directly, by some manner of action on the blood itself. But at all events it must enter into all our views on this part of pathology, and in this light I have spoken of it in another chapter.

would not wholly agree on the subject. But this is a point of difference upon which I do not enter; satisfying myself by taking for the argument those examples among the contagious exanthemata, respecting which no doubt can exist. The small-pox, measles, and scarlatina (admitting the latter name in default of any one more appropriate) are evidently the instances which best fulfil all the terms of the question ; and from which probably an answer will be drawn, if ever we succeed in obtaining it. I do not include the chicken-pox and cow-pox in this enumeration, seeing the dispute which yet exists as to their nature and relations. The typhus, and possibly other forms of simple fever, have connexion with the subject, and the plague a still closer kindred ; and illustration may be derived from all, though less definitely than from the three diseases named above. The booping-cough is placed in the class of contagious disorders occurring but once in life ; and comes therefore within the terms of the inquiry; yet with many diversities of character which would add to the difficulty of the research, were we called upon to include it.

The great problem to be solved is that of the change in the living body, effected by a given disease, which prevents the same cause of disease from again producing the same morbid actions, except in rare instances, or after a certain lapse of time. For, the fact being once known, it is a ready and natural suggestion that the train of actions, whence this singular change results, must be definite in course and character. And on the same grounds the presumption occurs, as more probable than any other, that the agent in every such disease must be a specific virus, received into the system from without, and evolving earlier or later the series of changes which ensue. The principle of contagion in these cases does not so directly suggest itself. Yet, when to the general statement of the problem we add the fact, that, in certain of these disorders, there is a palpable reproduction of the virus whence they were derived, it becomes a ready inference (however difficult of explanation) that in all of them the train of morbid actions must tend to diffuse, by some manner of infection, that which is the essential element of the disease.

Coming then at once to the main question, we have to inquire whether there be any known phenomenon, or physical analogy, which can illustrate, however generally, this remarkable influence upon the body. Or, specifying the inquiry more exactly, — in what parts of the body (if in any especial parts) do the changes take place producing these extraordinary effects? And, secondly, in what may the changes themselves be presumed to consist?

The former question is that in which we seem to make nearest approach to something like solution. I have stated the presumption that the blood is the portion of the body most directly the subject of these phenomena ; into which the material of infection is received, and through which the series of actions forming the disease is evolved and terminated. Were argument wanting to strengthen the probability, it might almost be found in the question whether any other part of the human frame can be conceived equally capable of fulfilling the conditions of the inquiry ? Unless we avow total ignorance, or seek to veil it under phrases which convey no real meaning, we must admit that here alone can explanation reasonably be sought for, however remote the discovery from our present attainment. An altered state may indeed be produced throughout every part of the circulating system, from local irritation of a particular tissue. But we can entertain no conception of other part than the blood being the agent in multiplying, by a long series of morbid actions, the virus or principle in which these actions commenced; and secreting it afresh, as would seem to be done in some of these diseases, from all surfaces of the body. This is one of the instances where it is easier, from the nature of the topic, to apprehend the conclusion than to express the reasonings on which it is founded. Language is forced to become hypothetical to meet the obscurity of the inquiry.

On this part of the subject, however, there is more direct evidence in the actual introduction of the materials of some of these diseases into the blood, and the production thereby of the specific maladies to which they belong ;—a result familiar to us in the cases of inoculation, and in two or three other disorders where an animal virus is obviously brought into the circulation; but proved also experimentally in the communication of disease by the blood of the person infected, even where there is no virus secreted in any palpable form.* Here the argument gains great weight by the double or reciprocal evidence thus afforded. And if the proof be sufficient to show in certain cases, that the blood is the seat of the combinations, as well as the active cause of the transferences, in which a disease consists, we can have no reasonable doubt in assuming this, where the facts are not yet equally ascertained.

These experiments also, if admitted, remove another doubt that may suggest itself, viz., whether the series of changes, constituting what is called the disease in these cases, is really completed in the blood ? or whether there are not specific actions of secretion going on upon the surfaces of the body, and connected with the eruptive part of each disease, by which its peculiar virus is reproduced, and becomes an element of fresh infection to others ? It must be owned that the question is burdened with great difficulties, the same in effect as those which belong to the general doctrine of secretion. They are enhanced by the peculiarity of this being a matter alien to the system, and morbid in its own nature ; yet, as we are obliged to suppose, generated or augmented in quantity, in the progress of the disorder, by some process for which we have neither

---

* Though the experiments on this subject are more limited and uncertain than might be desired, yet they afford considerable proof that the measles have been produced by inoculation with the blood of patients under the disease; and, further, that in other animals, glanders, canine madness, and the mange have been produced in similar way.

name nor conception. The chief problem here is the true order of succession in the events, or that which may justly indicate their relations of cause and effect. A fair examination into what we really know on this subject will show how scanty is the amount, even on points which seem essential to any reasoning upon it. In affirming the likelihood that the series of changes, from the reception of the virus to the complete evolution and decline of the symptoms, must principally take place within the blood, we are expressing all for which we have any argument either from observation or analogy.

The same difficulties, equally inevitable, and even multiplied in amount, affect the other part of the question proposed; viz., in what these changes actually consist? how, above all, it can happen, that a given series of actions, arising from a virus received, should thus preclude, except in rare or partial instances, the recurrence of similar effects from a similar cause applied? The bare statement of this question carries with it, we must admit, a sort of interdiction to the hope of solution. While avowing, however, that science hitherto affords us no definite answer to the inquiry, there are nevertheless certain facts and phenomena which seem to lie nearest the truth, or to furnish at least the most plausible methods of research. And upon these it is worth while shortly to dwell;— the rather as they have themselves great interest in the history of disease.

The topics they comprise may briefly be thus enumerated :— *First*, The leading fact already adverted to, that these diseases, in their proper form, have a determinate course, from the first reception of the virus to the complete reëstablishment of health. *Secondly*, The apparent insusceptibility of some persons to receive these infections at any time of life. *Thirdly*, The susceptibility not existing at one time, but renewed at another; sometimes without obvious reason, but in certain cases with general relation to periods of life. *Fourthly*, The deviations from the regular type of each disease; occasionally in the length of interval between the infection and the first appearance of symptomatic fever; more frequently in the interrupted and incomplete evolution of the symptoms. *Fifthly*, The occasional recurrence of each disease in the same person, in affect of this incompleteness of its first course, of change in that state which gives protection, or of other cause wholly unknown to us. And, *Sixthly*, The facts, partially determined, regarding the incompatibility of these several diseases, their degree and order of mutual interference, and their liability to be disturbed or prevented by other disorders existing in the body at the time;— points all of great practical importance, and involving some of the most remarkable questions in medical science.

These circumstances, moreover, may be regarded as the only elements we possess for inquiry on the subject. For it must be avowed that no analogy can be drawn from other branches of physics;—none even from the general doctrines of life, or the phenomena of other disease,—which will serve to explain the peculiar mystery of this case. We know, indeed, that incalculably small quantities of certain substances brought into the blood act as poisons there; producing occasionally trains of morbid actions of very definite kind. But these are wanting in the great peculiarity designated in the title of this chapter: nor do they, as in the instance of the diseases before us, reproduce a matter of the same kind, capable of perpetuating the disorder by communication to others.

Before commenting on the subjects just stated, a condition may be mentioned, necessary as it would seem, and perhaps obvious, on any view of the subject; viz., that the virus concerned in these phenomena must be in every sense of *animal* nature,—the product originally of animal actions or changes, as well as propagated and diffused by the same. No other conception than this can well be entertained, however difficult or impossible to apprehend the details; and the remark will probably apply to every case in which contagion is concerned. The regular period of maturation, the definite course of actions and metastases, the multiplication of the matter of the disease,—though not all equally cogent as reasons, strongly enforce the same view. The latter phenomenon especially, which has closest relation to some of the natural processes of life, seems insusceptible of other explanation. Admitting then that some animal poisons may enter into the blood without producing such effects, we cannot fairly contemplate the peculiarities of those in question, without seeing that they have their source, as well as actual seat, in the functions of animal life.

Reverting now to the several points stated above, a general remark occurs, that, under admission of the truth of the first, all the others have a natural, or even in part a necessary, dependance upon it. If the morbid actions ensuing upon a virus received are, from any cause, perfectly regular and defined in their ordinary course, it may be inferred as likely, that the susceptibility to undergo them will vary in different persons and at different times;—that any interruption to, or incompleteness of, the regular course of symptoms, may produce disorders of other kind, or liability to the original disease;—and that such diseases, for the most part, must be incompatible mutually, or with other maladies present in the body at the time. These circumstances are sufficiently connected for mutual illustration; though far short of showing in what that remarkable change consists, which, when complete, gives exemption for the remainder of life.

The different degree of susceptibility to these disorders, and their incompatibility mutually, or with other diseases, are points which have been much examined. On the latter subject I will merely remark, that we may in every case conceive incompatibility to depend, either on an inflammatory state of the blood existing at the time, or on some different virus of disease present in the circulation, and producing morbid actions there, which preclude, more or less, any other from coexisting with them. These general questions, important to every part of the subject, are peculiarly interesting in their relation to the history of small-pox, to the modifying action of the vaccine virus, and to the whole theory of inoculation. As such, indeed, they possess a practical importance which belongs to few others in pathology. They have been multiplied in number, and have acquired fresh interest of late years, by the increased spread of small-pox, simple or modified, even among those who have undergone vaccination; giving presumption thereby, that the influence of this preventive may be lost by time, or the vaccine virus itself be altered or impaired by unceasing use and transmission. In the next chapter will be found some remarks on the actual state of these questions; on the probability there may be of solving them; and on the practical deductions which arise out of our present knowledge on the subject. I do not, therefore, enter upon them here, further than to show their general bearing on the topic before us.

Its obscurity, in fact, would be in great part removed, were we ever to obtain an entire solution of these difficulties. If we could prove that the vaccine virus is but a modification of that of small-pox, and show distinctly in what the difference consists, and from what source it arises, we should be gaining a great step in advance. All assured facts as to the duration of the protection by vaccination, the causes which modify this, and the true nature of the varioloid diseases, are of equal value and similar application. The relation of chicken-pox to small-pox, whether a product of the same specific virus, modified by unknown causes in its effects, or of a different virus having some common principle of action,—is another question, less important in practice, but equally bearing on the history and true doctrine of these disorders. And, above all, a knowledge of the circumstances which practically alter the susceptibility to the infection of small-pox, give occasional liability to its recurrence, and regulate the mutual interference of this and other diseases, would seemingly bring us nearest to the principles in the economy of life, which govern these singular morbid phenomena, and determine their permanent effects on the body.

The measles and scarlet-fever afford similar illustrations, though less extended and less striking, from the absence of that singular connexion with another animal virus, which has become so essential a part of the history of small-pox. The scarlet fever, however, has peculiar relations of its own, which long obscured the views of the most observant physicians, led to a disjointed nomenclature of the disease, and even still perplex our opinions on the subject. Limited more than measles or small-pox to one portion of life, it nevertheless is subject to greater irregularities than either of them; appears more frequently in incomplete forms, and seemingly blends itself more readily with other disorders of the body. I have noticed some of these relations in former chapters; and need not recur to them now, except in as far as they are connected with the curious topic of the incomplete or irregular development of this disease.

In speaking of the methods of inquiry as to contagion, I have alluded to the influence which variation in the quantity or concentration of any given virus must have in determining its action on the body.   Among the contagious exanthemata, none illustrates this principle so well as scarlatina.   Looking at the disorders, among children especially, during the seasons when this disease prevails as an epidemic, we find many which strongly warrant the suspicion of their being derived from the same virus; yet so incomplete and irregular in aspect that it is impossible to define them as really forming part of the malady.   A great cause of perplexity here, as in every part of the history of scarlatina, is the peculiar form of cynanche attending it, which occasionally appears as the only distinct evidence of the constitutional disorder.   These deviations from the regular type, if we may thus describe them, occur in several different ways; all familiar to medical experience, though not always viewed in the connexion to which they belong.

One class of these deviations, and the most difficult perhaps to identify, is that of febrile symptoms, generally of adynamic kind, but very irregular in character and progress ;—sometimes a certain degree of angina alone ; often none that is obvious ;—occasionally partial eruptions ; frequently none whatsoever ;—a general disturbance and distress to the habit beyond what the appearances warrant or explain :—all these symptoms occurring during an epidemic, and lingering in the body for a longer or shorter time, but not exceeding the character just described.

A second class of anomalies is that, when succeeding to such irregular symptoms, and without any conformity to the wonted time of maturation, the usual appearances of the disease eventually come on, and pursue the common course, with no deviation sufficient to create doubt as to the identity of the symptoms.   It is frequently difficult in these cases to determine the time between the original infection and the full development of the disorder ; but the interval is occasionally long.   I have known instances where there was reason to suppose it from a month to six weeks.

A third deviation, in some degree a modification of the preceding, is that where the disease, having appeared at the ordinary time, is incomplete in some part of its character, or recedes before it has gone through the usual course ; reappearing some time afterwards without any fresh infection, and being often more regular in type in this latter occurrence than in the first.

A further description of anomalies, much more familiar and not less remarkable than the foregoing, are those where there has been an irregular or incomplete evolution of the disease ; succeeding to which a number of anormal symptoms show themselves; deviating greatly, it may be, from those which were wanting to make up the natural type of the disorder; yet sufficiently akin to them in time and continuity to afford presumption that they are due to the same morbid matter, not sufficiently extricated from the system.   Glandular swellings, abscesses in different parts of the body, eruptions

22*

on the skin, vitiated secretions from the kidneys and bowels, are frequent examples of this nature. Occasionally they take a graver form; affecting, and with fatal issue, organs already disposed to diseased action from other causes. These sequelæ of scarlet fever are familiar in practice; and few cases can be said to be altogether exempt from them. But in their more marked degree they become a distinct object of inquiry; and very interesting, in conjunction with the preceding anomalies, as an exposition of that principle which recognises variations in the action of a virus from quantity, intensity, manner and period of its application, and from the peculiar circumstances of the body at the time.

The illustrations derived from measles are less striking than those just cited as belonging to scarlet fever, but they are of the same character, and affording similar inferences. We have the same ambiguous symptoms, occurring during an epidemic, without actually reaching the authentic form of the malady. We have instances where the disorder supervenes upon these irregular symptoms, but long after the usual time of maturation: and other cases where, after distinctly appearing at the regular period, it recedes too early, and again breaks out after a certain time, without fresh infection, and occasionally more severely than in the first occurrence. Of the latter anomaly I have seen two or three remarkable examples. We have numerous instances again, where the sequelæ of the disease, either from incompleteness in its course, or imperfect separation of the morbid products, are various, protracted, and severe.

Following the subject in such manner of inquiry, we are led to that greater anomaly in these disorders, which applies most directly to the present question, viz., their occasional recurrence in the same individual, from fresh infection, at a time more or less distant· from the original access of the disease. I have already adverted to this in the instance of small-pox, regarded both alone and in its connexion with the practice of vaccination. Scarlatina and measles furnish examples, much less frequent, but often as undoubted in kind. In my own practice I have seen several instances of secondary measles, in which the proofs were unequivocal of prior occurrence; many more in which there was presumption without certainty.* In most of the former cases, evidence existed of some incompleteness in the first course of the disorder; and usually in the catarrhal symptoms, according to the common opinion on the

* Three of these cases happened in the children of one family. The disorder, brought from a school where it was prevailing, affected all three in succession. Though the catarrhal symptoms were slight, it might not have occurred to name any of the cases " *Rubeola sine catarrho*," but for the second appearance of the disease in all. In one it occurred about six weeks afterwards, and without any proof of fresh infection, in a very severe form. In the other cases there were intervals of five and seven years respectively, and proofs of new sources of infection.

In Chapter VII. I have noticed a singular case in which there was evidence of the measles and scarlatina having severally twice occurred to the same individual; the latter each time in close sequel to the former.

subject.   There is more difficulty in obtaining distinct proof as to scarlatina, from its greater variety of aspects, and from the singular manner in which angina sometimes takes place of other symptoms. The examples, however, are indisputable, and not infrequent.*   If we admit, as must be done, that the protection given by the first occurrence of the disease is often incomplete, it seems probable, from observation, that these affections of the throat are the most frequent form of the secondary disorder.   Were cases of this nature admitted, in which there is strong presumption of the same virus acting on a susceptibility lessened but not extinct, the record would become more frequent than at present; and, wherever authenticated, singularly instructive in this part of pathology.

These anomalies in fact (if they can strictly be called such), and especially that last mentioned, are the channels through which we seem to make nearest approach to the truth.   The exceptions, as in so many other cases in science, become the best exponents of the nature of the law.   Though failing to give intimate or exact knowledge, they point out the direction in which it lies, and the most expedient methods of pursuing it.

The same remark applies to another class of facts, already named as one of the bases of all reasoning on the subject ; viz., the varying liability of the same person at different times to these diseases; and the apparent insusceptibility of some persons to receive a particular disease at any time of life.   Medical experience furnishes daily examples of these facts, infinitely varied in form and degree.   In the case of the small-pox they are most distinct to observation ; testified by an hereditary disposition to receive the malady, and evolve it in the gravest form ; or even by fresh infection to undergo it a second time ; for so alone can we interpret those singular instances, where many children in the same family have been subject to recurrence of the disease.   The scarlet fever and measles afford similar instances, though more obscure from the causes already noted.

The admission of an hereditary tendency towards these disorders is a very important point in the question.   Extending, as it may do in strict accordance with the analogy of other hereditary affections, to communities as well as families, it solves many seeming anomalies in disease, by connecting them with the more general laws of life. And it helps us in some part to explain the insusceptibility, as well as the proneness, to the particular disorders before us.   Though without any distinct proof of protection being given to the child by the previous state of the parent, yet is it intelligible from analogy that this may have occasional influence through a part of life ;— and further, that the condition of habit giving partial immunity against a disease, or rendering it less violent in its symptoms, may extend even to races of men, and be widely diffused by descent.

* To some of my readers the instance may be known of a late physician, eminent for his learning, who underwent the scarlet fever three times ; probably from some peculiarity of habit in reference to the disease.

We are not entitled upon actual knowledge to proceed far in this speculation. The inference, however, in the first case is supported by the frequent insusceptibility during childhood; and, in the second, by the numerous and remarkable facts which show a varying liability, in different communities and at different periods, to receive these diseases, especially in their severer forms;—circumstances which cannot be adequately explained by changes in the virus alone. I need but refer to the evidence we have of their extraordinary virulence, when appearing for the first time in particular localities; and to the proofs (sufficient undoubtedly to reason upon) that the small-pox in particular had a more fatal character one or two centuries ago than at the present time.* Even the severe epidemic form which the disorder assumes in any community, at certain and often distant periods, is not without application to the argument, though depending chiefly perhaps on temporary causes.

Among other deductions from the above premises is the inference that the change from complete liability to immunity is not always perfected at once, but admits of great modification under the causes creating it; or, as may more explicitly be stated, from variations in that state of body in which the liability consists. This is manifestly an important condition in regard to the diseases we are considering; and insufficiently recognised in the ordinary manner of viewing them. Not two states alone are involved, but several probably, in passing between the two extremes. It may be that these states are continuous, graduating into one another; or we may regard them, on the contrary, as separate and definite physical conditions, each liable in different manner or degree to the action of a given virus of disease. There is no certain evidence on which to affirm either opinion. But, however the reality may be, we are obviously engaged here with those phenomena which form the foundation of the knowledge we seek for; a conclusion further arising from the concurrence of so many separate views in the same direction of research, and from the singular uniformity even in the difficulties they present.

---

* Striking examples may be found in the narratives we have of the first introduction of the small-pox and measles into some of the South Sea Islands. A melancholy illustration occurred to my own notice in the case of the King and Queen of the Sandwich Isles, and their seven native attendants, when they visited England fifteen years ago. I attended them, with Sir Henry Halford, during the measles by which they were attacked soon after their arrival in London. The disease in all showed a malignant violence of which the examples are rare in this country. Medical treatment was greatly impeded by the almost total want of means of communication; and in the cases of the King and Queen (both of whom died) was rendered utterly unavailing by the violence of delirium, which overpowered all those placed in watch over them, and led to excesses contributing doubtless to the event.

I may mention as a particular instance, not generally known, of the virulence of the small-pox when invading a country after a long interval of exemption, that in 1707 nearly 16,000 persons perished from this disease in Iceland, the whole population at that time not exceeding 65,000 souls. The measles, also, has occasionally been very fatal as an epidemic in this island.

We recur then now (with whatever aid these considerations may afford us) to the question; in what the physical changes consist which thus give protection,—partial or complete—temporary or lasting—against a particular disease, without producing obvious effect on other parts of the animal economy? Their reality must be admitted, for without them exemption or liability would become mere abstractions, and all other facts in the history of the disorders be equally annulled. Have we then any sufficient proofs by which to refer them to a particular part of bodily organization, or analogy by which to explain their nature, duration, or difference in degree?

It must fairly be avowed that no facts or analogies we possess will carry us beyond the views already attained. I have pointed out in succession those parts in the acknowledged history of these diseases which seem to bear most closely on the mystery they involve. But none of them go far enough to disclose it; nor are there other physical phenomena which can throw light upon changes, the result indeed of morbid action, but intimately blended with all the most essential functions of life.

If an opinion were hazarded on a part of this question, when the whole is so obscure, it might be one which looks to the blood as the actual seat of these singular changes. We have already seen the probability that this is the agent in the maturation of the virus received, and in the series of phenomena which form the obvious character of each disease. Though we cannot, even from such admission, derive any certain argument for the ulterior conclusion just named, yet does it find support, as a presumption at least, from some of the reasons previously employed. It is not unreasonable to suppose that the medium, through which this train of actions is carried on, may be that in which their effects are principally and permanently testified. All these circumstances which show varying susceptibility to a given infection, and the phenomena indicating a partial protection from a disorder imperfectly evolved, may best be thus conceived, however imperfect the inference when pursued into details. We are entitled, indeed, to put the same question as before.—In what other portion of the body the alterations, needful to the effect, can be presumed so likely to take place? We cannot suppose the skin, or other membranes, to have become impermeable to the infecting virus; since, in some at least of these diseases, the direct introduction of the matter into the circulation does not reproduce them after having once occurred. The eruptive part of the disorders, whatever its importance in a pathological point of view, affords no argument as to the seat of the changes in question;—or, rather, in the recognised fact that one or two perfect pustules may denote complete protection against small-pox, gives proof that these external textures are not to be so considered. No other organ or part of the body affords the slightest scope for explanation; nor can we shelter our ignorance under any vague appeal to the nervous influence or the powers of life, so often employed when no clear interpretation is at hand.

It must be owned that the preceding supposition as to the blood does not advance us a step beyond; or enable us, even remotely, to surmise the nature of an alteration producing this effect, and none other that is apparent besides. Nevertheless, if there be any portion of the living frame capable of answering to this condition, it is assuredly the blood; the remarkable composition of which fluid, its peculiar vital properties, its alteration at different periods of life, and its great liability to be affected by transient causes of disturbance,—all warrant the conception of changes in its state, numerous, definite, and even of long duration, though wholly inaccessible to our present means of research.

In the preceding remarks I have not adverted to that curious point in the history of diseases under review,—the question, namely, whether there is any certain record of them in the ancient writers on physic; or, if not, what is the earliest authentic date of their appearance amongst us? For obvious reasons the small-pox has chiefly given foundation to the inquiry. Without entering into details of a controversy so familiar, I must confess my own persuasion that we have no adequate proof of this disease having been known to the Greek or Roman physicians. Its specific and strongly marked characters,—the proportion of mortality it inflicts,—and its frequent diffusion under a virulent epidemic form,—would all seem to require a description more precise than any which have been quoted from antiquity. Admitting the account of Rhazes as the first that has any certain application to the disease, it is undoubtedly difficult to conceive why it should then have appeared in this part of the world for the first time, yet is the fact not really more obscure than many other points in the history of these contagious epidemics. Their original generation among mankind is the great mystery of the case, to which all others are subordinate.

Reviewing the whole of this inquiry, the following inferences, whatever their respective truth or probability, may be admitted, as giving a more distinct form to the various arguments it involves.*

First, That the series of actions or changes, constituting these diseases, have their seat in the blood, and are carried on throughout by the circulation.

Secondly, That, although we have no cognisance of the actual physical state or changes which give protection against their occurrence, or recurrence, there is more reason for seeking these in an altered state of the blood than in any other part of the animal organization.

---

* In stating these conclusions I still refer chiefly to the three great diseases of this class. The difficulty has already been mentioned of giving the hooping-cough any common place with them, even under admission of its infectious nature, and of the peculiar character which the title of the Chapter conveys. The fact of exemption from a second occurrence of the disorder is indeed much more doubtful in this case; and what appears such, may be often merely the effect of different time of life in altering the liability to the morbid cause; or giving it direction to other parts of the body, and thereby changing the whole aspect of the symptoms. The latter view, under a more general application, has been repeatedly noticed, as sanctioned by various facts, and leading to many curious inferences.

Thirdly, That the conditions which render one disease incompatible with another,—or produce the various results of their mutual interference,—or limit to man their production and development,—all probability depend on the same physical principles as the simpler fact of immunity, and have equally their source and seat in the blood.

Fourthly, That the state of immunity, on whatever bodily conditions it depends, is liable to fluctuation in various ways;—often partial and imperfect when first obtained,—occasionally diminished or lost by time, even where there is presumption of its having been most complete at first,—possibly affected in some degree, and after a certain lapse of time, in all;—the rate of such changes different in different persons, and modified also by the access of other diseases, or by the contingencies of life.

Fifthly, That a constitutional or hereditary tendency exists throughout all these phenomena;—modifying susceptibility,—determining, in conjunction with other causes, the regular or irregular course of the disease,—affecting its degree of virulence,—and giving liability to its recurrence; and that this habit of body is not limited to families, but extends even to larger communities.

Sixthly, That the several modifications, above named, depend further on the quality or quantity of the virus received in each case;—conditions admitting of being infinitely varied; and giving, in conjunction with the effects of season, locality, and human constitution, the peculiar character which every epidemic more or less assumes.

Other inferences might be specified; but the foregoing embrace all that are more important in the general view I have taken of a subject, thus endless in its details, and in the hypotheses to which it has led. Though speculative in several points, (an inevitable result of their nature,) yet will they be found applicable in various ways to the questions contained in the next Chapter; and these are by far the most important and interesting of the practical deductions to which they direct us.

CHAPTER XXV.

ON THE PRESENT QUESTIONS REGARDING VACCINATION.

Two classes of questions suggest themselves on this topic: those, first, which regard the history and theory of vaccination in its relation to small-pox;—secondly, those founded on the former, but of greater practical interest, which respect its manner of use, the sources of error or ambiguity, and the guidance which every medical man in his own sphere is bound to give to public opinion and feeling on the subject. So much has been written on these questions since the beginning of the century, that the only excuse for any addition is the need of keeping them clearly and constantly in view ;—at a time, especially, when the numerous and increasing failures in vaccination have brought public distrust on the practice ; and even led many medical men to waver in their judgment on the greatest of all the specifics yet discovered for the prevention of disease.

In the preceding Chapter I have alluded to the first of these topics, in connexion with a class of diseases of which small-pox is by far the most remarkable example. The questions arising here have hitherto been multiplied, rather than lessened, by time. They are of singular interest as a branch of medical history, involving points which great learning and sagacity have been directed to explain. That success has not yet been more complete, is less a reproach to the science, than an illustration of the difficulties which surround it, and of the peculiarity of the evidence needful to overcome them. Happily, however, for a subject thus important to human welfare, these difficulties are not of a nature insuperable by research. On the contrary, we have reason to presume that much which is of greatest practical concern will hereafter be solved, either by direct experiment, or by those averages of observation, the extension and increasing exactness of which have peculiar value in this manner of application.*

The physical relation of the vaccine disease to small-pox stands at the head of these inquiries, though of less practical moment than some of the rest. The question may be put distinctly, as one of identity or otherwise, and in this light it has for the most part been treated. A fair view of the whole evidence must lead us to consider the result as still undetermined. If it could be shown, even in a limited number of cases, that the diseases are thoroughly interchangeable,—the virus of small-pox becoming vaccine matter in passing through the cow, and the vaccine lymph producing a true variolous disorder,—the question would be closed in favour of those who maintain this identity, in accordance with the opinion of Jenner himself. But we must admit that these effects, though alleged to exist, are not uniform enough, or sufficiently verified by repetition, to authorize entire belief. An argument on the same side has been derived from the approach of the two disorders to a common character, both of eruptive and constitutional affection, when the small-pox has been modified by repeated inoculation, and the vaccine disease assumes its most virulent form. And such evidence may be enlarged by taking the varioloid disorder as another example of this common character, representing a state in which the protection against the small-pox has been imperfectly given, or is partially

* Those who desire to study these topics in their whole extent, and from the best sources of information, will do well on this account, as on every other, to peruse Dr. Baron's Life of Jenner, lately completed ; a very valuable addition to our medical literature.

worn away. These concurrences afford presumption, but do not reach to certainty.

The protection afforded by vaccination, though it may be admitted as another argument of identity, and was so received by Dr. Jenner, is far from amounting to proof of it. There is no reason to our comprehension why changes to this effect, but of the nature of which we are ignorant, may not as well be produced by a separate agent, as by a modification of that against which protection is sought. The true difficulty is in conceiving how the immunity should exist at all. Thus reasoning, we do not disprove the singular relation between the two forms of disease, so strikingly attested by the simple fact of this exemption given; but merely affirm that it does not amount to that unequivocal proof of identity of which we are in search.

The next question, not wholly settled, regards the nature of those disorders, termed varioloid or modified small-pox; chiefly occurring where vaccination has been previously undergone, and explained by supposing its original influence imperfect, or impaired by time. They have great interest, whether we look to the general theory of the contagious exanthemata, to the history of small-pox, or to the conditions which determine and attest the action of the vaccine virus on the human habit. The term of modified small-pox is probably just, as denoting a disease really altered in degree, and in the regularity of its progress, by certain previous changes in the body; which, if more complete, are capable of preventing its reception, or arresting it in the outset. The question, however, occurs, whether there may not be a true varioloid or modified virus, produced perhaps by the causes just named, but definite in itself, and proper to the epidemics which bear this character. Though it is not easy to obtain unequivocal proof, yet the presumption becomes strong against this view, from the facts, that the small-pox is actually prevalent during all such epidemics;—that the varioloid disease is produced by its contagion, and is capable frequently of reproducing it;—and that there is a regular gradation from the most severe forms of one disorder to the mildest aspects of the other.

That the varioloid matter does not always produce the small-pox by inoculation, in those liable to it, may be attributed to the different degree and rate of maturation in these cases making it requisite to select, not only the particular case, but even the pustule from which matter is taken. This circumstance well merits attentive discrimination; denoting, as it does, the conditions of which we are more particularly in quest, for the enlargement of our knowledge on these topics.

The relation of the chicken-pox, and some other pustular disorders, to small-pox, is a further point tending to complicate the subject, by adding another question as to identity, not yet finally settled. The prevalent opinion, influenced by that of Heberden, Willan, and other eminent physicians, is that of a specific difference between the diseases; and, notwithstanding some powerful advocacy to the contrary, this view seems, on the whole, the most probable.* All proofs, however,—whether from the results of inoculation, or from observations as to reciprocal protection, or from the relations of the two disorders as epidemics,—are still imperfect; and rendered doubly obscure by the introduction of the varioloid disease as a new element in the question. It requires singular sagacity in research, and a just appreciation of the nature of medical evidence, to discriminate among these pustular and vesicular disorders, which thus multiply before us; and to decide what is specific difference, what simple modification of a common cause. Not merely particular facts, but principles, are in question here; as universal as the doctrines of fever and inflammation in their application to pathology, and not less difficult of interpretation to our present knowledge.†

The questions already stated bring us to those which regard the completeness of vaccination as a preventive remedy,—the duration of its protecting power in the body,—and the changes its virus may undergo by long use and frequent transmission;—the most momentous by far of all the inquiries affecting the subject. The events of the last ten or fifteen years have forced them strongly upon us; while apparently at the same time preparing evidence for their final determination. Not only in Great Britain, but throughout every part of the globe from which we have records, we find that small-pox has been gradually increasing again in frequency as an epidemic; affecting a larger proportion of the vaccinated; and inflicting greater mortality in its results. I do not enter into any detail of these facts, as they are now generally admitted.‡ Even while writing these remarks, fresh testimonies occur to my notice, coming from different sources. We can no longer deny the likelihood that the protection given by vaccination is unequal in different cases, or that it may be lessened or lost by time. Experience has here confirmed a presumption, which some ventured very early to entertain, and which indeed was sanctioned, prior to experience, by

* Dr. John Thomson is well known as the most able modern advocate of the identity of these disorders. See his Historical Sketch of the Small-pox; published at a time when all opinions were perplexed by the varioloid epidemic, which had recently occurred with such severity in Scotland, and in many other parts of the world.

† The abstruse question as to what constitutes actual identity, and what specific difference, runs through every part of this subject; and the attempts at definition, as in so many other cases, have but more perplexed it. Variation in the degree of action of a given virus is intelligible, and we know it to be capable of producing a very different aspect of symptoms. But when diversity of aspect is not only well defined, but habitual and lasting, we cannot any longer rightly apply the term of identity; and it becomes needful to interpret the occasional appearances of this, rather as exceptions than proofs.

‡ The evidence furnished from some of the German States, from Denmark, and Sweden, has peculiar value in its completeness, and in the statistical form given to all the results; conditions which, from various causes, are much less easy of attainment in this country.

various considerations. Among the latter may be mentioned the seeming impairment from time of the intensity of certain other animal poisons, and even of that of small-pox itself;—a circumstance, if rightly established, of great interest to the subject, and illustrating many obscure points of general pathology.

The early enthusiasm for the great discovery of Jenner swept these doubts away; and they returned only tardily, and under the compulsion of facts. Other questions, intimately connected with the preceding, went through a similar course. The variations in the vaccine lymph itself, at first only partially seen or understood, became more strongly attested by frequent irregularities in the vesicle, and by failures of protection, before the influence was likely to have been weakened or lost by time. Whether the result of casual causes, or of more general changes affecting its action on the body, it could no longer be doubted that the immunity given was less generally perfect in kind and degree. Any explanation of the fact, from the ignorant or imperfect performance of vaccination in the outset of the practice, was found insufficient to meet the number and variety of the proofs. And, though more palpable at one time than another, according to the greater or less prevalence of epidemic causes, yet every succeeding year has multiplied them, and every statement from other countries attested their truth.

These facts in the recent history of vaccination are familiar; but they need to be kept distinctly before us, in a matter of such deep concernment to human welfare. No causes can well be conceived for the changes just denoted, and still apparently in progress, but the two already specified;—either an alteration taking place in that state of body, whatever it be, which constitutes the protection originally given;—or some diminished efficacy of the vaccine matter in general use, from time, repeated transmission by inoculation, or other less obvious causes. These conditions, indeed, are not mere alternatives to each other. They are perfectly compatible; and, as far as we can see, likely to act concurrently in a great variety of cases. Each manner of change is highly probable, not merely in the explanation it affords of the remarkable results in question, but even as naturally according with other facts in the animal economy and history of disease. In the last chapter I have dwelt more at large on these general relations. They bring testimony to one point, very important in the argument, viz., that the small-pox itself furnishes analogy for both the conditions we are examining;—its recurrence giving cause to suppose the state of protection to be occasionally altered or effaced by time;—and the virus itself being liable apparently to similar changes; though perhaps, from its greater intensity, less frequent in occurrence, or slower in their rate of progress.

Impossible, indeed, though we have found it to understand, in what this physical state of immunity consists, there is equal difficulty in conceiving it to remain unaffected by the changes which age, habits of life, and diseases bring upon the body. This argu-

ment professes no explanation, and leaves undefined the time requisite for such changes.   It simply affirms as more likely, from
analogy, that the protective influence should gradually decay, than
remain ever complete as at first.   Recognising the principle, long
averages of observation may decide the question as to time; with
admission always that, even where protection is continued generally
for the whole of life, the same principle of decay may yet be in
operation; though too tardily to show itself, as in other cases, by
the recurrence of the disease.   The latter point, though but a presumption, requires notice in the argument.

Some authors have ventured surmises respecting the duration of
the vaccine influence in the body, but on grounds hitherto insufficient for proof.   The inquiry, indeed, is made more difficult by the
doubts existing as to the lymph now in common use; but, if happily
hereafter the sources of vaccination should become better assured,
we may reasonably hope to generalise what is now a broken series
of perplexing and contradictory facts.   There is cause to believe
that in some instances the protection has been extended over a
period of thirty-five years; but the average duration of that which
is completely effective must be rated far below this mark.*   It has
been a question naturally occurring, whether its diminished influence is in any general proportion to the interval of time succeeding
vaccination.   The documents obtained in England and elsewhere,
as well as the results of revaccination, favour the idea that such
proportion exists; probably not with any exact uniformity of rate,
but determined in part by causes intermediately affecting the body.
These documents concur in showing a maximum in the number of
small-pox cases after vaccination, from the age of fifteen to twenty-
five;—few before ten years of age;—and a diminishing number.
after twenty-five, as might be inferred- from other considerations.
This at present seems the utmost extent of our knowledge on the
subject.†

Respecting the second presumed cause of failure, viz., that arising
from changes in the general quality of the vaccine virus itself, this
has already been mentioned as an inference strongly supported by
all the facts and analogies we possess.   We cannot, it must be
owned, explain how a long series of transmissions through the
human body should alter its qualities or enfeeble its power. But,
in our ignorance of these conditions, it is easier to conceive their
occurrence, than that the active cause should continue unaltered,
through circumstances so various and multiplied as this transmission implies.   We have argument to the same effect in the fact that

* Dr. Copland, whose medical learning gives great value to all his opinions,
early entertained belief of the temporary influence of vaccination; limiting the
time of entire protection to seven or eight years, and that of partial protection to
somewhat more than twice this period.

† The table published by Dr. Gregory in 1823, very valuable as a document at
that time, has since been confirmed and greatly extended by similar documents
from other parts of Europe. .

the eruption is more strongly marked, and the constitutional affection greater, where vaccination is performed with lymph fresh from the cow. And, to this conceivable degeneration from what may be termed natural causes in the body, we have to add the perpetual casualties of matter incompletely matured, vitiated by the concurrence of other disease, inadequately preserved, or imperfectly applied;—all obvious sources of change in the material agent of protection; and sufficient, in conjunction with the other cause assigned, to explain the diminished security by which our opinions and practice are now perplexed.

The second class of questions before us relates to the practical methods which may best be employed to obviate these evils, and to restore and sustain the influence of vaccination; making it better correspond with the anticipation which attended its early reception in the world. That this object is attainable there is much reason to presume. That it is most desirable none can doubt, but those who look vaguely over the surface of events, or allow themselves to be confounded by difficulties, without the will or ability to obviate them.

Some authors, indeed, have argued against vaccination, not so much from its failures, but because they regard the protection it affords as merely giving greater scope to the ingress of other contagious diseases, coming into action to fill the void of mortality thus made. I know nothing which can sanction this gloomy inference. It is true that the press and struggle of a crowded world may generate various evils, of which disease and mortality are the earliest and most certain effects;—these circumstances (now closely weighed by political economists) demanding occasional legislation, as well as the more general discipline of social life. But we have no reason to suppose the express substitution of one set of diseases for another in this case; nor any just motive for relaxing in our efforts to eradicate an evil, of which experience has so thoroughly defined the nature and amount.*

The argument for the continued use of vaccination would indeed be valid, even had we no hope of raising its benefits beyond their present limit. While yet we can protect in the majority of cases, and so greatly modify a dangerous disease in the rest, we are not entitled to disparage this certain good, or to neglect the means of preserving it. But we have assurance here, better warranted than in most other parts of medical science, that our progress may go further; restoring the higher security which has been lost, and probably suggesting methods of maintaining it more perfectly for the future.

Of the means for this end, four may distinctly be cited as the most important and specific. First, the obtaining fresh and genuine

* The opinion of some German physicians, that the scrofulous diathesis has taken place of that of scurvy in the general character of the European constitution, would have important application, if well founded, to almost all diseases ; but no especial reference to the view stated above.

vaccine lymph from its source. Secondly, revaccination at certain periods, and the determination of the times best fitted for this. Thirdly, improvement in the methods and tests of perfect vaccination. And, fourthly, the influence, moral or otherwise, which is needful with the world, to obtain a more complete and exclusive use of this preventive remedy.

The first of these objects in order is perhaps so in importance also. The facts to which we have referred, as multiplying everywhere around us, make it highly expedient, or even necessary, to replace the vaccine matter now in circulation; which has certainly lost the uniformity, and perhaps, to a great extent, the purity essential to the highest degree of protective power. Unhappily, the means of attaining this object have not corresponded with its urgency, or with the common impression prevailing on the subject. In England, as in other parts of the world, there has been found an unexpected difficulty in recovering the genuine vaccine lymph. The disease is not only rarer among cows than it was presumed to be, but blended in them with other pustules and vesicular diseases: several of these affecting the human subject with a spurious pock; others incommunicable; but all adding to the embarrassment of the research.

· These diversities of eruption, as well as those separately occurring in the human subject, place us in what may well be termed a wilderness of such disorders, from which nothing but the most exact observation can wholly extricate us.* With the certainty, however, that the true cow-pox still exists, (and in some countries, it is alleged, more frequently than other particular diseases of the cow,) it is clear that we may with care eventually refresh or replace the stock of lymph now in use. It has, in truth, already performed a vast and wonderful work among mankind;—far more remarkable in the amount and continuity of success, than from the anomalies or failures which have occurred to interrupt the progress of its effects.

It seems desirable that the supply of new lymph should be from several separate sources, provided each of these is thoroughly authenticated by observers and experiments worthy of credit. The need of the latter caution is obvious; particularly at a time when conviction of the importance of the object is likely to lead many into the research. An error in ordinary vaccination may be of little import, and limited in its effects to a single case. But here, where the great object is to identify and obtain in its purest form the subtle agent with which we have to work, ignorance or incaution may bring in a wider and more serious mischief. This suggestion is further warranted by the actual difficulty of all such experiments, proved in those recently made for the purpose of comparing the effects of lymph direct from the cow with that taken from man. The conditions to be observed are so numerous, the diversity of

---

* The sagacity of Jenner led him to foresee some of these eventual difficulties, as well as to distinguish certain spurious forms of vaccine disorder, checking and embarrassing the course of his own researches.

results so considerable from slight deviations in the manner of experiment, that none but those possessing experience and sagacity can be trusted with these observations. The greater difficulty of obtaining proper pustules by lymph fresh from the cow, than by that which has passed through the human body, is itself an unexpected source of perplexity or error. And the case altogether is one where results obtained from dubious sources are more likely to retard than advance the great object in view.*

The second of the objects that have been named, revaccination, though unquestionable as a source of security, yet labours under some of the difficulties which belong to this subject in every part. The principle of the practice is obvious, and applying expressly to those deficiencies which we have cause to suspect in the results of vaccination. The value of the protection given by the latter is the argument for whatever may make it more certain and permanent through life. Whether applied as a general test, or to remove some more explicit doubt, or to sustain a security supposed liable to decay, equally is revaccination admissible or expedient. And in reference to the latter point, if the fact is admitted on the grounds before alleged, expediency rises into necessity, as expressing the sole means we possess for obviating this decay, and restoring the protection originally given.

The doubts connected with revaccination arise in part out of the circumstances which authorize and give value to it. The most obvious of these regard the time and frequency of repetition, and the nature and certainty of the tests thereby furnished. For the former of these points, especially, large averages are needful; such as it is difficult, from various causes, to obtain in this country; and which presumably require to complete them, a longer time than has yet elapsed since the discovery of the remedy. The general rule must clearly be founded on the duration of the protective power, in whatsoever way determined; and the results already mentioned are consistent enough to warrant their being appealed to in this view. It is obviously, however, the maximum of interval we are to consider as thus indicated. Revaccination should precede the time when protection has ceased, or is so far diminished as to allow the access of the varioloid disease. Nor have we any assured reason to give why it should not be performed still earlier, and repeated at stated periods, as many have proposed. , Some hypothetical objections may be entertained on physical grounds; and averages show that it rarely takes effect within a certain period after vaccination. But the only motive of much weight against the practice is the expediency of establishing such distinct relation between the object in view, and the means of attaining it, as may

* It is gratifying to know that the sedulous endeavours of my friend Mr. Estlin, of Bristol, to obtain fresh vaccine matter from the cow, have been successful in the event. His letters in the Medical Gazette of September 15th and October 20th, 1838, are very valuable; not solely in the statement of the fact, but also in that of the proofs by which it has thus far been substantiated.

best insure the general adoption of the remedy. In the state of society in this country, revaccination, if often called for, would incur much risk of being omitted altogether.

On the latter consideration, omitting others, it becomes of consequence to define the best period for a practice unequivocally desirable at one time or another. And, reviewing all that has yet been learnt on the subject, I am led to believe that where there is fair proof of the original vaccination being perfect in kind, the period best to be selected for repetition is that from ten to twelve years of age ;—a time anterior to the more explicit changes of puberty, and preceding the age at which the liability to small-pox is shown by averages to be again most frequently renewed. Future facts may modify or alter this view ; but meanwhile it appears to be sanctioned by the evidence we possess, and is liable to no risk of inflicting injury, even if hereafter found to be less expedient than some other yet undetermined. And it may be added, that revaccination, securely performed at the period named, might possibly render any further repetition needless ; such inference being drawn from the tables in our hands, and from the general fact of liability to small-pox diminishing as life proceeds. It must be admitted, however, as still more open to future corrections than the former, and can only indeed be determined by time.

In the case of adult revaccination, a caution occurs as to the further use of lymph derived from this source, under the contingency of its being vitiated by other animal poisons or morbid humours which have been evolved in, or obtained previous access to, the body. The point is one not easily solved, seeing our ignorance of the nature, connexion, and possible combination of these subtle agents. I am not aware of any proof of positive evils thus produced ; but, as we know the action of the vaccine lymph to be impaired or prevented by various morbid causes present in the body, we have reason to consider it an expedient general rule that its supply should be maintained from the vaccination of early life, rather than from that of adult age, when more disturbing causes may be presumed to exist.

The third object pointed out for further research is very comprehensive as well as important; including all that relates to the actual practice of vaccination, the modes of rendering it most complete, and the tests of its being so. The limited purpose of this chapter will not allow more than a mere specification of the principal points ; each one of which has been the subject of much discussion ; and many, it must be owned, without any result determinate enough to satisfy the doubts from which controversy has arisen.

One of these doubts regards the time when the first vaccination may best be performed. It has been held by some that the full susceptibility to the disorder does not usually exist in early infancy, but is gradually developed ; on the same principle as at later periods of life it declines in various contagious diseases of the same class. If this be true, it is so only under numerous exceptions; and experience, I think, shows that we cannot greatly err in taking the age of two or three months as the fittest;—avoiding thereby, on the one hand, the rashes and bowel disorders which often occur in the first weeks of life;—on the other, the period of teething and the various febrile irritations which attend it;—while at the same time not unduly exposing the child to the intermediate risk of small-pox.

This practical question, as to the particular time of vaccination, requires to be carried into many details upon which our knowledge is yet imperfect. If there are states of the body which wholly prevent the disorder, it is clear that there must be others, varying perhaps only in degree, which permit a certain development, but make the result imperfect for protection. We have reason to suppose that this modified cow-pox may occur of different kinds and degrees. Its existence implies the need (not simply for the individual, but for those to whom in succession the lymph is conveyed) that much watchfulness should be given to vaccinate only when the body is free from obvious disorder. A febrile condition, from whatever cause produced, might be conjectured, and appears actually to be, the state most interfering with the completeness of the changes sought for. Hereditary temperament, such as that of scrofula, cannot of course be submitted to the above rule, further than as prohibiting vaccination at any time when showing itself in the form of actual disease.

All these views are familiar, but they require constant enforcement in practice. And experience shows that we are not to disregard conditions seemingly much more remote: such, for example, as the influence of a hot season in producing an irregular acceleration of the course of the disorder, of which sufficient testimony has been given as an occasional occurrence.

From the same cause of their familiarity I need not dwell on other details belonging to the practice of vaccination; viz., the selection of lymph from right sources;—the proper methods of its preservation;—the particular manner of its insertion;—the tests to be taken during the advancement of the pustules, and the marks by which to prove their completeness;—the time for obtaining lymph from them, and the proper limit to the quantity so removed;—the indications to be derived from the vaccine cicatrix, &c. We have by no means acquired equal certitude on these several points, but all are open to exact observation and averages of effect; and they are so connected, that attainment of knowledge in one point will generally facilitate it in another.

Among the questions, yet uncertain, we may reckon that of the number of punctures and insertions of matter best fitted for security. There are other objects, perhaps, not sufficiently adverted to; such as the importance of securing at least one pustule perfect in all its characters;—the presumption that it is desirable to leave one untouched by the lancet;—and the uncertainty of the proofs derived from the marks of former vaccination as to any present state of immunity.   On all these points, however, our practice in vaccination is gradually perfecting itself; and there is much cause to hope that eventually none will be left uncertain either in principle or application.

The summary given of the principal objects now present to us, on the subject of vaccination, leads to the fourth consideration proposed; viz., how most effectually, under present circumstances, the medical man may use his influence with the public around him, in maintaining and extending the practice, and thereby preventing the impairment of the great good that has been gained to the world.

The circumstances of late years have greatly changed the aspect of all that relates to this question.   Opinion needs to be retrieved, and new views to be suggested, under the disadvantage of recalling in part those formerly enforced.   For a certain period the profession and the public stood in a sort of opposition to each other; the former seeking (conscientiously at all events, and perhaps rightly, while the proofs were still thus incomplete) to erase the impression made by frequent failures in vaccination, and the increasing spread of small-pox.   The argument, strong at first in plausible explanation, became gradually more equivocal; and at length so reduced by concessions, as greatly to impair its influence on the public and even to react unfavourably on the minds of those who employed it. This change of relative position, and the increasing certainty as to facts before ambiguous or but suspected, require an altered dealing with those whose conviction must be obtained to insure the good in which they have such deep concern.   It is no longer expedient, in any sense, to argue for the present practice of vaccination as a certain or permanent preventive of small-pox.   The truth must be told, as it is, that the earlier anticipations on this point have not been realised.   And if fairly told, with the just conclusions annexed to it, the result is likely to be far better than can arise from a lingering dispute, on grounds no longer tenable even by the most zealous in the cause.   For the argument on behalf of vaccination, though modified, is in nowise forfeited.   The evil to be overcome is the same; still present among us; and capable of being more widely extended.   The protection given by the first vaccination appears liable to decay with time, and the vaccine lymph itself is probably susceptible of change and deterioration. But for these defaults we have remedy at hand in revaccination duly performed, and in fresh matter obtained from the cow;— means adequate, as far as we can see, to repair the deficiency, and render more lasting the immunity, which, even in its partial form, has been, and yet is, so great a blessing to the world.

Greater knowledge of the facts, and the habit of weighing them has familiarized the minds of intelligent medical men with this view; but it needs judgment and perseverance to convey it clearly and effectually to those around.   No long or laboured argument is of much avail here.   The points must be put simply and concisely; in such way, if possible, as not merely to convince at the moment, but to be readily retained and made instrumental in carrying the conviction to others. Were I to suggest any manner of reasoning, most generally effective for these objects, and best according with the truth of facts, it would be some such as the following:—" Your child is at this moment liable to a dangerous and loathsome disease. If you inoculate him for small-pox, you give the disease in a milder form indeed, but always distressing, sometimes fatal, and not absolutely certain as a safeguard against recurrence. If you vaccinate, you afford him, without pain or risk of any kind, protection probably complete for a period of years; capable of being readily renewed; and, when failing of completeness, greatly mitigating the severity of the disorder."

To some persons the motive may be added, that by inoculation for the small-pox they become a party to keeping this poison still in the world. But practically it may be found better to limit the reasoning as stated above. And the argument for revaccination, as the facts now stand, may be enforced in the same sense. " Your child has had perfect protection for a certain period of life. There is cause from experience to presume that this protection is now drawing to an end, or perhaps is altogether lost. By revaccination you renew it, if renewal be required, without risk, suffering, or the confinement of a single hour."

In this country, where legislative enactment and civil authority cannot be employed to insure vaccination, we have no effectual way of dealing with the great body of the people but through the intervention and example of the upper classes;—another sufficient reason for seeking by every means to procure their conviction, and on grounds which may not be shaken by occasional failures in the object. Whether through increase of this influence, aided by the successful pursuit of the objects before adverted to, the small-pox may ever be wholly eradicated, is a very doubtful question, and the probability on the negative side. But this does not alter the course to be pursued. We are bound to strive after as much good as we can; with the almost certain assurance of its being capable of extension beyond the present limit, and of being rendered more secure by improved methods of practice.

In these remarks on the questions which now exist respecting vaccination, I have sought to follow the inquiry even to the most recent period; having regard in this to the numerous researches which are continually in progress. Of late, indeed, attention to the subject has been singularly awakened; and even while writing, I observe new sources of information opened, and the results of more extended averages brought before the world.* They authorize, as

* Some of the most valuable of these documents we owe to the active zeal and intelligence of our German brethren. The work of Dr. Heim on the state of vaccination in the kingdom of Wirtemberg is the subject of an excellent article in the British and Foreign Medical Review, from which its importance, as a part of this inquiry, may safely be inferred. The Prussian Reports on re-

far as I can judge, the method of viewing the subject adopted above, and the practical conclusions I have sought to enforce. These are not new, and they may have been urged before with greater weight of details.   But, if they have just foundation, the importance is obvious of keeping them before us in a single and connected view; and to this point I have chiefly attended throughout the foregoing observations.

CHAPTER XXVI.

ON THE USE OF OPIATES.

THE manner of employing opium in modern practice might, until very lately, have been cited among the many examples of perverse changes of fashion as to particular remedies and methods of treatment.   All that tended to increase the credit and use of purgative medicines lessened for a time, in the same ratio, the reputation and employment of this remedy. A contradiction was presumed, greater than actually exists, between the two modes of treatment. The fear of confining the bowels and checking the secretions, constantly present to the mind of the practitioner, readily imbued the patient with the same alarm.   And thus was prevented the adequate use of a medicine, having power of mitigating pain, of relieving spasm, of procuring sleep, of producing perspiration, and occasionally even of aiding the natural action of the bowels, by obviating the disordered actions which interfere with it.

I speak of this as having been, because it is certain that opiates are again more largely employed, since the introduction of morphia, as a common preparation, has furnished new methods of administering the remedy, and revived attention to the principles of its action.   Yet even now it may be affirmed that there exists a distrust both as to the frequency and extent of its use, not warranted by facts, and injurious in various ways to our success in the treatment of disease.   This is the more singular, seeing the boldness of our practice in other points ; that we have in the sleep produced a sort of limit and safeguard to its effects; and that we possess remedies of easy application for all injurious symptoms that can arise.   To the insufficiency indeed of the quantities given, may be attributed in some part the comparative disregard into which the

vaccination, as practised on a great scale in that country, have much authority and value.
    The prize questions proposed by the French Academy of Sciences, to be answered in 1842, though not required to stimulate research on this subject, yet may aid in better defining the points of inquiry, and directing public attention to the results.

remedy fell during a certain period. Half a dose might disturb and distress the night which a full dose would have made one of perfect rest; or perplex the aspect of symptoms which a larger quantity would have alleviated or removed.

Yet medical experience does but follow common observation in recognising the inestimable value of sleep in sickness; of the suspension of pain, and the check to all disordered actions, thereby obtained. For pain and sleeplessness, though strictly but symptoms of other ailment, may often in practice be viewed as disorders in themselves, the removal of which is essential to the success of our general treatment.* How frequently do we see a nervous restlessness come over the patient, the consequence of protracted sickness or other causes,—retarding cure, by preventing the due effect of remedies, and receiving no relief itself from the means employed for the disease. In such cases the physician is not to submit himself to names or technicalities. The regular course of treatment must be suspended till the hinderance is removed; and even seeming contradictions to this course may safely be admitted for the attainment of the object. Here opium is the most certain and powerful of the aids we possess; and its use is not to be measured · timidly by tables of doses, but by fulfilment of the purpose for which it is given. A repetition of small quantities will often fail, which, concentrated into a single dose, would safely effect all we require.

On this subject we must refer to a fact regarding opium, singular in itself, and affording many curious inferences. I mean, the frequent absence of its ordinary effects in producing constipation, headache, and nervous symptoms, when given for the relief of acute pain or spasmodic actions in some part of the system. It would seem, however vague the expression, that the medicine, expending all its specific power in quieting these disorders of the nervous system, loses at the time every other influence on the body. Even the sleep peculiar to opium appears in such instances to be wanting, or produced chiefly in effect of the release from suffering. Though certain analogies may be quoted in illustration of these facts, nothing like explanation of them is furnished by our present knowledge. Their reality, however, cannot be doubted as matter of medical experience; and the instances are further remarkable in the large doses which may frequently be given in such cases, with impunity as to all the ordinary effects of the medicine.†

---

* A physician of large practice, whom I knew but in the latter days of his life, acted not unwisely, perhaps warily, in carrying about with him a box of small opium pills; with which he often gave relief, or made preparation for it, while yet in the house of his patient.

† An instance is just now before me of a young lady of fourteen, who had never before taken opium in any form, but to whom from 140 to 160 drops of laudanum were given daily for many days in succession, to relieve the acute pain arising from inflammation of bone. Here, beyond the relief thus afforded, for which these large doses were essential, there occurred no obvious effect on any of the functions, bodily or mental, nor any need of counteracting remedies. Little

The power of this remedy in checking various morbid actions in their earliest stage, even such as have no direct relation to the nervous system, is too much neglected in modern practice. In common catarrh, for instance, twenty or thirty drops of laudanum, or an equivalent dose of some other opiate, given with a warm diluent at bed-time, and followed in the morning by whatever laxative may be required, will often arrest altogether a complaint, which the later use of purgatives, antimonials, and saline medicines would only tardily remove.

Nor is there, except in some cases to which I shall soon refer, any such risk as might seem likely from this sudden effect of opium in checking the train of morbid actions, even in cases of more import than that just mentioned. The recommendation of its use, fairly attested by experience, in the treatment of the paroxysm of ague, may be cited as an instance in point. Where the check is given by the removal of irritation, or of that which John Hunter has termed " alarm to the nervous system," or by the procuring of sleep, the effect is almost always safe and beneficial to the patient.*

In truth, the injurious effects of this substance as a medicinal agent are altogether overrated ; a natural consequence of the mental and bodily evils resulting from its abuse when otherwise taken. I have seen the distresses produced by this excess, too frequently and too impressively, to allow me to offer a word in palliation of it. But there is nevertheless reason to say, respecting the general action of opium on the animal economy, that no agent of equal and similar power produces its peculiar effects with less detriment to the constitution ; nor is there any which admits of such extension of use, if gradually made, without fatal result. The excess in it is a hurtful intoxication, enfeebling both mind and body ; but scarcely more so than the habitual excess in wine and other alcoholic compounds, with which we too largely and familiarly deal as a part of diet. Every sound and sufficient reason must lead us to limit its use strictly to medicinal purposes. But so limiting it, and in cases where it is rightly admissible as a mode of treatment, little apprehension need exist regarding the amount of dose ; and inconvenience is at least as likely to arise from deficiency as from any ordinary excess.

assistance even was required for the bowels, though confinement of posture was added to the effect of the medicine. As the pain abated, the peculiar influence of opium came to be more felt, and furnished further reason for lessening the amount employed.

* It may seem strange, that while Lind strenuously recommends opium at the commencement of the hot stage of an intermittent, other authors have as strongly advised it at the beginning of the cold stage. We do not yet know enough of the mode of operation of the medicine through the nervous system, to be enabled to affirm that these opinions are incompatible, though it is probable that both cannot be just. It is a curious evidence how much is yet wanting to fixed principles of practice, even in the most familiar disorders, that the same contrariety exists as to the use of the powerful remedies in the cold and hot stage of agues

In some cases there is doubtless an idiosyncrasy regarding opium (as with respect to mercury, ipecacuanha, and other substances, whether in medicine or food) rendering it, even in minute quantity, a source of much injury to the nervous system. Instances of this kind occur, where the fact can no more be doubted than can the analogous ones of the effect of tea and coffee upon some constitutions. Within the last three months I have seen two cases, in each of which there was distinct proof that opium, in the ordinary dose, produced a great enfeeblement of voluntary power for some days; in one of these instances affecting the right side only, and so powerfully as to give alarm of hemiplegia.

There seems also reason to believe, in conformity with the remark of some authors, that the effects of opium are proportionally greater on young children, whether owing to the facility of absorption at this age, or to the greater susceptibility of the brain and nervous system;—a point, if well established, of obvious importance in practice. But all cases of idiosyncrasy regarding opium require scrutiny, lest we bring under this head the mere errors of fancy or prejudice, or the effects of the medicine partially and injudiciously employed. I recollect many instances, where I have had occasion to correct at a later time an opinion thus conceived, or assented to on insufficient proof.

It cannot be doubted that opium is one of the most certain and beneficial means we possess of exciting general perspiration. This is probably an effect of its power of allaying inordinate action in the vascular system throughout the body; but there may be other causes also concerned, which are less obvious to us. I have spoken on this subject when treating especially of sudorific remedies; but I revert to it here, as a point scarcely enough regarded in general practice. In fevers, indeed, the use of opium for this purpose is often prohibited by the other conditions of the malady; but there are many cases of slighter kind, where the perspiration and tranquillity, conjointly resulting from its use, suffice to arrest a disorder, which experience tells us might go much further were no such aid afforded.*

The employment of opiates in inflammatory diseases, and especially in such as affect the chest and head, offer many difficult points to the judgment of the practitioner. Here are morbid actions going on, of which we cannot safely for any length of time conceal from ourselves the amount. To stupify the sensibility to pain, or to suspend any particular disorder of function, unless we can simultaneously lessen or remove the causes which create it, is often but to interpose a veil between our judgment and the impending danger. However beneficial sleep and ease, they may be purchased at too dear a rate in such cases; and we must seek them rather in sequel to those more active remedies by which the power of the disease

* The usual doses of Dover's powder, the form of opiate most frequently prescribed with this view, are too small for the object desired. Nor is there sufficient cause for the preference given to this preparation over other opiates as a sudorific.

is met and subdued. Frequently, indeed, no art can procure them before.

Yet it is certain that there is a character of some inflammatory diseases, and a time probably in all, where this remedy may safely and beneficially be admitted.. In certain forms of peritoneal inflammation, whether puerperal or otherwise, attended with extreme pain and restlessness, and passing very soon into the typhoid state, relief to the condition which thus rapidly exhausts the vital powers is at all events to be sought for; and no appearance of distended bowels, or disordered secretions, can come in contradiction to this rule of greatest safety. Happily, the two modes of practice are not so incompatible as the more general use of the purgative treatment would seem to imply. The combination of calomel with full doses of opium is admissible and beneficial in most of these cases; and, where more express laxatives are required, they are usually best employed when the urgent irritation is removed. It is, for the most part, very difficult to render them effective before.*

Again, in cases of inflammation less special than the preceding, there is a period in each, succeeding to the early and more active treatment, when opiates have their appropriate value; not merely in giving rest, but also, as is probable, in lessening what remains of excess in vascular action. A right judgment as to the symptoms which indicate their use at such times, or even at intervals between the active remedies, is one of the best proofs of the ability of the practitioner; for no written rules, however plausible in show, can really minister certainty to this part of practice.

The use of opium needs discretion in another class of cases, which have not, I think, been sufficiently adverted to in this light. I mean those instances, where the heart and organs of respiration are in a state so critical as to enfeebled power, that the condition induced by opiates may suffice to turn the balance against them. This may happen either directly, by its influence on the nerves of these organs; or indirectly, by preventing the voluntary aids which a patient can render to himself, when the respiration is labouring and distressed. In an aged person, for example, suffering under chronic bronchitis or catarrhal influenza,—and gasping, it may be, under the difficulties of cough and expectoration,—an opiate, by suspending these very struggles, may become the cause of danger or death. The effort here is needed for the recovery of free respiration; and, if suppressed too long, mucus accumulates in the bronchial cells, its extrication thence becomes impossible, and breathing ceases altogether.

This caution is not unnecessary. I have known more than one case, where there was cause to believe that the fatal event had at least been hastened by an opiate indiscreetly given at bed-time; either from anxiety in the practitioner himself to relieve obvious

* In the valuable treatise on Puerperal Fever by Dr. Ferguson, just published, I find a strong attestation of the success with which he has employed opiates in this dangerous disorder, and some excellent comments on the subject.

distress, or from the solicitation of those around that something should be done. Instances of this extreme kind are happily not frequent. But the medical man is bound to be prepared for them; and to have in readiness, not his judgment only, but his firmness and power of forbearance. For the feelings are often invoked, as well as the reason, and he has to balance a certain present distress against a doubtful and contingent danger. No technical rule can be laid down for such cases: experience, and the discretion of the moment, must alone decide what should be done, and what refrained from.

The employment of opiates in cerebral affections is another question of much interest and various difficulty. It might be conjectured that there are some cases where the benefit is great; others, where injury alone can result: and experience fully confirms this presumption. Though it would be easy to detail particular cases in which one or other of these results is likely to ensue, I know no single principle, yet ascertained, by which they may be classed and distinguished. Perhaps one of the best practical tests might be found in the state of the pupil; known to be differently affected by opium, by belladonna, and certain other narcotics. Where contraction of the pupil is one of the symptoms of the disease, it may with some reason be supposed that opium is contradicted as a remedy; and a like inference might lead to the use of the opposite class of narcotics in its stead; transposing these methods, where the disease habitually produces a dilated state of the pupil. As far as my experience goes, it partially confirms the accuracy of the test, but is by no means sufficient to allow me to speak of it with certainty. We are still obliged to act here upon the suggestions of the time and symptoms present, or upon the experience which partial trials may afford.

There is great scope for further research on this subject, as on all that relates to disorders of the brain; and a strong presumption that opium is capable here of larger and more beneficial application than has yet been given to it. In certain cases of insanity especially, where much active irritation is present without inflammation, its employment, not by partial and irregular doses, but by keeping the patient for some time steadily under its influence, is often attended with a good attainable in no other way. Here, as in so many cases of physical pain and irritation from other causes, the maintenance of repose is a summary advantage, giving time and power to the functions of mind to resume their natural state.*

The latter remark applies strongly also to certain states of fever, where the typhoid character has come on; and, with it, much disturbance in the functions of the brain, delirium, or intolerable restlessness. Here opiates may often be used with singular benefit, and without any of those ill effects which might be presumed from a

* Dr. Seymour has well distinguished these cases, and made other valuable remarks in recommendation of opium, in his treatise on these disorders.

hot skin, a dry tongue, suspended secretions, and disorder of the head. The removal of cerebral irritation, especially if sleep ensue, is a good which might weigh against many inconveniences, even if they occurred: but, in point of fact, they are much less likely to happen where the opium directs itself specifically to the relief of irritation of this nature.

It is needful to add, that there are other cases of fever of typhoid kind, and where seemingly the same cerebral irritation is present, yet where opiates appear to act injuriously, by producing a comatose state rather than sound sleep. Unless distinction be found in the different state of the pupil noticed above, or in the hepatic symptoms which perhaps are more marked in these cases, and injuriously influence the state of the brain, I have no practical test to recommend, beyond that careful observation of the first trial which may give guidance for the future. It is an important point in treatment, and deserves explicit attention.

In many of these cases of disturbance of the brain, opiates may very advantageously be combined with the use of the tartarized antimony. And I would further observe, that morphia, in one or other of its preparations, may usually be preferred here to any other form of the remedy. Without entering into questions as to the separate action of narcotine and other principles contained in the common opium, I think it is proved that the effects of morphia are more explicit, more secure, and freer from injury or inconvenience than those of any other opiate. It is in some sort the gain of a new agent in medicine; giving us not only less equivocal results, but also the power of a nicer adaptation of means to the peculiarities of each case. This is an acquisition of especial value, where the functions and disorders of the brain are concerned ; and we have probably not yet ascertained all the good to be derived from it.*

The three topics I have thus slightly touched upon,—the employment of opium in inflammatory diseases, in disorders of the heart and respiratory organs, and in affections of the brain,—involve some of the more difficult questions as to the use of this remedy. Many others would occur were the subject treated in detail; and particularly those which relate to its effects in disorders of the liver and alimentary canal. Here again there is need of much discrimination ; and it may be affirmed that these are especially the organs, the action of opium upon which is liable to most suspicion of injury or failure. Except in cases of simple morbid irritability or spasm in some part of the canal, where it becomes a fit adjunct to other means, its general and certain tendency is to impede or disorder all the processes of digestion, and the secretions therewith connected. And in complaints of the liver and its appendages I scarcely know

---

* In like manner, the discovery of aconitine and veratria provides us with other agents on the nervous system of great and singular power ; and capable, in their chemical form, of much more definite use than under the previous method of employing these narcotics.

one, unless it be the painful passage of a gall-stone through the ducts, where opium may not be said to be hurtful in its single effects, though occasionally and indirectly useful when combined with other means. I have alluded to affections of the brain, in which the liver is concerned in aggravating at least the symptoms; and here too its influence is for the most part injurious, and always to be regarded with suspicion.

In those cases generally, where a course of purgative medicine is distinctly needed for the relief of the portal circulation, or of congestions about these viscera, opium can rarely be used without direct injury, or delay in the progress of cure. Where relief to irritation is needed, it is better sought for in these cases by a temporary suspension of the active remedies in use; and the physician shows his skill by steadily maintaining the principle of treatment which he has seen cause in the outset to adopt. There is much greater dfficulty in laying down rules for that large class of disorders to which the name of bowel complaints is applied ;—some of them symptomatic of the more general states just mentioned ; others, the effect of irritation or disease of the mucous membrane in some part of the alimentary canal ; others produced merely by improper or undigested food. The second class of cases, including dysentery, is that in which opiates seem most frequently admissible; either conjoined with, or interposed between, the laxative medicines which are more obviously essential. But it must be owned that the general course of treatment in all these disorders is vague and inconsistent; and that no divisions or descriptions have yet been adopted, determinate enough to define its proper direction, or to supersede the particular judgment in each case. While seeing, however, in this and other examples, how far medicine is from being an exact science, we may recognise the ample scope it affords for sagacity and watchful observation, and the eminent value of these qualities in every part of practice.

The external application of opium is not sufficiently brought into use, nor is there a due appreciation of all that may be attained in this way. That certain of its specific effects are conveyed through the skin to other parts of the body is unquestionable from experiment; though the action, so produced, is less strongly marked than that of belladonna and some other narcotics. These effects are distinctly augmented by removing the skin; so as to bring it into more direct action on the nerves of the part, if topical causes are concerned ; or within reach of readier absorption, if more diffused effect be sought for.* In many cases of painful affection of par-

---

* The experiments of Sir B. Brodie (*Phil. Trans.* for 1811), and the more recent researches of Muller, show that both these agencies of opium must be admitted, but render it certain that the action of absorption into the blood is much the most important in kind and degree. All modern inquiry tends to show the facility and extraordinary speed with which substances may enter into the circulation by means of imbibition, not before known to exist. Even since the remarks in this chapter were written, the endermic method of treatment, as it is called, has acquired a remarkable extension and increase of repute ; justified

ticular nerves I have found great benefit from a strong opiate ointment on a blistered surface; or a little of the muriate of morphia
sprinkled over it.   In the more complex case of gastrodynia, so
trying to the skill of the practitioner, though the cause cannot thus
be obviated, yet much relief to suffering may often be given by
similar means applied to the epigastrium, or other more especial
seat of pain.   I have found no remedy more beneficial in those
irritable forms of local psoriasis, which are so distressing from
their obstinacy, than the application of poultices, prepared with a
small proportion of a solution of opium, and continued until the
state of the skin is thoroughly changed.

In many nervous and spasmodic affections, as in some forms of
asthma, when we have reason to suppose that the medulla spinalis
is the chief source of disorder, the same remedies may be applied
along the course of the spine : and often with singular good, when
all methods of depletion or counter-irritation have proved utterly
unavailing.   If opium might be supposed capable of good in hydrophobia, after the many fruitless trials of it, this is the manner of use
most likely to succeed.   And the general method of practice is one
which I feel assured, on experience, may beneficially be carried
much further than we have hitherto pursued it.

Resources of this kind ought ever indeed to be present to the
mind of the practitioner.   If insufficient for cure, they yet are ad-
juncts of great value to other more active means of treatment. But
often the relief they afford is more speedy than that from internal
remedies ; and, what can never be too highly appreciated in medicine, with much less ambiguity of result.   Cases indeed are related
of serious mischief from opium applied externally to wounds, or ex-
coriated surfaces ; but the instances are rare, and probably to be ·
qualified by facts regarding the peculiar temperament of those so
affected.*   The more common cause of failure in this remedy is its
insufficient use ; either from the proportion of opium being too
small, or from the careless manner of application common to this
with most other external remedies.

———◆———

CHAPTER XXVII.

ON SLEEP.

It concerns not less the physician than the metaphysical inquirer,
to learn all the conditions of this remarkable function of life, and

on the whole by present experiment, and sanctioning the hope of much future
benefit from this modification in the use of remedies.

* I have seen one or two remarkable instances of the noxious effect of belladonna, thus applied, upon the sensorium. In one of these, delirium, continued
for more than thirty hours, was the consequence of dressing a blistered surface,
by mistake, with belladonna ointment.

the causes by which they are modified. Remarkable it may fitly be called; for what is more singular than that nearly a third part of existence should be passed in a state thus far separate from the external world!—a state in which consciousness and sense of identity are scarcely maintained; where memory and reason are equally disturbed; and yet, with all this, where the fancy works variously and boldly, creating images and impressions which are carried forwards into waking life, and blend themselves deeply and strongly with every part of our mental existence.* It is the familiarity with this great function of our nature which prevents our feeling how vast is the mystery it involves; how closely linked with all the phenomena of mental derangement, whencesoever produced; and, yet further, how singularly shadowing forth to our conception the greater and more lasting changes the mind may undergo without loss of its individuality.

I am not sure that the subject, in its medical relations, has even yet received all the notice it deserves. Much knowledge indeed has been gained of late. by looking more closely into the physical connexions of sleep with other actions of the body; and particularly with those functions of the nervous system to which it is most intimately allied. But there is still scope for a few remarks; having reference partly to the physiology of sleep, partly to its connexion with the various forms and treatment of disease.

It is singular that in a state thus familiar, and filling so large a portion of the term of life, it should yet be difficult to distinguish that which is the most perfect condition of sleep,—the furthest removed from the waking state. No certain proof can be had of this from our own recollections, nor from the feelings on awakening. Both depend more or less on the dream or other condition immediately antecedent, or even on the manner in which we are aroused from it. The best proofs, though ambiguous, are derived from the observation of those around. That may be presumed generally the soundest sleep, in which there is most complete tranquillity of the bodily organs commonly dependent on the will. Sensation, the other great function of the brain involved, furnishes evidence to the same point in the varying effect of stimuli applied to the senses when thus closed. And this test might perhaps be the most certain, were it not that we have cause to believe the different senses to be unequally under this state, even at the same moment of time: and further, that there is ambiguity from the passage of sleep into coma, through gradations which cannot be defined by any limits we are competent to draw.†

* " Half our days we pass in the shadow of the earth, and the brother of death extracteth a third part of our lives," says Sir Thomas Browne; a writer whose genius and eloquence give him a high place in English literature, as well as in that of the profession to which he belonged.

† Aristotle, towards the end of his Book, Περι ενυπνιων, has some curious remarks on the subject, well illustrated by examples. The whole of his writings on this and other collateral topics deserve much more frequent perusal than is given to them at the present day.

Evidence by ready tests as to the soundness of sleep is often of value in practice; both in reference to the point last mentioned, and because the physician is very liable to be misled by the error of the patient himself on the subject. The best proof which the latter can give is the absence of consciousness of having dreamed. This, however, does not render it certain that dreams have not existed. The observation of others, and the recollections often suggested afterwards of those of which there has been no memory at the time, prove it to be wholly otherwise. The question as to this point, indeed, is one that has been much debated, and a decisive answer is very difficult. But I hold it as more probable, that no part of sleep is without some condition of dreaming;—that is, without images present to the individual consciousness, and trains of thought founded thereon; however vague and unreal in themselves, and however slight or null the recollections they carry on to our waking existence. To believe it otherwise is to suppose two different states of sleep, more remote from each other than we can well conceive any two conditions of the same living being;—one, in which sensations, thoughts, and emotions are present in activity and unceasing change;—another, in which there is the absence or nullity of every function of mind; annihilation in fact, for the time, of all that is not merely organic life. Though we cannot disprove the latter, and must admit the difficulty of explaining the sleep of a newly-born infant in any other sense, yet is it on the whole more reasonable to suppose that no state of sleep is utterly without dreaming; the diversity being testified chiefly, (though imperfectly, as far as consciousness is concerned,) by the varying recollection of what has passed through the mind during the time in question.*

However this be, it is important in all our reasonings, practical and theoretical, upon sleep, to keep in mind that it is not a unity of state with which we are dealing, but a series of fluctuating conditions, of which no two moments perhaps are strictly alike. It may be affirmed that these variations extend even from complete wakefulness, to the most perfect sleep of which we have cognisance, either by outward or inward signs. In the symptoms, as well as treatment of disease, attention to this point is often of material consequence; and it assists us, far beyond any other view, in explaining many of the seeming anomalies in this great function of life.

Looking to what may be termed the passage between sleep and waking, it is singular with what rapidity and facility these states often alternate with each other. Every one may verify this upon his own experience. One familiar instance, among many, is that

* This question is noticed expressly by Aristotle: Διὰ τίνα αἰτίαν καθεύδοντες, ὅτε μὲν ὀνειρώττουσιν, ὅτε δὲ οὐ· ἢ συμβαίνει μὲν ἀεὶ καθεύδουσιν ἐνυπνιάζειν, ἀλλ' οὐ μνημονεύουσι. Περὶ ὑπνου. Lord Brougham, in his Discourse on Natural Theology, holds an opinion the reverse of that stated above; and vindicates, with his wonted power of argument, the belief that we dream but during the time of transition into and out of sleep; when the two states are graduating into each other.

of being on horseback when much wearied for want of rest. Here, at every few moments, the mind lapses into sleep, from which the loss of balance of the body as frequently and suddenly arouses it. In this case, and in all of like kind, neither the sleep nor the waking consciousness is perfect; but the mind, if we may so express its state, is kept close to an intermediate line, to each side of which it alternately passes. No such line, however, really exists; and it is merely a rapid shifting to and fro of conditions of imperfect sleep and imperfect waking, giving varied and curious proof of the manner in which these states graduate into each other.*

It is, indeed, in this passage from one to the other, and especially from waking into sleep, that we may best authenticate our knowledge of these phenomena. The most ordinary incidents here are full of instruction, if observed with this view; but their very familiarity is an obstacle to our gathering it from them. Watch, for example, the loss of voluntary power in a person sinking into sleep;—how gradual it is,—how exact a measure of the progress of the state coming on. An object is grasped by the hand while yet awake,—it is seen to be held less and less firmly,—till at last all power is gone, and it falls away. The head of a person in sitting posture gradually loses the support of the muscles which sustain it upright; it drops by degrees, and in the end falls upon the chest. Here, too, we have another proof of the singular rapidity with which the loss and recovery of voluntary power may alternate on the confines of sleep. The head falls by withdrawal of power from particular muscles. The slight shock, thence ensuing, partially awakens and brings back this influence, which again raises the head. It is well known how often this may be repeated within a short space of time, each such motion implying a difinite change in the state of voluntary power.

The gradual changes which occur in the perceptions from the senses, while sleep is coming on or departing, afford the same curious notices of the condition of the mind in its relation to the world without. The eye is least open for experiment here; but, in the senses of hearing and touch, the progressive lessening of sensibility may be made obvious through every stage of change, with the same fluctuations which attend those of the voluntary power; and giving the same proof that the state of sleep is ever varying in degree as respects all the functions engaged in it. There is, for example, one condition of sleep so light, it may fitly be termed, that the person can manifestly hear questions addressed to him, and even sometimes make partial or broken reply; and it is an old trick to bring sleepers into this state by putting the hand into cold water, or producing some other sensation, not active enough to awaken, but sufficient to draw the mind from a more profound to a lighter

* Exact estimate of time is obviously difficult here; but I have frequently, when in a carriage, obtained proof that this alternation of the loss and recovery of waking consciousness must have occurred at least three times within a minute, by knowing the distance gone over while the observation was made.

sleep. The application of facts of this kind to explain many of the appearances of Mesmerism is very obvious.

It would seem that these two faculties of sensibility and volition are sometimes unequally awakened from sleep. The familiar case may be taken of a person sleeping in upright posture with the head falling over the breast, in whom sensibility is suddenly aroused by impressions from within or without, but who is unable for some time to raise his head, though the sensation produced by this delay is very uneasy or even distressing to him.

The same mode of observation may be followed as to the higher mental faculties to which these functions severally minister. The mind kept for some time, as often happens, in a state intermediate between sleep and waking, is capable of recognising those rapid and repeated changes by which it shifts to each side of the imaginary line; and the moments of waking consciousness frequently afford distinct notice of the temporary aberrations which have intervened. It is a sort of self-analysis, which better shows than any reasoning, how completely these states graduate into each other, and to what extent the acts of the wakeful mind interpret those of the most perfect sleep.

Bichat, whose observations on the subject have all his wonted originality of thought and language, more distinctly propounds this view of the relations concerned in sleep. The phrase, " Le sommeil général est l'ensemble des sommeils particuliers," expresses his conception of the nature and complexity of this state; as one in which each separate sense and mental faculty may be at the same moment in very different conditions, even so far that some may be termed awake, while others are wholly wrapt in sleep. With some qualification, particularly as to the latter point, this opinion must be admitted as best accordant with facts, and indeed almost needful to the explanation of many of the phenomena. It comes nearest to what may be termed a just theory of sleep; and any seeming deviation from simplicity in its first aspect is speedily obviated by the facility it is found to give to all reasoning on the subject. The proofs are numerous through instances of the kind already stated; and in all such examples, the simpler and more limited the circumstances, the clearer is the evidence they afford.

Sleep, then, in the most general point of view, must be regarded not as one single state, but a succession of states in constant variation;—this variation consisting, not only in the different degrees in which the same sense or faculty is submitted to it, but also in the different proportions in which these several powers are under its influence at the same time. We thus associate together under a common principle all the phenomena, however remote and anomalous they may seem;—from the acts of the somnambulist, the vivid but inconsequent trains of thought excited by external impressions, and the occasional acute exercise of the intellect,—to that profound sleep in which no impressions seem to be received by the senses, no volition is exercised, and no consciousness or memory is left of thoughts having existed in the mind. Instead of regarding many of these facts as exceptions and anomalies, it is sounder in reason to adopt such definition of sleep as may practically include them all. And this, which can be done in perfect accordance with just physiological views, has been the course and tendency of modern inquiry on the subject. The principle is one, not merely sound and sufficient in theory, but beneficial in many points of practice, by solving difficulties which often occur in the aspect of symptoms and treatment of disease.

In following the various states and acts of sleeping through their relation to those of waking existence, tracing the gradations of one into the other, we obtain results of the same precise and practical kind, as those derived from pursuing the healthy functions of mind into the different forms of mental derangement. Each part of these topics, thus considered, illustrates every other; furnishing suggestions which cannot equally be drawn from any other source.

In this manner, again, of viewing sleep,—not as one, but a series of complex and ever-varying states,—we find best explanation of those singular conditions of trance, magnetic sleep, catalepsy, &c., which have served at all times to perplex the world by the strange breach they seem to make between the bodily and mental functions, by their unexpectedness in some cases, and by the peculiar agency producing them in others. The latter circumstance especially serves to disguise from us their real relation to other familiar affections of the nervous system. As respects more particularly magnetic sleep or trance, in all its alleged shapes, there is no well authenticated fact making it needful to believe that an influence is received from without, beyond those impressions on the senses, which are capable, according to the temperament and other circumstances, of exciting disordered as well as healthy actions throughout every part of the nervous system, and especially in the sensorial functions. The whole scope of the question is manifestly comprised in this single point.

Another circumstance regarding sleep requires notice here. Though admitting it to come on by a series of gradations from the waking state,—and to be in itself not one but many states, in the various degrees in which the mental and bodily faculties are submitted to it,—the consequence by no means follows that all these gradations must be gone through in the passage from one stage of sleep to another. The time occupied in the transitions is doubtless very different in different cases; and in many instances, particularly in certain nervous disorders, it seems that the changes or alternations between two states, remote from each other, may take place with extreme suddenness. There is yet a further question, whether there are any of these intermediate conditions, so far defined, that under certain influences they can be anticipated or produced, or sustained when actually existing? The inquiry is one deserving to be pursued; but it would too much lengthen these remarks to enter upon it in this place.

All that relates to dreaming is of course subordinate to this general idea of the nature of sleep. In another chapter I have spoken of the connexion between dreams and certain morbid states of mind, particularly those of insanity.* I do not here enter into other details on a topic upon which so much has been written. There is but one question to which I will allude, from its connexion with the inquiry into the physical conditions of sleep, viz., why are some dreams well remembered; others not at all, or much less perfectly? Two causes at least may be conjectured here. One is, that, in the former case, the sleep is really less perfect in kind;—that peculiar condition of brain less marked, upon which the imperfection of memory, if not also the exclusion of sensations, appears to depend. Another is, that the images and thoughts forming some dreams are actually stronger and deeper in impression than those of others;—an expression too vague for use, were it not that we are obliged equally to apply it to that ordinary diversity of waking states, upon which the memory so much depends for its degree of promptitude and completeness. The combination of these circumstances, with others perhaps less obvious, affords as much explanation as we can attain without more complete knowledge of the proximate causes of sleep. To the first probably we may look for interpretation of the old notion of the "*somnia vera*" of approaching day. The physical state of sleep is then less perfect;—trains of thought suggested,. follow more nearly the course of waking associations;—and the memory retains them, while earlier and more confused dreams are wholly lost to the mind.†

The power often gained of awakening at a fixed hour depends obviously on that law of habit which governs so largely the course of all our functions, and particularly those of animal life. The time in these cases cannot be altered without creating by especial means a new habit. When on any single occasion the need of waking early produces the effect, it is merely because the sleep itself is disturbed by the dominant idea of this need, and is broken at repeated intervals, without relation to the time required.

* See Chapter XV. (On Insanity, Dreaming, and Intoxication.) Bichat says of dreams, "Ils ne sont autre chose qu'une portion de la vie animale échappée de l'engourdissement où l'autre portion est plongée."

† Such dreams, however, though lost at the moment, leave traces which, like the memory of waking acts, are capable of being restored at a more remote time by new associations. There are few who have not occasionally felt certain vague and fleeting impressions of a past state of mind, of which the recollection cannot by any effort take a firm hold, or attach them to any distinct points of time or place;—something which does not link itself to any part of life, yet is felt to belong to the identity of the being. These are not improbably the shades of former dreams; the consciousness, from some casual association, wandering back into that strange world of thoughts and feelings in which it has existed during some antecedent time of sleep, without memory of it at the moment, or in the interval since. A fervid fancy might seek a still higher source for this phenomenon, ("Des tels faits embarrassent plus les esprits forts qu'ils ne le témoignent,") and poetry might well adopt such; but the explanation is probably that just given.

The question as to the physical causes of sleep, remote and prox-imate, has been so much discussed, that I advert to it only for the purpose of simplifying what we know on the subject. The great object in view is manifestly the reparation of exhausted power. This need extends, in the most general sense, to life in every form; but applies peculiarly to animal life, and bears some proportion here to the higher organization and faculties of the species.* The law of intermittence, more distinct as we thus rise in the scale of func-tions, depends upon, and provides for, this necessity; showing itself most expressly in that periodical repose to the two great functions of sensibility and volition which we name sleep; and which, so estab-lished, links itself closely with every other part of our mental and corporeal existence.

Considering the proximate cause under this general law, it seems certain that it is to be found in some particular state of the nervous substance, having close relation to these functions;—a state different from that of waking life, yet graduating into it;—incapable, per-haps, of being ever ascertained by observation, yet not the less real as a change on this account. We have proof, partly in the nature of the functions affected, which depend immediately on this part of the organization, partly in the nature of the causes tending to produce sleep. These are all such as have influence more or less direct, on the nervous system;—fatigue of body or mind; the absence of strong impressions on any of the senses; exhaustion by pain or other strong impressions previously sustained; the action of various narcotics; particular conditions of the blood, and of circulation through the brain; certain stages of digestion; and other causes acting still more explicitly on the nerves alone. The latter involve some of the most curious conditions of the animal economy, such as have at all times tended to perplex the human understanding, and beget opinions far overstepping the bounds of human research.

In looking to these various causes which act on the sensorium to the production of sleep, we find again the advantage gained by viewing this state as one of unceasing change; not only in general intensity, but further, and more remarkably, in the degree in which different functions and faculties are involved in it. This is especially true as respects the influence of the circulation; the most important of these causes, and that with which we have greatest practical concern, from our power of modifying its action. Knowing what we do of its singular and rapid changes in waking and healthy state, it is easy to understand how similar inequalities may so act on the brain and nervous system as to produce every gradation of sleep, and every variation in the particular functions submitted to it. Whether quality of blood, or the mechanical effects of quantity and rate of movement, be most concerned (and there is reason from

* The hybernation of some animals must be regarded as an exception to the principle; this state obviously depending on other causes than the mere need of rest.

observation to admit both), equally will any such inequalities tend to produce the effects in question.

And here too we must seek explanation of many of the irregularities of dreaming. It is certain that these greatly depend (probably much more than the variations of the waking state) on the fluctuating circulation through the brain. We have much curious proof how slight a difference of pressure, partial or general, on this organ, is capable of producing the most singular effects on its functions, and disturbing not only the perceptions of the senses, but all the higher operations of mind. Dreams are the most striking evidence and interpreters of this fact.* Yet is the order of circumstances not wholly known to us here. The actions and reactions between the nervous system, and that of the circulation, are so numerous and complicated, that it is impossible to decipher them in any detail; or even, in many cases, to indicate which is cause and which effect. This, indeed, forms one great difficulty in tracing out the steps of the physical causes of sleep. There is no cause, however, to suppose it insuperable; though a more certain limit lies beyond, common to all researches of this nature, and stopping every further progress in this direction.

In investigating the nature of sleep, we must advert to the causes which prevent, as well as those which favour or produce it. They of course are chiefly the converse of the latter; but some of them deserve notice from the further illustrations they afford. The peculiar effect of certain substances, even of common articles of diet, as coffee and green tea, may be mentioned among these.† Though by

* Where dreams have been singularly vivid and consecutive through the night, I believe it will generally be found that there is some concomitant heaviness or oppression of head, indicating congestion or other disturbance of the vascular system there. And that this operates mainly as cause (though perhaps itself reciprocally acted upon) may be inferred from the previous conditions likely to disturb the circulation, and also from the frequent repetition of the same vividness of dreams, with intervals of waking between.

† In speaking of the effects of coffee on the nervous system, I may mention a statement I have heard from one or two West Indians, that the aroma of this berry, strongly concentrated and long applied, is capable of producing delirium, or some degree of aberration of mind. This account I first received in the case of a young man, a native of St. Domingo, who arrived in this country in a state approaching to mania, and died soon afterwards. His illness was attributed by a friend who accompanied him, (and who assured me he had known similar cases) to his having slept during the voyage in a cabin half filled with bags of coffee. I have had no means of ascertaining the truth of this opinion; which, in fact, was disproved in the case in question, by cerebral disease actually discovered, and presumably of a date anterior to the voyage. The influence of coffee and tea, in relation to sleep, seems to depend upon some similar cause in each case, whatever this may be. Even the peculiar sensation about the præcordia (the effect, it is to be supposed, of the state induced on the coats of the stomach) is very much alike in both cases. This sensation, familiar to persons who are thus affected, often continues for six or eight hours, and bears proportion apparently to the influence of these liquids in preventing sleep. It is certain, and easily to be understood, that all such effects are much modified (increased, perhaps, as well as lessened) by conjunction with other articles of food, and especially with wine.

no means invariable, and often blended with other effects, yet are they distinct enough to furnish the same inferences as those we derive from opium in its action as a soporific. In both cases we have to presume a direct change of state, though of different kind for each, throughout a great part of the nervous system. Any influence these agents produce on the circulation, is wholly inadequate to explain the phenomena. We know that opium, and other narcotic substances, have effects, locally applied, on nervous sensibility and the action of the muscular fibre; and there can be little doubt that in sleep it is the same singular influence, extended more widely over this part of organization; and reaching, through the cerebral part of it, the higher faculties of our being.

The length of time during which maniacs, in restless or violent activity, sometimes continue without sleep, is among the facts which seem to baffle all speculation. If venturing any hypothesis on the subject, it would be, that in some kinds of mania there is an actual excess in the production of that nervous power, by the exhaustion of which, under ordinary circumstances, sleep is produced. Were this view, for which there are some plausible reasons, capable of being proved, it would explain why the intervention of such state (designed to give time for reparation) should be so little needed in these cases. And, even without explanation of this curious anomaly, we may take the fact in illustration by analogy of various lesser cases; in which we observe diminution of sleep for considerable periods, without any proportionate waste of power. There are seemingly differences in the capacity of the sensorium at different times for the performance of its functions; similar action being attended with greater and more speedy exhaustion at one time than another. This is a fact familiar to the consciousness of every one; and which must be referred to physical variations (appreciable only by their effects) in the state of the nervous power ministering to these actions.

It is a point worthy of note, though familiar, that whereas moderate mental occupation and excitement tend to produce sleep, excess in degree or duration of this state has the effect of preventing it. And this is true, not only as to strong emotions of mind, the influence of which is often painfully proved, but even as to simple intellectual exertion, where the effort is earnest and too long protracted. Many singular instances have occurred to me of habitual loss of sleep from this cause. Such effect is never to be neglected; as it is a token of what may become danger in various ways. The practical admonitions of the physician are as necessary here, as in the treatment of fever or inflammatory disease; the brain invariably suffering in the end from exertions which produce this result. The slighter inroads of the habit can only be detected by the patient himself; but he must be led to a right estimation of their consequences.

The influence of the previous state of mind in procuring or preventing sleep is curious in every way. Minute observation here

25*

offers many incongruities, which cannot adequately be solved
without knowing better than we do its physical causes, and their
relation to the sensorial functions.   What seems most needful for
attaining it is the disengagement of the mind from any strong
emotion, or urgent train of thought.   Great anxiety to bring on
sleep implies these very conditions, and is therefore more or less
preventive of it.   The various artifices of thought and memory
used for the purpose often fail from this cause.   When they succeed,
it depends either on the exhaustion becoming more complete, or on
the mind being rapidly carried from one object to another; a
desultory state of this kind, without emotion, being apparently one
of the conditions most favourable to the effect desired.

A great source of inequality and disturbance in sleep is doubtless
to be found in the state of the viscera; and especially of those by
which digestion is performed,   This process, going on during sleep,
carries the ingesta through successive stages of change, and through
different parts of the alimentary canal; every such change, even
under the healthiest action, altering in some way the state of the
body, and the impression upon the sensorium; indirectly, through
the circulation;—or directly, by excitement to different parts of the
nervous system;—or mechanically, by hindrance to the flow of
blood in the great vessels, from pressure upon them in the
epigastrium.

Out of this general view many particular questions arise.   Such
are those which regard the cause of the sleepiness directly following
a full or ill-digested meal; or of the disturbance to sound sleep
which often occurs in the middle of the night, six or seven hours
after dinner, and is obviously connected with some part of the
process of digestion.   The first effect depends probably on the loaded
stomach itself; and is testified by that *laborious* and unrefreshing
sleep familiar to most persons at one time or another.   The latter
effect may depend on the colon becoming loaded about this time
with what is received from the small intestines; performing its
functions with difficulty; and from the recumbent posture creating
disturbance by pressure on the great vessels and other surrounding
parts.   All such effects of digestion upon sleep are strikingly
attested by its influence on dreaming; and they are of course
greatly varied in kind, and augmented in degree, from any disorder
of the organs concerned.   Restless nights form one in the long
catalogue of distresses of the dyspeptic patient, and aggravate
greatly the evils out of which they arise.   Medicine in its dietetic
part may do much here; nor is the physician to disregard any means
as trifling which can minister to so great a good.

Whatever of wholesome change in diet may have been made in
this country of late years, there is cause to think that we deal injuriously with the night by bringing the time of dinner so closely
upon it.   The interval of four or five hours between the heaviest
meal of the day, and the time of going to bed, is by no means that
most favourable to sound rest.   The early stage of digestion is

passed over, during which there is natural tendency to repose; and we seek it at a time when the system, as respects the influence of food, is taking up again a more active state; and when exercise, rather than the recumbent posture, is expedient in forwarding healthily the latter stages of this process. The old method of supper at bed-time, in sequel to dinner in the middle of the day, was better in regard to the comfort and completeness of rest at night; and the habit of good sleep may often be retrieved by adopting a plan of this kind, when every anodyne has failed of effect. With all the facility the human body has of adapting itself to change of circumstances, there are cases where this can never wholly be done. And the connexion of digestion with sleep is so important and unceasing, that we have every cause to infer some relation as to time between the two functions, better fitted than any other to fulfil healthily the purposes of both. This it is the business of the physician to ascertain; and though he cannot change the course of worldly habit in these matters, the knowledge so gained may at least become an important aid in the treatment of disease.

The close dependence of sleep on the state of the alimentary canal makes it probable that evil is often incurred by giving purgatives habitually at bed-time. The custom is a common one; and not least so in dyspeptic cases. Yet here especially everything ought to be avoided which by irritation can disturb the soundest of rest;—a consequence often inevitable of the action on the membranes which aperient medicines produce. Advantage may often be gained in such cases, by changing the time of using these remedies, where they cannot be dispensed with altogether.

The relation of sleep to perspiration is a point of importance in the animal economy. It seems certain that this secretion or transudation, however it be termed, is augmented by sleep, as a general state of the body, independently of the influence of external causes.[*] The facts is connected with and illustrates certain of the phenomena of fever; and is capable in various ways of practical application. There is reason to believe that this is the cause of perspiration in many cases, where medicines given to procure it receive credit for the effect.

The influence of different diseases upon sleep, as well as the reciprocal effects of disturbance in this function, form a curious subject; but withal so complicated, that it can scarcely be pursued on any general principle. An important part of the inquiry is the relation of sleep to disorders of the brain; with some of which it has close kindred both in the functions affected, and in the apparent manner

[*] The multiplied observations of Sanctorius and Keill on this subject are confirmed by the more recent inquiries of Dr. Edwards. The labours of Sanctorius in these parts of physiology are scarcely enough regarded at the present time. Two or three particular results are quoted and requoted from him; without due notice of the vast mass of observations he collected; with singular diligence and fidelity, and often by very curious and instructive means of research. The modern method (for such it may be termed) of applying averages to results of this kind is very valuable, or even indispensable, where the conditions are so numerous, and so complicated with each other.

in which this takes place.   There are instances here in which it would be difficult to recognise any other distinction than that of duration; though, from the difference of cause which this presumes, we may infer that other variations really exist.   It is certain that the states of sleep and coma frequently graduate into each other, in such a way as to show that the proximate physical conditions are nearly the same in both.   Either name may be given to the state produced by moderate pressure on the brain, when a portion of the cranium is removed. In a remarkable example of this kind, which I saw in one of the English military hospitals at Santarem, when travelling in Portugal in 1812, there was cause from observation to infer, that the patient went through every grade between these conditions, in proportion to the pressure applied.   And instances are probably common to the same effect, though always liable to some doubt in their interpretation.

The judgement of the physician is often embarrassed in these cases; and practical injury may be the consequence of error.   It is an observation of Dr. Wilson Philip, in his valuable paper on this subject in the Philosophical Transactions, that no sleep is healthy but that from which we are easily aroused.*   And though the remark requires to be qualified by the consideration that sleep may be too light in kind to fulfil its purposes in the animal economy, it justly points out the opposite excess, and a state too closely verging on the conditions of brain which endanger apoplexy.   Changes of circulation in the head, however produced, are doubtless concerned in all these variations.   One degree of pressure seems essential to perfect and uniform sleep; while a greater degree, without other alteration of state, assumes more or less the character of disease. The best inferences, in relation to practice, are generally to be derived from notice of other symptoms; particularly from the degree of sensibility present, the state of respiration, and that of the action of the heart.†

Connected closely with this subject is the further practical question as to the proportion of sleep best fitted for health, and more especially for the well-being of the sensorial powers.   It is obvious that this can be answered explicitly only for individual cases.   One temperament undoubtedly requires more than another; nor can the sufficiency of the function be measured merely by number of hours, varying as it does in all that may be termed its intensity and completeness.   The remarks, already made, clearly point out these distinctions, to which the mind and body have equal and similar relation.

The effects of deficiency of sleep are more familiar to us than those which belong to its habitual excess.   Yet this excess, as a habit may unquestionably exist.   The brain may be kept too long, at each successive period of sleep, in a state which, though strictly

* On the Nature of Sleep, *Phil. Transactions* for 1833.

† The aid frequently got in bringing on sleep by placing the head low and the difficulty of sleeping in an upright posture, are familiar proofs how much the state of the brain in sleep is determined by the manner of circulation through it.

speaking as natural as waking, is equally liable to be unduly extended; and which, as we have seen, may pass into disease by gradations scarcely to be defined. The expressions of Aretæus, υπνος πολλος παχυτης, αργιη, ομιχλη της αισθησιος and again, υπνος πολυς ναρκα τας αισθησιας της κεφαλης· are just in every part of their application. For the state of the sensorium produced by excess of sleep, appears, in a strict sense, to be one unfavourable to its powers of perception and action. Such state may, with some fitness, be described as a chronic disorder of the brain; affecting more or less all the functions of the body, but particularly those of animal life. It belongs to old age, as an effect of natural changes, and a part of the dispensation of human existence. But the growth of habit and self-indulgence may prematurely bring it on; and the physician is bound to have regard to this contingency, as well as to the opposite condition of sleep deficient in amount.*

It would appear that, independently of any abridgment of proper rest, there is somthing of ill effect to the brain in the sudden interruption of sleep, often repeated. Whatever the physical difference of the states of sleeping and waking, it seems that the change from the former to the latter ought to be gradual, as are the approaches of sleep on the opposite side. The action of the heart becomes quickened, or otherwise disturbed, by such interruption. The same emotion of mind occurs as from any sudden surprise, and frequently there is a painful and difficult effort in recalling the entire consciousness of the waking state.

Among the causes which influence sleep and dreaming, I doubt whether changes in the state of the atmosphere have been sufficiently noticed. My attention having been casually drawn to this point some years ago, I have since made many observations upon it, and with more uniformity of result than could be expected, seeing the many other causes which act concurrently; as time, quantity and kind of food, excitement or fatigue of mind or body, habit as to times of sleep, and the variations due to actual disease. Removing these ambiguities as far as possible, I have found that any very sudden and considerable fall of the barometer produces in many persons a sort of lassitude and drowsiness, followed by restless and uneasy sleep, or frequently a state of laborious dreaming. It may be doubted whether this influence depends on changes in the balance of circulation thus produced, or on alterations in the electrical state of the air concurring with its change of weight, and affecting (as we have often cause to suppose likely) certain functions of the nervous system. However this be, I cannot doubt the reality of the fact as one of frequent occurrence. It is indeed merely an example, among so many others, of the partial subjection of the phenomena of life to the agents which are ever in movement around us.†

* Ύπνος, αγρυπνιη, αμφοτερα του μετριου μαλλον γενομενα, κακον.—*Hippocrat. Aphorism.* The " vigilans stertit " of the satirist describes what is often a reality in life.

† During the month preceding the time when I am now writing (April, 1836), there have been two or three very singular and sudden depressions of the barometer

CHAPTER XXVIII.

ON THE INFLUENCE OF WEATHER IN RELATION TO DISEASE.

AMIDST all the opinions and phrases current on this subject, it is singular how little real knowledge has been gained, or applied to practice. The difficulties of the inquiry are great, both from the complexity of the agents concerned, and from that of the organs and functions acted upon. Yet with the certainty we have of the extent, variety, and unceasing nature of this influence, it is manifestly a field of research, where patient observations and averages cannot fail of affording the most valuable results.* ·

On this topic, as on many others in this volume, the remarks which follow do not profess more than to give a certain degree of method to its several parts; and to suggest the conclusions, chiefly practical in kind, which appear to have engaged least attention. Some of the points, only touched upon, or briefly treated, might well furnish material for separate volumes, from their importance, and the scope they give to experimental research.

The subject, taken in its whole extent, admits of being distributed into several separate objects of inquiry.

The history of the diseases of particular climates, though still deficient in many respects, and altogether wanting for many important localities of the globe, is perhaps that part which has hitherto been most successfully cultivated. For this object, however, observation is not to be limited to the effects of different meteorological states on the animal economy. It of necessity extends to many other local conditions, not fitly coming under this head, yet blending with and modifying all those which depend on climate alone; and requiring to be specified before inferences can rightly be drawn from the latter.†

(one of more than an inch within a few hours, from a point already low), attended by gales of unwonted violence on the southern and western coasts of England. It has occurred to me on all these occasions, but particularly on the latter, to observe similar influence, as respects sleep, on myself and many different persons; taking for evidence those in ordinary health, rather than such as were suffering under malady at the time.

* Nor is attention to this subject always solicited by the sick themselves. Besides the accustomed looseness of inference on every point regarding health, it is singular how averse many patients are to attribute any effect to the influence in question. Every other cause is invoked rather than this very powerful one.

† The want of exactitude in noting these local conditions, which I have often had occasion myself to observe, has been most judiciously commented upon by Dr. James Johnson, in his work on the Diseases of Tropical Climates. Inferences, for example, can never be useful or admissible, which apply to the vast regions and various surface of India, as if it were one locality and a single climate. This is a strongly marked instance; but the comment applies to many others, where medical description partakes of that vagueness and want of attention to specialties, which belongs to all popular opinion on the subject.

The same may be said of that part of the subject which respects the climate of particular places, and their relative fitness as residence for invalids. Research here has been chiefly confined to the case of those labouring under pulmonary disease; and the observations with this view directed to averages of temperature, comparative quantity of rain, and prevalence of particular winds. Even, however, where it has been possible to attest these facts by averages of sufficient length, the difficulty remains of comparing other local circumstances less obvious; but which modify, and are often more than equivalent to, the direct effects of climate. And it must be added, that this is a subject on which fashion, hasty observation, and mistaken methods of inference in the world at large, have very great influence. Accordingly we find that our knowledge here, though extended and better assured by two or three valuable works, is still wanting in certainty; and the practice founded upon it often singularly vague and of doubtful benefit.* The truth of the avowal will be admitted by every physician, who candidly looks to this part of the treatment of disease.

Another view of the subject, less exclusive than either of the preceding, is that of the relation of the several states and changes of atmosphere to the various functions of the body; a wide topic, abounding in curious results, and these of equal interest to physiology and pathology. Those which especially concern the former, though more or less at all times matter of popular observation, have only of late been taken into the domain of science. The researches of Dr. W. F. Edwards and others, while adding greatly to our knowledge both in extent and exactness, show how much is yet to be learnt, before we can appreciate the influence even of the most familiar agents around us. Every part of the history of disease affords the same inference. We feel these agents to be in perpetual operation;—some of their more obvious effects in producing disease are currently understood by all;—medical knowledge has registered a few others, in which certain disorders are manifestly produced, or rendered epidemic, by particular states of weather;—but there still remains behind much more than has yet been acquired. Scarcely is there a single branch of science which in its progress may not be brought to contribute to this object. And without claiming any present certainty for the connexion which some physiologists affirm between electrical and nervous agency, it must be allowed that this part of science, in particular, is likely to explain hereafter some of the more singular effects of the atmosphere on the human body.

The foregoing observations apply to the several modes under which this subject may be viewed; each having its peculiar objects, while all serve for mutual illustration. The remarks which follow, have reference especially to the influence of certain states of air or weather in producing morbid conditions of the body; either in their

* I may name as the best work we have on Climate, that by Sir James Clark; very valuable in local details, and in the practical inferences founded upon them.

immediate effect, or indirectly by evolving or giving greater activity to other causes. The latter distinction must be kept in view, as far as our knowledge will allow; since, doubtless, many of the diseases of season and climate are derived from such secondary causes, rather than from those more obvious to common remark.

With this exception (under which we must include the exanthematous and certain other fevers), the prevailing diseases of each season, as a class, are to be referred chiefly to the continuance, or more frequent repetition, of the causes by which particular cases of these diseases are produced. I need not, from their familiarity, enumerate those which are usually cited, though not perhaps with much precision, as severally predominant at different seasons of the year. Taking them collectively, they furnish certain average results of mortality, which form a very interesting and important branch of medical statistics, and have been greatly extended of late years in number and exactness; promising for the future various conclusions of more general application than any we now possess.

On this subject more is often to be learnt by carefully and continuously noticing the phenomena of one locality, than by diffusing the research over many. Each mode of inquiry has its value, separately and for mutual illustration; but that perhaps is most instructive, which connects the prevalence, type, and change of disease on a single spot, with corresponding conditions in the atmosphere around it. Observations of this kind, spread over a long period, disclose relations discoverable in no other way. They are valuable also, because more or less within the reach of every practitioner; and in their aggregate they furnish material for those general conclusions, upon which alone reliance is to be placed.*

But besides the recognised diseases of certain seasons, there are others not in general so considered, which nevertheless are frequent

* Some of the German reports, as those in the " Medicinische Zeitung " of Berlin, afford valuable examples of such research; the more so, from their associating the epidemic disorders of other animals with those of man. The latter is a source of knowledge and illustration not perhaps adequately regarded in our own country.

With all their imperfections in physical knowledge, and deficiency of instruments for exact observation, the ancient physicians gave greater attention to the influence of weather on disease than has been commonly done at later periods. There is much that merits notice in their maxims as well as practical conclusions on this subject, drawn from a climate more definite in its periodical changes than that of the more northern parts of Europe, and furnishing therefore more ready and certain inferences. Some of those found in Hippocrates are admirably descriptive in themselves, and apply with singular exactness to facts every day present to our observation. I transcribe his account of the northern and southern winds, as an example of this vigour and accuracy of description.

Νοτοι βαρυηκοοι, αχλυωδεες, καρηβαρικοι, νωθροι, διαλυτικοι·—'Hν δε δυναστευη βορειαν, βηχες, φαρυγγες, κοιλιαι σκληροτεροι, δυσουριαι φρικωδεες, εδυναι πλευρεων, στηθεων·

Still better proof of his eminent faculty for such observations will be found in the remarkable books on Epidemic Diseases; the cases in which well deserve study, not on this point alone, but as models for every part of the history of disease.

enough, at particular times, to make it probable that atmospheric influence is concerned. My notes furnish me with many instances of this kind; some of them, indeed, liable to question, as being possibly the result of casual or unknown causes; yet deserving notice in the suggestions they afford for future observation. It cannot be doubted that affections of the head, depending on disturbed balance of circulation through the brain, do at some periods much exceed the common average of these cases. The same remark I would extend, on my experience, to various neuralgic disorders; including under these some affections, usually termed rheumatic, which are thus, however, most correctly classed. Lumbago and sciatica are undoubtedly more prevalent in certain states of atmosphere; and we may recognise a similar effect in the familiar instance of pain renewed in old sprains, or in joints affected by former inflammation. Further, though more doubtfully, I have found reason to think that attacks of gout, in patients having this habit of body, are more common than usual at certain periods, without other cause to which this can reasonably be assigned.

With respect, again, to disorders of the internal membranes; while many of these are noted as prevailing at particular seasons, there are others not thus described, yet which observation shows to depend greatly on external causes, giving them frequently an epidemic character. Every physician must have noticed a class of bowel disorders, almost specific in kind, which prevail extensively at one time; while, at another, there is the tendency, not less marked, to different forms of cynanche, or to erythematous inflammations of the fauces, palate, and gums. Erysipelas evidently prevails more generally and severely under particular states of weather, and these not connected with any regular occurrence or character of seasons. The infantile fever, however it be classed in our nosology, is clearly the subject of external influences, to the same extent, and possibly in the same way, as the exanthematous disorders. And with respect to gastric fevers in general, whatever name they assume, we have evidence of their becoming epidemic under certain continued states of weather; and apparently alike at different periods of their occurrence.

Hooping-cough may be further mentioned, as obviously partaking in the same liability. The different affections of the membrane of the air-passages—catarrh, croup, asthma and bronchitis,—though not all depending on this cause solely or equally, yet are greatly under its influence; and rendered more frequent or severe as particular conditions of atmosphere are present, or prolonged in duration. Even bronchocele, a disorder of which it is so difficult to render any plausible account, seems to afford another example of this influence.* Other glandular affections are much more frequently and certainly submitted to it.

* One or two instances are known to me, where the ordinary prevalence of bronchocele in a particular locality has been suddenly augmented by many new cases; sometimes numerously in the same family. The cynanche parotidæa is

In specifying these instances (to which many besides might be added), it is impossible to affirm that they are all attributable to those atmospheric states, which are familiarly understood under the name of weather.   Other causes, to which I have already alluded, may be the more direct agents on the body in many of the cases named ; and in some are undoubtedly so.   But as we know the production and diffusion of these agents to be greatly determined by variations of the atmosphere, and have little cognisance of other conditions affecting them, we may justly note and classify the various cases in which the state or changes of the air appear to act, as producing these disorders in the human frame.

Setting aside, then, what directly relates to incidental miasmata in the atmosphere, whether gaseous admixtures, animal or vegetable products, or other matters still less within our knowledge, any inquiry respecting the influence of weather in the production or modification of disease, must include four principal objects:—*first,* the temperature of the air ;—*secondly,* its hygrometrical state :— *thirdly,* its weight ;—and *fourthly,* its electrical state and changes. The agency of winds may obviously be referred in great part to one or other of these conditions.   That of light, though the facts are sufficient fully to prove its existence, is too subtle to be well defined in the present state of our knowledge.   Nevertheless, seeing what has been done by science in expounding the physical conditions through which this great agent operates, and its effects on other forms of living organization, particularly on the growth and economy of plants, there is cause to believe that some of its relations to the body may hereafter be brought more expressly within our reach.*

While stating separately these conditions, it is manifest that none of them can really act singly upon the body ; and this com-

much more familiar as an epidemic at certain periods, in which effect weather may also be concerned ; though it is more probable, from the specific and infectious nature of the complaint, that this is only partially the case.

* Dr. Reid, of Edinburgh, has inferred from experiment, that the effects produced by an atmosphere, loaded with excess of carbonic acid, are more speedily removed when the patient is placed under a strong light, than when merely brought into fresh air.   In conformity with this, it has been found that there is greater proneness to disease in those parts of crowded buildings, such as barracks, from which light is most excluded ; a fact of which Sir James Wylie's experience in Russia affords some striking examples.

Even while arranging this chapter for the press, I observe announced certain new facts regarding light ; expounding, it may be, other relations of this great agent to the more ordinary forms and combinations of matter which surround us ; and, if strictly chemical in nature, furnishing another remarkable instance in addition to those we already possessed.   I allude to the separate discoveries of Mr. Talbot and M. Daguerre (differing in details, but probably identical in principle), of materials affording a surface of such kind that images or pictures, given by the camera obscura, or solar miscroscope, are permanently impressed thereon, nor liable to be effaced by subsequent exposure to light.   The testimony of Arago and Biot authenticates the fact that the light of the moon, hitherto so little amenable to experiment, has yielded an image by its action on the delicate test discovered by Mr. Daguerre.

plexity of effect is a main difficulty of the research.   Excess or deficiency in relation to a medium state, or the mere fact of change in any one of them, must presumably have influence, direct or indirect, greater or less in degree, on all the rest.   Meteorology, itself only beginning to take place among the exact sciences, has hitherto done little to meet the perplexity of these questions.*   It is a difficulty greatly enhanced by the variety of the living tissues upon which these agents have severally or conjointly effect; and, it may be, by other relations of their action to the laws of life, of which our knowledge is limited at present to a few general intimations.

For, in considering this subject, a foremost point for notice is the susceptibility of other animals to atmospheric changes, which we are altogether unable to appreciate ; a phenomenon often so remarkable as almost to warrant the notion of other senses than those possessed by man.   Instances of this kind are too familiar to need recital.   They are furnished numerously from every part of the animal kingdom : and many doubtless exist, especially in insect life, more singular than any of which we have knowledge.   Strictly

---

* Evidence of what is yet wanting to this branch of science may be drawn from the extent and variety of research now directed to remedy its deficiencies. The direction, velocity, and physical causes of winds and hurricanes ;—the phenomena of evaporation and dew, and the nature and manner of formation of clouds ;—the causes of the deposition of water as rain, hail, and snow ; and the relative quantity of rain in different localities and at different heights ;—the averages of heat under every variety of climate and locality ; its distribution by isothermal lines, its degree at different elevations, and under the various influence of reflection and radiation ; and the temperature of space ;—the barometrical states of the air ; and their irregular or periodical changes, as produced by heat, electricity, the lunar attraction, or the ocean tides ;—and the electrical or magnetic conditions of the atmosphere, in their wide and various scope ;—all these phenomena, as well as their mutual actions and dependencies, are now the subjects of active and successful inquiry.

We have remarkable proof, in several recent discoveries respecting winds, temperature, and rain, of the ignorance or error before prevailing as to some of the most familiar of these facts ; and even the most striking of the discoveries thus made, give larger view of what remains behind for future attainment.   The theory of hurricanes, so successfully developed of late, and rendered capable of such important practical uses, leaves it yet uncertain whence are derived these vast and violent whirlwinds,—what is their connexion with other winds,—what their relation, of cause or effect, to the remarkable electrical appearances which usually attend them,—and how they produce such sudden and extreme barometric changes.   There are few topics in this branch of science which do not afford illustration of similar kind.

It is a part of the sagacity of true genius to interrogate nature in her most familiar workings, seeking for causes and relations among phenomena, which others disregard from their seeming simplicity.   The Memoir on Thunder and Lightning, by M. Arago, composed for the *Annuaire du Bureau des Longitudes*, 1838, is an eminent example of this method of philosophy ; and singularly attesting at the same time the truth of what has just been stated.   Of the variety of phenomena comprised under this title, whether purely physical, or such as affect organized life, there is scarcely one which can be regarded as altogether solved ; and the greater number have barely been touched upon by speculation, without actual experiment or proof.

considered, however, they assure us of nothing more than a higher power and keener susceptibility of the ordinary organs of sense. Without denying the possibility of others, we cannot regard the exquisite perfection in which many animals possess from nature the senses of smell, sight, hearing, and touch—or even the extent and exactness which these attain in man from constant and earnest exercise—without admitting the likelihood that new phenomena both of sensation and action may arise from this greater acuteness. It is in some sort an ingress to a new sphere of life, where particular avenues are thus enlarged; and perceptions admitted, inaccessible to organs otherwise constructed, or less exercised.

Some of the phenomena of animal instincts clearly lie in this direction. The conditions and changes of weather are so urgently important to a vast number of species, connected as they are with the great instincts of food, shelter, and propagation, that provision was to be expected to meet these necessities; and such is actually found in an organization capable of being affected by changes, of which man is wholly unconscious. Acts, which seems to us altogether to anticipate the need, are in them the result of sensations already received, and leading to this result.

In considering the separate qualities of atmosphere already mentioned, in relation to their morbid effects on the human body, the same remark applies, as in so many other parts of the history of disease; viz., that the agencies are all natural, or even salutary, in degree: and that it is only the excess of state, or of change, which becomes a source of disorder. And further, that the susceptibility to be acted upon by each, varies greatly in different individuals:— conforming in this to the diversity in degree of all other impressions, as determined for every one by his respective idiosyncrasy. We have much here still to learn; and it is a subject where there is reasonable prospect of future success.

The influence of temperature is the most familiar of the conditions we have to examine, and that which has been chiefly studied; in its direct effects on the body, and indirectly through the diseases of climate. As respects the former, it seems certain that changes, sudden or frequent, are principally concerned in these results.* The power of accommodation in the body, depending on the generation of animal heat, and on the functions of the lungs and of the skin, provides in the healthy state against all which are not in excess. But where these functions are impaired, or the body otherwise disordered, every such change has influence; either by disturbing the balance of circulation between the external surface, and the membranes or different glandular structures within the body;— or by checking or augmenting the discharge of perspirable matter; —or in part, it may be, by more immediate action on the nervous system; though of this we have less certain proof.

* Αι μεταβολαι μαλιστα τικτουσι νουσηματα, και αι μιγισται μαλιστα.—*Hippocrates.*

The degree in which external cold may alter the balance of circulation,—directly, by contracting the capillaries and smaller arteries of the surface; or indirectly, by the effect of this altered balance upon the action of the heart itself,—is scarcely enough regarded in its various details.*   It is to be presumed, on the most common grounds of estimation, that the difference thus made may vary, (according to the degree of cold and the powers of reaction from within) from the smallest assignable amount, to that of several pounds of blood, changed in its manner of distribution through the vessels of the body.   The importance of such fluctuations must be obvious on the most general view.   And they include, it may be added, not merely the repulsion of blood from the surface by the contraction of the capillaries, but also the effects of the reaction and return of blood to the part; the latter consequences often very remarkable in their influence on the bodily functions.

The tendency of sudden changes of temperature to produce topical inflammation, is doubtless owing chiefly to these disturbances in the balance of circulation, which arise from changes, general or partial, in the capillaries of the surface.   Rheumatic affections, whether inflammatory or not, are usually attributed to the same cause; rightly, as respects some states which bear the name; not so, as to others, which are undoubtedly of different origin.   Many disorders of the serous and mucous membranes, of the lungs, of the alimentary canal, and other viscera, depend more certainly on changes in the distribution of blood thus made; either suddenly, or by continuance and repetition.   And these also are among the changes which have direct influence on the brain; the result of various averages showing that apoplectic seizures are most frequent when either heat or cold are severe in degree;—the mode of action doubtless different in the two cases; yet in each depending principally on disturbance excited in the movements of the blood.†

The influence of external temperature on the functions of the skin, whether those of transudation or simple evaporation, is scarcely yet fully estimated; though the researches of Dr. Edwards and others have done much to extend our knowledge on the subject. The changes so made, either in augmentation or diminution of the natural discharge, are obvious and often very great.   Without reciting the observations directed especially to these points, it may be remarked that a natural provision against injury exists here, as in the case of the temperature of the body, in the diminution of

---

* The experiments of M. Poiseuille, in his treatise on capillary circulation, confirmed by those of M. Magendie, show the effect of a low temperature in retarding or preventing the passage of blood through these extreme vessels.

† Regarding the *coup de soleil*, usually cited as one of the most striking examples of the effects of heat on the brain, we have some recent evidence (though hardly decisive), to show that the change, thus suddenly induced, belongs rather to the pulmonary circulation, than directly to the head.   This is contained in a paper by Mr. Russell, surgeon of the 63th regiment, at Madras; read before the College of Physicians two years ago.

other excretions, and in the relation of absorption to the matters perspired;—a remedy inadequate, indeed, to repair extreme or continued losses, but sufficient, for all the ordinary occasions of life. This subject belongs, subordinately with that of heat, to the general doctrine of climates; the influence of which on the animal economy is regulated, in part, by the provisions just named; in part, by actual changes in the state and texture of the integuments of the body; exclusively of those modifications which depend on the usages of life in each country or community.

The effects of perspiration suddenly checked by external cold, are the subject of general apprehension, and influence many of the details of medical practice. Though in some instances mischief may arise from this source, I believe the alarm to be unwarranted in degree; and many of the effects, so attributed, to be due to other causes acting concurrently; such as exhaustion from fatigue, the perspired fluid left on the body, and the influence of cold itself in suddenly changing the balance of circulation between external and internal parts. The latter effect may equally happen, independently of perspiration; and there is no ascertained reason why this, previously occurring, should alter or change its amount. The customs of some countries and the necessary habits of particular avocations, show how suddenly these changes may be made without any injury, if other causes of mischief are excluded; and prove the uselessness or wrong selection of many of the cautions current on the subject. This is a point on which just views are very desirable to the practitioner. It is in every case important that his judgment should be unfettered by common opinions, exaggerated or unproved;—and though here, as in other instances, it may be well to concede sometimes, yet must he ever maintain the prerogative of applying his better knowledge, when circumstances require it.

To the more common results of variations of temperature, hitherto noticed, may be added those which depend on extremes of heat or cold, suddenly, or continuously, applied to the body; the observations regarding which have been much extended of late years. The recent voyages of northern discovery furnish many as to the effect of high degrees of cold, of great interest to physiology; but as these are now familiar, and do not apply to practice, I merely allude to them as one portion of the inquiry.

There are other parts of this subject, more practical in kind, which, though better considered now than formerly, do yet not receive all the notice they deserve. Such are the direct applications of cold as a remedy; possessing certainly great value, and admitting of much more general and defined use than is made of them. Common prejudices, fostered to a singular degree on this point, are not only a great hinderance to the physician, but often do much to pervert his own views and practice. Accordingly we find that the effect produced for a time by the writings of Dr. Currie, on the application of cold in fevers (exanthematous as well as others), has been only partially sustained; and that the common course of treatment scarcely goes beyond the removal of the old and noxious errors of close atmosphere, hot rooms, and thick clothing;—doubtless a very beneficial change, but not precluding the more direct and extensive application of cold to the surfaces of the body.* Whatever the theory of this action, the benefits gained are incontestible;—familiar to all who have fairly employed it, and well recognised by patients themselves.   Almost may it be taken as a rule, that wherever there is a hot and dry skin, cold in one degree or other may safely and expediently be applied to change its state. The benefit of simple abstraction of heat is great in such cases; and the fact is not sufficiently adverted to, which I have often put to thermometrical test, of the extent to which this influence is diffused beyond the surface to which the cold is immediately applied. There is no real risk here to countervail the good gained.   We are sedulous in providing for and varying the application of heat to the body; while, from one cause of alarm or another, little provision is made for the opposite remedy, though not less capable of being actively and beneficially employed.

A point subordinate to this, which has had less notice than its practical importance deserves, is the influence of cold or hot air respectively, upon wounds or open surfaces.   The greater sensibility of parts so exposed, and the more direct actions on their vascular texture, make this condition a very important one.   And accordingly we have much proof in private practice—still more from the experience of hospitals and military campaigns—of the effects produced by heat and cold severally, or by changes from one to the other.   I have seen this remarkably in the army hospitals in Portugal; where, in summer, the general rate of recovery from wounds was accelerated or retarded, as the temperature became suddenly cooler, or the reverse.   It is singularly attested in the instance of the wounded, left exposed on the field of battle.   Though the better understanding of ventilation has contributed towards this object, yet might much more benefit be derived from the direct effects of cold as an antiphlogistic means; either through the atmosphere, or by immediate application to parts affected.   The employment of cold water externally, as a dressing to fractured limbs, gives one proof among many of the benefits of the latter practice; and we have reason to infer, that the liquid form is the best in which such application may be made for the relief of inflammation in open wounds, or other inflamed surfaces.†   Here also prejudices are to be overcome; the best assistance towards which is often derived from the sensations of the patient himself.

* I say *surfaces*, because in fact cold acts remedially on the lining of the alimentary canal, as well as on the outer skin; is often as imperatively required by the sensations of the patient; and not less sanctioned by the good obtained.

† Dr. Macartney, of Dublin, in his Treatise on Inflammation, has largely and ably illustrated this practice, both as matter of history and present experiment; connecting it with his own doctrine as to the general nature of inflammation.

While thus briefly referring to some of the effects of temperature, and chiefly on points of practical import, it must be repeated, that we can rarely view them separately from the other conditions before noticed. Every change as to heat or cold in the atmosphere must either be the effect of, or produce, other changes of atmospheric state; and none of these, it may be affirmed, are wholly indifferent to the body. Even in the simple case just mentioned, of the influence of warm or cold weather on open sores, though the atmosphere be admitted as the source of change, the effects are probably not due to temperature alone. Still less can it be supposed in regard to certain winds of our own climate; such as those from the east and south; the relations of which to the body are in nowise interpreted by the thermometer. The same remark extends more remarkably to the Sirocco of the South of Europe: and generally, perhaps, to the dominant or more peculiar winds of every locality over the globe. Where any one is especially noxious in producing epidemics, or in its effects on the general health, there, probably, is the direct influence of temperature on the body least in proportion to the other causes concerned.

Even in the endemic diseases of particular climates, the same view may be entertained. We have no certain proof that the fevers of the West Indies, or the Guinea coast—or the dysentery, remittent fevers, and liver diseases of different parts of India—or the malaria-fevers of Italy and Greece, are owing to the heat merely of these several climates. Hepatic disorders, indeed, generally, may be considered as having closest connexion with this influence; but in others of the above examples, the best evidence we possess leads us to causes, in which temperature is only indirectly concerned.* And though this evidence be notoriously imperfect, yet is it valuable in the direction thus given to further inquiry. We have no direct cognisance of those miasmata, whether of animal or vegetable origin, or simply chemical in kind, which form the material of epidemic disease; but we know that such material emanations exist; that they differ in different localities; and that variation of temperature is the condition seemingly most essential to their several forms and various activity. We have evidence, both experimental and of natural occurrence, of the effects of a certain degree of heat in producing or evolving these agents; and of a higher degree in destroying them, or suspending their action. Such results might be inferred as probable, from what we have cause to presume of their nature; looking here, as the nearest analogy, to

* Here I may again refer to Dr. J. Johnson's book on the Diseases of Tropical Climates, in which he shows how vaguely these relations of disease and locality are often considered, and made the subject of inference. We speak of hepatitis and remittent fevers as diseases of India, without adverting to the fact that the true hepatitis (or that which is not a sequel to fever) is ten times more prevalent on the coast of Coromandel, than in the plains of Bengal;—intermittent and remittent fevers in an equal ratio more frequent in the latter locality. The medium annual temperature of Madras is known to be amongst the highest on the globe; (88° Fahr.) that of Calcutta about ten degrees lower.

the chemical constitution of the known poisons, whether of animal or vegetable origin,—to the feeble affinity by which their elements are generally united,—and the facility with which they are decomposed, and enter into new combinations from slight changes of temperature alone.

I need not refer to the many illustrations of this subject furnished by the history of disease. They are continually multiplied, as observation becomes more exact; and it is likely that the estimate of effect from this source will enlarge in proportion to our knowledge. The unequal influence of equal averages of heat in different localities might itself suggest doubts whether too much is not attributed to its direct action, too little to its operation through other agents. All examination of particular local conditions, such as soil, elevation, general humidity, quantity and kind of vegetable growth, manner of culture, and extent of running or stagnant water, shows the singular importance of these circumstances, as determining the endemic disorders and average health of different localities, exclusively even of the habits and employment of the people in each. Every country and district furnishes such instances; and all concur in proving that we must estimate the influence of temperature upon the body, and especially of heat, subordinately in great part to these more varied conditions. Isothermal zones would afford a very uncertain measure of the character or prevalence of disease.*

But it is a further question here, whether variations of atmospheric temperature may not induce a state of body, rendering it more liable to receive specific infections, however generated by agents without? That there are such differences of bodily condition, however vaguely known to us by external signs, must be admitted. And it is perhaps not a rash inference from the temporary effect of exposure to great heat, in quickening the circulation and augmenting the animal temperature, that continued exposure to the same cause, even much less in degree, may keep the constitution in a state prone to morbid actions, when the exciting causes are present. The uncertainty in this case depends in part on our ignorance of the equality of the causes, and of the relative degree of exposure to them; and can only be met by strong presumption, or actual observation of change in the bodily state. But I think it improbable, seeing especially the small increase of animal temperature from elevation of that without, that heat alone is concerned in producing such alterations: and, if depending on atmospheric

* Many excellent papers on this subject have appeared of late in the Transactions of our provincial Medical Associations, based on that statistical method, which alone is capable of affording sound results. They all show the intimate relation between the nature of the surface and the prevalence or infrequency of particular diseases in given localities ; a point in which external temperature is only indirectly concerned, but where the effects are of singular importance in a practical view. Long and careful averages can alone be effectual in expounding them, by removing gradually all extrinsic or accidental circumstances.

causes, it is likely that these are of mixed kind, and blended with other actions more peculiar to the body itself.*

The action of cold, regarded in the same general light of locality or season, is perhaps less remarkable than that of heat, as not equally involving those physical agents which become the direct causes of disease. But besides its effects on the balance of circulation already noticed (and which, though more strikingly shown by sudden changes of temperature, are also a result of continued cold), we have to notice its indirect influence in producing certain habits and necessities of life which variously affect the health ; and more especially the alteration it makes in all that relates to food in those countries, where it gives the predominant character to the climate.

The same manner of reasoning on the morbid effects of heat and cold, whether immediate, or such as depend on long exposure, must lead us to make large allowance for the momentary condition of the body, and the general habits of life. A man under strong exercise, or with habits of such, is very differently affected from one in repose. Protection from, or exposure to, the causes which augment the direct influence of temperature, as the open sun, wind, and rains,—comfort or privation in the manner of life,—habits of temperance or sensual excess,—even the different occupations and temper of mind ;—all these conditions modify more or less the effects of heat and cold on the body ; and some of them, in particular cases, so powerfully, as almost to invert the accustomed results of such exposure.

In practice also, and for a rule in the habits of life, regard is not sufficiently paid to the different power which different individuals possess, of generating animal heat. This function, whether depending on changes in the blood and manner of circulation, or more directly on the nervous system, is as various in its power and exercise as any other of the body, and requires to be dealt with as such. Each age, too, has its changes in this respect, as well as every condition of health; and precautions founded on them cannot expediently be neglected, provided they are not so minute as to interfere with other parts of the economy of life, equally essential to the welfare of the whole.

In a brief outline like this, it is needless to particularize instances. They are familiar to common remark ; cited in medical works (though not always so specifically as the subject requires); and are very striking in the more extreme cases, where the struggle between

---

* The best observations we possess, show that the change of temperature in the human body, made by extremes of natural climate, does not exceed one or two degrees. The experiments of Berger and Delaroche, on the effects of exposure to higher and more sudden heat, prove that a temperature of 80° Fahr. above that of the body may raise the animal heat eight or ten degrees ; a grade still below that evolved in some fevers, and under particular lesions of the nervous system. It is important to notice, that the same conditions produced different results in the two experimentalists ; an effect that might have been anticipated, seeing its probable dependence in part on the excitement to circulation, which is so various in different individuals from the same causes.

the agency from without, and the powers of resistance from within, is most strongly marked. For we must ever revert to those great provisions in the constitution against all extreme or sudden changes of external temperature, by the laws which govern the production of animal heat ; the action of the exhalants of the lungs and skin; and possibly also the secretions of other organs.* No correct results can be obtained as to the agency of heat and cold upon the body, without keeping these powers of balance constantly in view ; and as they again are perpetually undergoing modifications from the various conditions of life, so is there a circle of relations, tending altogether to equality of average, though greatly broken and interrupted in its several parts.

We have no evidences of equal provision, as respects the second of the general conditions of the atmosphere; viz., its hygrometrical state.† But, on the other hand, there is every reason to infer that no similar need exists for it. The simple agency upon the body of dry or humid air, is doubtless much more limited in every sense than that of heat and cold ;—restricted, as far as we can see, to certain organs, and less powerful in its influence on these. It is still more difficult also to detach it in observation from the influence of other causes. Sudden and considerable changes do not occur in the hygrometrical state of the air, without corresponding changes in its temperature, weight, and electrical condition. Even the common fog, or mist, is far from being a single or simple phenomenon. In some instances it is the cloud already formed, and brought by currents of air or other causes to a lower level;—in other instances, as in the fogs which occasionally intervene between thunder-storms, the result apparently of a change going on in the electrical relations of the earth and atmosphere at the spot, producing alterations in the hygrometrical state of the latter. Science has not yet assigned their proper place to these several changes, as regards the relation of cause and effect. But however this be determined hereafter, the complex nature of their action on the body still remains, and will long retard any certain conclusions on the subject.

Another source of ambiguity, in considering the effects of different degrees of humidity of the air, is the influence of local circumstances of soil and surface in modifying this ; especially in that lower stratum of the atmosphere, with which man has chief concern :—and this modification regards not merely the quantity of water taken up by the air, or precipitated from it, according to the several conditions of the surface, and the action of external sources of temperature ; but also the various miasmata disengaged, or other-

---

* Taking the record, seemingly well authenticated, of the two extremes of temperature of the human body, as determined by diseases affecting the blood, we find them to include a range of nearly 40° of Fahrenheit.

† Unless, indeed, we admit as partially and indirectly such, the apparent relation between perspiration and absorption ; the latter process balancing, by its increase or diminution, any changes the former may undergo from the different conditions of the atmosphere as to moisture or dryness.

wise acted upon, by the same processes. I have already adverted to these material causes of disease, in their more particular relation to heat. Whatever their nature, (and we have everything still to learn here,) it seems certain that the presence of moisture, either on the surface or near it, under the form of vegetation, damp air or soil, and acted upon by a certain degree of temperature, contributes much to their production, if not indeed essential to it. And to these conditions, conjoined perhaps with the electrical state of the atmosphere, we may chiefly attribute the greater unhealthiness of the rainy seasons in tropical climates, which the mere quantity of rain falling will not equally explain.

But further than this, there is some cause to presume that aqueous vapour in the atmosphere, whatever its mode of combination, is much concerned in giving activity and spread to these miasmata as the cause of disease. It is idle to speculate upon physical relation here, (whether that of solution, or of independent elasticity, according to Dalton's theory of vapours,) while so entirely ignorant of the chemical constitution of these agents. We can only affirm that the conditions which concur to their production, are likely to aid their diffusion and action on other bodies: and though the proofs are by no means assured, yet there is evidence that a foggy and humid state of atmosphere is that in which contagious or epidemic diseases are most readily and extensively spread. Other causes, however, doubtless operate, and produce many apparent or real exceptions to the fact.*

Recurring to the more direct influence of air, loaded with moisture, on the body, we have reason to expect it to be greatest on the functions of respiration and of the skin ; and observation, as far as it goes, confirms this view. The effects in each case are probably owing chiefly to the altered amount of discharge from the exhalant vessels of the organs concerned ; in part also, especially when the external temperature is low, to the greater effect of cold, conjoined with moisture, on the capillary vessels and sentient extremities of nerves of the surfaces exposed. The difference to the feelings between a temperature of 45° Fahr., in dry or in damp air, is one which cannot escape the most ordinary attention. It is a difference equally marked as that between steam, and air heated to 212°, in their respective application to the body. The membrane lining the air passages is obviously most liable to these effects, and to disorders depending upon them ; as the experience of patients suffering under asthma and bronchitis, however varying in details, painfully testifies in its general results.

For the reasons already given, we are rarely indeed entitled to speak of humidity alone as a morbid cause; but it undoubtedly concurs with and renders others more effectual. And in the case of very damp air received into the lungs, it is probable that it may

* Dr. Macculloch's views, in his work on Malaria, are carried beyond what facts will justify ; but they bear the impress of that acute observation which distinguishes all his writings.

act expressly by retarding or impairing the changes made in respiration; and especially those depending on exhalation, which forms so important a part of this process.   Modern research, in showing the facility with which these changes take place, (not merely by vascular structure, but through intervening membranes, and in dependence on more general physical laws,) exposes in the same ratio their liability to be altered or impeded by causes, which before scarcely came into our view.

The action of very dry air on the body is even less certainly known to us.   There is reason to believe that the effects of the Simoom wind (exaggerated, perhaps, in common narrative) are due in part to this cause;—in conjunction with its singular heat, the quantity of minute sand it conveys, and above all, the electrical condition of the current of air.   There are more familiar reasons, however, for presuming that the atmosphere may occasionally be too dry, (becoming so either naturally or by artificial means,) for the healthy state of the functions of the skin and respiration.   Without referring to the question, still undecided, whether absorption of atmospheric moisture through the surfaces of the body does occasionally or habitually take place as a natural process,—and without affirming that the effect is derived from pulmonary evaporation unduly increased,—we have various proofs that a state of air is often created by artificial heat, insalutary to the body; and that this condition may be removed by means which restore to it a certain degree of humidity.   Houses or apartments heated by stoves, (particularly under the style of domestic architecture in England,) are liable to suspicion on this score; and if the fact be ascertained, which is not difficult with the better hygrometers now in use, it becomes expedient in every case to remedy it; either by exposure of a surface of water for the benefit of slow evaporation, or by other means.   What is merely an inconvenience for the hour or day, may pass into a serious injury to the health, when there is long-continued exposure to it.*

The influence of the atmosphere in producing morbid conditions of body, through its changes of weight, is a curious subject of inquiry in many points of view.   It is chiefly and most familiarly noted, in disturbances of the balance of circulation throughout the body; and particularly in that of the head and lungs; from obvious causes as respects the economy of these organs.   The functions of the lungs, indeed, are subject to this influence in several ways; even the mechanical part of the process being in some part concerned; as well as the balance between the external air and that

---

* In a paper read before the Royal Society in 1836, on the ventilation of the Custom-House of London, Dr. Ure states the peculiarities of atmosphere in the Long Room, warmed with hot air, and where 200 persons are always present, to be its extreme dryness (sometimes 70 per cent of Daniell's hygrometer), and negatively electrical state;—the general effects produced being vertigo, with a sense of fulness and tension about the head; a quick but feeble pulse; and deficient circulation in the lower extremities.

within the bronchial cells; and the relation of the whole to the quantity of blood in the pulmonary circulation. While the action of the heart must necessarily be affected by all which thus tends to disturb the equal movements of the circulating fluid.

Another consideration again regards the relative effect of air of different density, in producing the proper changes on the blood. It is clear that there exists a point of rarefaction, at which this quantity of oxygen is insufficient for the purposes it has to fulfil. Or, giving the statement its most general form, there must be a particular specific gravity of air (concurring probably with the medium barometrical pressure), which is best fitted for the necessities of the function; and all deviations from which, in one degree or other, interfere with the completeness of its performance.

These effects, however, under ordinary circumstances, and in healthy state of body, are slight or inappreciable in amount; limited by the range of barometrical variation, and by the usual slowness of the changes taking place. They are augmented of course when the variation is more rapid and of greater extent;—still, however, depending on changes in the state of respiration; and on irregular distribution of blood, from the altered balance of pressure between the external and internal parts of the body. The latter cause might be expected to affect most the vascular system; seeing its structure, functions, and the mechanical principles which in part determine the motions of fluids, even in the vessels of the living body. The common observations with the air-pump and cupping-glasses show the facility with which these vascular textures, and the contained fluids, yield to any such change of balance; and the effects in the diving bell, on the head more especially, produced by an increase of only one-fifth, or one-sixth, in the atmospheric pressure, may be received as proof, though less obvious, of the same fact.*

But in less peculiar cases than these, notable effects may occur, when the changes in the weight of the air are frequent, sudden, and considerable, even within the ordinary range of atmospheric variation. Regarding merely the average pressure upon the whole body, it is to be supposed that any very sudden fluctuation, to the amount perhaps of one-thirtieth, may produce temporary changes in the balance of circulation between external and internal parts, of much moment to the latter. And these are particularly to be looked for, when there is individual liability to certain diseases, or close approach to them at the time; a point requiring to be kept in mind more than it usually is, in estimating the influence of exciting causes, whatever their nature.

This observation, as I have already stated, appears especially to apply to affections of the brain. I have made note of two or three

* The suggestions of Sir James Murray (*Report of the British Association,* 1835), for the use of artificially rarefied or condensed air, in application to the surface of the body as a remedial agent, deserve much attention. The cases are numerous, where changes in the local distribution of the blood, thus readily made, would be of much value in the treatment of disease.

periods, since I began practice, during which there has been a more than wontèd frequency of apoplectic or paralytic seizures within my immediate knowledge; so marked as to make it difficult to attribute the fact to mere casualty, notwithstanding the many circumstances which tend to invalidate such results when not verified by large averages. The same fact, observed by others, has generally been attributed to external heat alone. But allowing what has already been assigned to this cause, the particular character of the weather at these times will scarcely support the inference; nor has the result in question been equally apparent even under higher degrees of atmospheric temperature. While, on the other hand, I have observed at these periods frequent and rapid changes in the barometer, often with great depression of its level; and have noticed at the same time the very common occurrence of lesser affections of the head,—vague and uneasy sensations, oppression, vertigo, and what may be termed a feeling of want of proper balance to the frame—all indicating some cause present which tends more or less to disturb the equality of circulation through this organ.

In fact, the ordinary phrases of heaviness and lightness of air (however misplaced or even inverted their use) prove the general consciousness of these changes in their slighter influence on the body. It may be difficult to say through what organ or function this feeling is chiefly conveyed; but probably it is a compound effect of the changes in circulation, in which the sensorium, the lungs, and the muscular system, all participate. Even the organs of digestion seem to be affected, directly or indirectly, by the same causes. Without referring to the doubtful instance of vomiting produced in highly rarefied air, I think I have observed frequent disturbance both in the sensations and functions of the alimentary canal, under any rapidly diminished weight of the atmosphere, or where its changes were more frequent than usual. I have remarked in the preceding chapter on the indications of disturbance to sleep from the same cause.

All these inferences, however, are rendered uncertain by the great difficulty of simplifying the conditions which belong to them, where the physical causes concerned are so unceasingly blended in their operation. It may be, for instance, that what is attributed to changes of weight of air, really belongs to electrical changes in the atmosphere, producing or attending the former. Another more familiar case of ambiguity, is that of the sensations experienced in reaching a high mountain-summit. Though often attributed to rarefaction of the air breathed, I doubt not (on my own observation as well as that of others), that they are chiefly owing to the expenditure of bodily power that has been incurred by muscular action, hurried breathing, and quickened action of the heart. These sensations in great part subside, when the immediate causes of lassitude and disorder are removed. Or, if we yet need explanation of that singular sense of fatigue in the limbs, which is alleged to occur when walking in elevated regions, even without the toil of ascent, we may perhaps find it in a suggestion of Humboldt; whose sagacity is ever awake to all natural phenomena, even such as pass unheeded by others from their seeming familiarity.   He conjectures that this sensation may depend on the mechanism of the joints and equipoise of the bones being disturbed by the low atmospheric pressure; and the experiments of the two Webers, recently made at his suggestion, have afforded a singular confirmation of this idea.*

The observations in ascent by balloons, now become so familiar to us, show, even unexpectedly in degree, the extent to which the body can undergo the most sudden changes of atmospheric weight, without any very obvious effect, where the health is unimpaired, and no causes of bodily fatigue are conjoined.   In the note below, I have stated some facts derived from the best authority we now possess on this curious subject.†

These observations lessen any surprise at the great powers of accommodation by habit to a constant high degree of rarefied

* Poggendorff's Annalen für 1837, No. 1.   These experiments, made upon the hip-joint after the two bones had been detached by cutting the capsular membrane through, show that the pressure of the air will still retain the head of the thigh-bone firmly in the socket, from which it sinks down when the air is artificially rarefied underneath; the joint thus becoming a sort of air-pump, in which the head of the thigh-bone acts as a piston.

† I have been recently favoured with these observations by Mr. Green, whose boldness and ability as an aëronaut have given him such general and well-merited reputation.   Having now ascended in balloons with more than 400 persons, under every possible variation of height, rapidity, and state of atmosphere at the time, his evidence on the points in question is far more complete than any other we possess.

Mr. Green informs me that he has found none of these individuals sensibly affected, otherwise than by the sudden change of temperature and by a noise in the ears, compared by some to very distant thunder; the latter sensation occurring only during rapid ascent or descent of the balloon, and, when greatest in degree, far less distressing than that produced by descent in a diving bell. He has never felt his own respiration hurried or oppressed, except when exerting himself in throwing out ballast, or other management of the balloon, or when suddenly passing into a very cold atmosphere.   His pulse is occasionally quickened ten or fifteen beats, but this only when some such exertion has been sustained.   He mentions to me expressly, that in no instance have his companions experienced vertigo or sickness; thus rendering doubtful one of the statements current on this subject, and showing how little the two great functions of circulation and respiration are disturbed, under circumstances where much effect might have been anticipated.

Though the inference is limited to two persons, yet it may be worth while to mention the great experiment made by Mr. Green and Mr. Rush in September 1838, in ascending to the height of 27,136 feet, or 5¼ miles above the level of the sea; the greatest elevation ever reached by man, and very exactly corresponding with the highest ascertained summit of the Himalaya mountains.   The barometer fell from 33° 50′ to 11° during this ascent; the thermometer from 61° to 5°. The first 11,000 feet were passed through in about seven minutes.   Yet, under these remarkable circumstances, Mr. Rush suffered no inconvenience but from cold; and Mr. Green little other than from the toil of discharging ballast and gas at different intervals, which hurried the respiration during the time.

atmosphere. The city of Mexico stands 7,460 feet above the level of the sea; and there are inhabited points in the Andes of Peru even 6,000 feet still higher.* It must be admitted, however, that we have no sufficient knowledge of the diseases in these localities, or of the average rate of mortality, to justify inferences as to effects on the body derived from this single physical cause, when forming what may be termed a constant condition of climate.

Of a general view of the circumstances stated, there is reason to conclude that the influence of the different degrees of atmospheric pressure in disturbing the bodily functions and general health, is rather derived from the frequency of fluctuations, than from any state long continued, either above or below the average standard; —that, of the two conditions, suddenly incurred in any extreme degree, the human frame is better capable of withstanding a rarefied than a condensed atmosphere;—and that, in every case, the previous health, and proneness to disorder in particular organs, are greatly concerned in determining the results on the body.

Little though its influence has yet been defined, I believe that the electrical state of the atmosphere is that of all its conditions which has most important and diffused effects on the animal economy; more rapid and pervading than any other; and, as one of the vital stimuli, more intimately allied to the functions of the nervous system. It is that, further, which most closely blends itself, either as cause or effect, with all other meteorological changes; producing thereby many of the difficulties already noticed in estimating their relative amount of influence. When modern science has shown us that every chemical action is attended by, if not identical with, electrical change;—that the processes of vegetation, as well as those of animal life, involve unceasing alteration in its states;—that no two bodies can be present to each other of different temperature, nor even separate parts of the same body be differently heated, without evolution of this agent;—that every act of evaporation or deposition of water on the surface of the globe has similar effect of change, even the spray of a waterfall sensibly altering the balance of electricity around it;—we may well understand how wide is the circle of these mutual changes, and how important in the economy of nature, including in this the existence and functions of organic life itself.

It is difficult to advert to the effects of atmospheric electricity on the body, either as a vital stimulus or cause of disease, without noticing the question, whether this great natural agent is not itself directly engaged in the functions of the nervous system? If this were eventually determined to be so, the relation of the actions without, to those of the same agent within, would become of still more complex kind, and little amenable to our present means of research. But, taking at present the simplest view of the influence

* Mr. Pentland, in 1826, ascertained the height of the town of Potosi to be 13,260 feet above the Pacific. Humboldt mentions inhabited places on the Cordilleras at equal elevation.

of electrical states of air on the human frame, many circumstances occur, well deserving notice, though yet wanting the certainty needful to give them a place in science.

The natural history of the animal kingdom through its whole extent, furnishes numerous examples (exclusively of those in which there exists an especial organization for electrical purposes) of the singular susceptibility of different animal species to electrical changes in the media which surround them; and many particular cases of instinct, hitherto unexplained, may doubtless be traced to this source. In man the effects are generally less marked, yet nevertheless certain. Without adverting to those singular cases in which the balance of electricity with external objects seems altered by the production of an excess of it within the body, it is obvious that changes of atmospheric electricity have much influence both on the sensations and voluntary powers, producing results variously analogous to those which attend certain morbid states of body more familiar to us.* A few may be noticed in illustration from among those most easily recognised.

An atmosphere, proved by other phenomena to be highly charged with electricity, produces in many persons sensations resembling those of slight incipient fever; vague alternations of chill and warmth on the skin, general languor of the frame, debility and aching of the limbs, oppression or other uneasiness about the head. In other instances, the feelings created in the muscles of the trunk and limbs have more of rheumatic character; the resemblance being such as to justify a suspicion that some of the muscular affections, often so termed, are actually derived from this cause. In some persons the susceptibility is so great, that even the approach of a thunder-cloud produces bodily feelings akin to those just described, together with a sense of fulness and pricking about the eyes, and a slight tingling over the whole body, which I have often noticed in such cases.

The effects of electricity, artificially applied, may be brought into illustration here. The feelings of numbness or aching that remain for some time in the muscles or joints, after the electric current has been passed through them (whether derived from the machine, from voltaic, or electro-magnetic combinations), much resemble those which occur in the early stage of fever, or under other morbid conditions of the body; while the sensations on the skin which some persons feel in the vicinity of a powerful electrical machine in ac-

* Of the various instances on record of the curious fact alluded to above, the most remarkable and best attested is that related in the American Journal of Medical Science for January, 1838. A lady, without any adequate cause, passed suddenly into a state in which she threw out electric sparks to any conductor around her, sometimes to the distance of an inch and a half, with the ordinary sensations attending electrical action; this state continuing for several months, and subsiding by gradual diminution of the power. Other singular details of this case are given, on authority which appears to be good, and without any obvious sources of fallacy.

tion,—or by being electrified on an insulated stool, with much conducting material around,—-are very similar to others of familiar occurrence, observed especially in certain states of the atmosphere, while electrical changes are going on. And in cases of this kind, there is also a certain degree of languor, or even diminished frequency of the pulse; varying in different individuals, but still uniform enough to prove the reality and nature of the effect.

One of the best tests of the actual operation of atmospheric electricity on the body is, as I think, that mixed sensation of heat and cold which most persons must recollect at some time to have felt,—or rather, the consciousness of sensations which cannot clearly be defined to be either.* Concurrently with such state of atmosphere, which the thermometer does not in any way interpret to us, there generally occurs more or less of the lassitude before described; the muscles are readily fatigued ; some degree of headache is often felt ; and other vague uneasiness of the bodily feelings, varying much in different habits, and doubtless influenced by the condition of health at the time.

Though these effects are in general more distinctly experienced previously to, or during thunder-storms, yet are they also sometimes attested in other states of weather where no such storms occur. Certain winds, very common in our own climate, will sustain, even for weeks together, this peculiar character of atmosphere; in degree sufficient to be marked by the results just described, and having still more singular and obvious influence on other animals inferior to man, and on vegetable life. These winds, which may be described generally, as coming from all eastern points of the compass, but more especially from the quarter lying between north-east and south-east, deserve inquiry under all the aids which modern science can afford. Their various effects on the human body, and on all living organization, are in nowise explained by the temperature or weight of the air. The great dryness of some easterly winds may give better reason for certain of the phenomena, but will scarcely explain the peculiar sense of muscular aching, uneasiness, and languor, they produce in many habits ; the almost instant perception of their effects by some, even without any exposure to the external air; and as rapid consciousness of change when they cease. Such sensations belong much more to what we know of electrical agency than to any other cause we can assign ; but they need observations more exact than have yet been made, and a careful comparison of these with the physical properties of the winds in question, which future research may also better determine.

Whatever the natural causes which render some of our easterly

---

* It is certain that the sensation of itching depends on several different causes acting on the extremities of the sentient nerves ; and it seems probable, from various familiar instances, that one of these is the state of electricity on the skin, in relation to that of the air or particular articles of clothing without. If the assertion of Donné be correct, that there is an opposite electrical state of the two surfaces of the skin, it might lead to further inferences on the subject.

winds thus peculiar, that from the south-east may certainly be considered to have direct connexion with the Sirocco, as it sweeps with greater or less intensity over the southern half of Europe. This very singular atmospheric current, which on its more distant border has probable relation to the Simoom and Harmattan, the hot winds of the African desert,—and passes over the Mediterranean Sea under the names of the Levant wind and Sirocco,—reaches England on the opposite side,—its peculiar qualities much mitigated, yet still showing the same origin in its general direction, in its hygrometrical conditions, and in what I believe to be its electrical influence on animal life. No sufficient explanation has yet been given of these peculiarities, nor are they perhaps definite enough as facts to warrant much theory on the subject. I cannot doubt, however, from my own observations, that the electrical state of these great atmospheric streams, whencesoever derived, is that to which their effects are mainly due. I have witnessed in different parts of the Mediterranean such singular and repeated proofs of this as to give assurance of the general fact, though there are yet wanting the exact determinations required to fix its place in the history of physical phenomena.*

* In my Travels in Albania, &c. (2d edition, 1819), I have related two occurrences of this kind, in which the electrical phenomena attending the Sirocco, as seen at night, were very striking. One of these instances I cannot readily forget. It was when approaching the coast of Ithaca, under the obscurity of a dark evening in October, after a still and sultry day, the wind arose suddenly and strongly from the south-east, kindling, almost instantly every part of the sky with gleams and flashes of electric light; vivid enough at intervals to allow the reading of the smallest print; and giving outline, not only to the cliffs of Ithaca closely above us, but even to the distant mountains of Santa Maura and the Acarnanian coast. As in almost every instance in which I have witnessed such appearances from the Sirocco, dark masses of cloud speedily began to gather in the north-west, the quarter towards which the wind blew; and amidst these the electrical discharges or interchanges were singularly splendid in effect, continuing until a late hour in the night. No thunder was heard during any part of the time, nor did rain fall; but I found, from observations on this and similar occasions, that the quantity of moisture in the air was very great, and have generally noticed the wind to subside with a fall of rain.

In other instances, where the Sirocco began to blow in the evening or during the night, I have observed appearances of the same kind, though none equally striking. They are generally, according to my experience, more marked at the beginning of the wind, as might be presumed likely from the blending of different portions of atmosphere unequally charged with electricity, or in different states. Though unable to speak with assurance from imperfect observations, yet I believe the current of the Sirocco to be usually one of negative electricity.

In the work just alluded to, I have mentioned the position of Malta as very favourable for a series of observations on this remarkable wind. Its effects on the barometer and thermometer require to be noticed; still more those which indicate its electrical and hygrometrical states. The latter, too, need the comparison of inland observations (which must be obtained elsewhere) with those made by the sea. Though Dolomieus's assertion that the atmosphere of the Sirocco contains less than the due proportion of oxygen, is liable to much doubt, yet ought the air to be examined eudiometrically also. And to these notices should be added others, as to the frequency, periods of occurrence, and duration of the wind; the exact points from which it blows, and the changes in these;

· Our knowledge of atmospheric electricity is, in truth, still in its infancy. What was written on the subject by Mr. Luke Howard and others, at a comparatively early period in the history of the science, is still an authority to which little has been added, in proportion to its progress in other parts. The causes of production, distribution and change;—its relation to that electricity which circulates in magnetic currents, or otherwise appertains to the earth, or may possibly exist in space beyond the atmosphere ;—its connexion with atmospheric heat, moisture, or weight; with the formation of clouds; and the phenomena of wind, thunder-storms, and rain ;—and above all, the relation of its positive and negative states—each one of these conditions is still largely open to inquiry. The latter especially, which has most assured and closest relation to all the rest, is the great mystery still hanging over electrical science ; the solution of which would not merely determine these particular questions, but probably, in its connexion with the general doctrine of polarity, enlarge our whole view of the attraction and combinations of matter, whether in atoms or masses throughout the universe.

What has been thus far said regards chiefly the influence of electrical states of the atmosphere on the sensations and muscular powers. Unless justified in considering as such the occasional effects of lightning on the body, I know no express example of disease which we can affirm to be produced by this agency. Some authors, indeed, have attributed to it certain epidemics of singular character, and not easily referrible to any known cause. But in this opinion they have hardly defined, whether it is to be considered as directly producing the disease, or merely a state of body predisposing to receive it; leaving open still the third contingency of its simply evolving from other sources the virus or material cause of disease. I have elsewhere shown that it is difficult, if not impossible, to connect these erratic disorders with any state of weather or known quality of the atmosphere ; and the reasons derived from their history, apply as distinctly to electricity as to any other property of the element which surrounds us. We must, however, admit the possibility, both as to these and other disorders, of the two latter contingencies just stated. Electricity may be concerned in favouring the generation of malaria, whatever its nature; or it may induce a state of body more liable to be affected by this, or by other

the external appearances attending it; and its effects in producing bodily disorder, whether of the sensations, voluntary power, or vital actions.

A conjecture of Colonel Reid, in his very valuable work on the *Law of Storms*, would, if verified, afford a plausible account of the properties of this wind, hitherto so little explained by any local circumstances. He supposes, in conformity with his general doctrine, that the Levanter or Sirocco may be the south-west wind of the great Desert of Sahara, sweeping round so as to become an easterly or south-easterly wind in the Mediterranean, and still retaining qualities which it has acquired in passing over this vast region of sand. Any future observations in Egypt, or other eastern parts of Africa, which might show strong southerly winds, corresponding in time with the Levant winds of the Mediterranean, would furnish much confirmation of this conjecture.

causes of disease in activity at the time. We have no proofs on which even to approach towards assurance, but presumption from several sources that this great agent cannot be wholly inert as respects either of the conditions in question.

Though unable then to affirm any one disease to be actually produced by electricity, yet, considering the subject in its whole extent, it is impossible not to see the likelihood of its influence on the body in many ways hitherto undistinguished, or not understood. If a stroke of lightning can in an instant destroy muscular irritability throughout the system,—prevent, in great part, or altogether, the coagulation of the blood,—and hasten putrefaction,—it is clearly to be inferred that lesser degrees of the same action must have definite effects, bearing proportion to the intensity of the electrical changes or transferences taking place. The conclusions, best warranted by the facts we possess, would direct us towards the blood and nervous system generally, as the parts of the animal economy most liable to be thus affected. The influence of atmospheric electricity on the latter is shown in the various effects, already mentioned, on the sensations and muscular power; and the proof is greatly strengthened, though indirectly, by the numerous experiments which prove the influence upon these two functions, of electric action from different sources, applied directly to the nerves themselves.* The quantity or tension of the agent, as affecting the body through the air, may be less, and its application not so direct on the nervous system. The low average intensity of animal electricity, as ascertained experimentally, must also be taken into account. But with all these allowances it is impossible that the effect should be wholly absent or different in kind; and circumstances may often greatly augment its degree, disordering in the same ratio that balance which is most conducive to the general well-being of life.

The same reasoning applies equally to its influence on the blood; and though this part of the subject is even more obscure, yet is there presumption that here the effects occur which are of greatest import in the history of disease. All that chemistry has recently done to determine the nature and relation of parts in the blood (concurrently with that great result which Faraday has established of the identity of electrical and chemical action) justifies the belief that every material change of balance between the electricity without, and that within the body, must have effect on the state of the circulating fluid; transient and wholly inappreciable, it may be, in the great majority of cases; in others, possibly, of longer duration and more extensive in degree. The general relation of acid and alkali, as important in the chemistry of life as in that of inorganic matter;—obvious, not only in the blood itself, but in the

* The researches of Humboldt, Müller, Prevost and Dumas, Dr. Wilson Philip, Becquerel, and other physiologists, might be referred to in this place;—not equally certain in results, nor conducting their authors to the same conclusions, but concurring to show the remarkable nature of this agency as a stimulus on the nervous and muscular systems, if indeed it be nothing more.

materials and processes by which it is formed, and in the secretions and excretions derived from it,—this relation is one in which we have peculiar and constant evidence of electrical agency. The coagulable property of the blood, in whatever it consists, is closely affected by the same cause, even when acting through various intervening tissues. Though we have no equal proof as to the globules, yet their definite form, size, and other peculiarities (necessary as it would seem to the existence of each species), make it probable that they are liable to alteration from an agent, which seems more than any other to determine all definite combinations and changes in the material world.*

The tenor and extent of the argument here must be rightly understood. We have no proof of the action of atmospheric electricity, in any of its ordinary states, upon the blood. But the effects of lightning, and the influence of the same principle, proved by experiment in other modes of application to this fluid, warrant the belief that such action may exist; and, if existing, that it must be a frequent cause of disorder· throughout every part of the animal economy. We cannot trace diseases with certainty to this source, but how rare are the instances in which we can affirm their real causes! The actual void of knowledge justifies our seeking them through all the new agencies which physical science may disclose; and none is more likely to afford successful results than that now before us.

Two classes of facts, neither of them yet sufficiently examined, are obviously very important to the inquiry. The first includes the indications which diseases themselves may give, in their progress, of alteration of electrical state in the body. The second involves the more general question as to the development of electricity in the animal frame; its natural variations from age, sex, temperament, and connexion with particular bodily functions; and its manner of relation to the electricity of the air without. With the exception of some curious observations of Humboldt and Pfaff on the electrical state of rheumatic patients, we have nothing that approaches to certainty on the former subject. On the latter we possess more results, but all requiring revision and extension by further experiment. We still have no averages sufficient to show the relative frequency of positive or negative states of the body;—still less what determines this difference, or the changes taking place in the same

* The action of electricity on the blood has been the subject of the same zealous research as its influence on the nervous system ; and directed ultimately to the same question, whether it is not itself the most essential principle in this fluid, ever present, and determining all the changes which take place within it ? The reasoning of Müller (*Handbuch der Physiologie,* p 128), in refutation of the singular experiments and inferences of Dutrochet, may be consulted as an example of the ingenious and minute inquiry given to this subject, as well as of the ambiguity which still surrounds it,—both as respects the chemical changes, usually so termed, in the blood, and the action of voltaic electricity in promoting or modifying them. The question concerning the relation of animal electricity and animal heat is a very curious part of this subject.

person.* And this involves directly the question as to manner of relation with the electricity of the atmosphere; one made less difficult, perhaps, since the sagacity of Faraday has reduced all the phenomena of induction to functions of the conducting power; but still requiring much care and research for its complete solution; and a regard, not merely to the changes of state within the body, but to those also ever occurring in the positive or negative conditions of the atmosphere without; of which the comparative excess of positive electricity during the day may be taken as a well marked example.

I have dwelt so far in detail on this part of the subject of the chapter, as being that on which our knowledge is most deficient; and from persuasion also of its future importance in solving many obscure questions in pathology. I might further plead its obvious connexion with all the uses, which may eventually be ascertained of electricity as a remedy in disease; a point where it must be owned that much successful research is needed, to remove that imputation of failure which has been the result of the partial and often abortive trials hitherto made.†

* The experiments of my friend Professor Pfaff of Keil, in conjunction with Ahrens, are more complete than any others I know on this subject.

† It must be admitted, indeed, as singular, that an agent so general, so variously excited, and so powerful as a vital stimulus, should hitherto have lent such slender and doubtful aid to the physician. For this, however, some probable causes may be assigned. Applied chiefly as a stimulus to palsied limbs or torpid organs, or often with less definite purpose to cases where all other means have failed, it has had also the disadvantage of a general method of use, too gross, as it would seem, for the subtle nature of its action on the living economy. The only conception of its effect would seem to have been that of a stimulus, and this in the least defined sense of the term. Any action upon particular functions is either unknown, or so partially determined, as still to afford no assured inferences for practice. The important researches of Dr. Wilson Philip, on the influence of voltaic electricity, transmitted through the pneumogastric nerve, on the function of digestion; and the cases he has published in proof of its beneficial effect in certain dyspeptic disorders, in asthma, &c.; may occur as the most striking exception to this statement. But even here much is wanting to the certainty of the inferences; and repetition is needful to give assurance to the practical results.

The application of electricity to paralytic cases is a remarkable proof of the vagueness of all notions on this subject. Because the muscles of a limb, palsied from some affection of the brain, are convulsed under electric shocks, or when made part of a voltaic circuit, it is inferred that their action under voluntary power may be restored by this agency. An opposite practical conclusion might almost as reasonably be drawn from the same premises.

In other cases, where electricity is passed through organs presumed to be in a torpid state, as the uterus in amenorrhœa, the practice is merely tentative, more frequently failing than succeeding in result; and the failure readily explained (even allowing the principle to be just), by the manner in which alone the electricity can be supposed to make its passage through the organ. The same general remarks apply to its use in cases of deafness, stiffened joints, and other disorders of still less determinate kind.

In relation to future inquiry on this subject, the application of electricity as a medicinal agent may best be viewed in the three following ways: first, in its action on the nervous system; secondly, on the blood; and, thirdly, on particular organs under disease. The first two topics are the most important; and all that

Throughout the whole of this chapter, I have been considering the influence on the body of those atmospheric conditions which are commonly termed *weather;* exclusively of all chemical changes in the air itself; of the admixture of other gases; or of the presence of ingredients of animal or vegetable origin, forming the miasma of disease.   Even with these exclusions, and merely touching on the several parts of the subject, it will be seen how vast is its extent, and how important its relations to the history of disease.   My principal object has been to indicate the latter; and to suggest some of the topics on which more complete knowledge is to be desired. Here, as already remarked, the progress of physical science is ever lending fresh aids to that of pathology; and the unexpectedness of some of the results is the best augury of what may be looked for in future, from the enlarging scope of the inquiry, and the new instruments and means with which it is pursued.

CHAPTER XXIX.

ON TIME AS AN ELEMENT IN MENTAL FUNCTIONS.

In many cases of affection of the sensorium,—as in the progress of recovering from apoplectic seizure, or generally in cases of partial coma,—a certain and often considerable time may be observed to elapse, between a question asked of the patient, and his reply. And this, seemingly without any uncertainty as to the answer to be given, or any apparent fault in the act of articulation, except slowness and greater effort ; but rather as if the mind received the perception more tardily than is natural, or more slowly put itself into action through the external organs in reply.   Occasionally, though aware of the fact from former experience, I have been led by the length of the interval to ask a second question before the first was answered ; this answer following afterwards as if nothing had intervened.

has been stated above tends to show that we may look to these as a basis of future discovery.   Many results already obtained (as those recently published by Dr. Addison, in relation to chorea, and the successful experiment of Matteucci in tetanus), make it probable that the use of electricity in nervous and spasmodic disorders, even when depending on the sensorium, may be greatly extended ; and though its action on morbid state of the blood seems much less within our reach, seeing the multiform conditions of this fluid, and the practical difficulties of application, yet is the object one well meriting diligent research.   In each of these cases future success will probably be due to new and more refined methods of use, better according with the natural actions of this principle within, and upon, the human frame.   Various suggestions to this effect arise out of recent discovery in electrical science, and the whole question of methods of application is one of great importance in the inquiry.

The fact I have stated will be recognised as familiar by all who have been observant of such cases. Yet I doubt whether this element of time, in its relation to the different mental functions, both in healthy and morbid state, has been sufficiently adverted to by physiologists; fertile though the topic is in curious results, and almost forced upon us for inquiry by common language and feeling on the subject.

Is there not, in fact, a material variation in the time in which the same mental functions are performed by different individuals; depending on different organization, or on other causes of which we can give no account? And this, not merely in complex acts of association, or continued trains of thought, (where the notion of difference is most sanctioned by phrases of common use, and can scarcely be rejected,) but also in the rapidity with which perceptions are received from the senses, and volitions carried into effect on their appropriate organs? or in other words, both in acts purely mental, and in those functions by which the mind is associated with material phenomena?

If there be cause to infer this from comparison of individuals, the inference is yet more distinct and remarkable from comparison of states in the same person, and from that examination of consciousness which every one may make for himself. It will be felt that there are moments when the perceptions and thoughts are not only more vivid, but seem to pass more rapidly and urgently through the mind, than at others: and the same with respect to acts of the voluntary power.* It is possible, indeed, that these two conditions of time and intensity may have close relation together, so that one forms a sort of measure of the other; but this would carry the description into points too subtle and metaphysical to be dealt with here. The application of the element of time to mental phenomena, though it may seem simple at first view, from their being all actually included under it, does in truth involve much of abstruse inquiry; well fitted, however, to repay those, who love the indulgence of such speculations.†

* Locke intimates something to this effect in saying, "There is a kind of restiveness in almost every one's mind. Sometimes, without perceiving the cause, it will boggle and stand still, and one cannot get it a step forward; and at another time it will press forward, and there is no holding it in."

† The hypothesis which best perhaps accords with, and explains, the relation of time to the mental functions, is that which regards the mind as a series of states or feelings, succeeding to each other from the first moment of life to the last, and no two of which are strictly coincident in time. However it may seem to contradict the old notion of the νους κυκλος, this manner of viewing the mind has much of reality to recommend it. It obviously includes the idea of time,—that is, of possible greater or less rapidity in the succession of states,—and illustrates more happily than any other hypothesis the numerous phenomena (making up, it may almost be said, the totality of life), in which the mind is wholly occupied with one perception or thought,—or, as it might better perhaps be expressed, one subject of consciousness,—to the momentary exclusion of every other, even of those which come most closely in precedence or sequence to it. Every psychical theory, as well as every deduction applied practically to the purposes of life, must be brought into relation with this view, to render them justly admissible.

I would notice in connexion with this subject the question, lately raised or revived, as to the velocity of nervous action in its simplest sense; and the possible difference of rate in different persons, and even in different nerves of the same individual. An apparent sanction has been given to the reality of such differences, by the singular facts which M. Nicolai, of the Manheim Observatory, records respecting the variation of time in the observation of a simple and single astronomical fact, (the transit of a star across the micrometer thread of a fixed telescope,) as noted by different observers on the same spot. The inequality, however, indicated by these observations, is far too great to admit of its being supposed dependent on unequal rate of transmission by the nerves of vision and hearing;—and Müller's solution is probably correct, which supposes the perceptions from the eye and ear in this case to be distinct and successive states of mind, with varying interval between them in different individuals; a solution which accords with the views just given, and with all that we know of mental phenomena.*

Pursuing the subject into details, we find many facts to illustrate it in the state of health; as many (and more striking from being less familiar), under morbid conditions of the body. During extreme old age, which in such various ways expresses by gradual change the sudden anticipations of disease, there appears to exist, not merely an impairment of the powers of perception and volition, but also of those functions upon which association or suggestion depend. The train of thought may be just in every sense, but it is more slowly pursued. A longer time, in the strict meaning of the phrase, is required for those combinations and changes which are involved in every such continuous action of mind. Here too, as in disease, there is more of toilsome effort in all acts of association and thought. The mind speedily becomes fatigued; the chain is broken; and confusion ensues. Observation shows these changes, occurring in every possible grade, in the cases which medical practice brings before us; and they often afford the most curious and unexpected analysis of conditions of thought, which in their more perfect and healthy state are indissolubly blended together.

It has been supposed by some that the state of dreaming involves a more rapid course of ideas through the mind;—a vague notion, however, as everything that relates to the ἔθνος ὀνείρων seems destined to be; and seemingly incapable of proof. All we can affirm here is, that the transitions are more frequent and abrupt than in the waking state, when the regulation of the will is present; and that, as respects rapidity in the succession of thoughts, it is probably as various during sleep as at other times. The evidence of such variation, while we are awake, is much more decisive. We derive it from consciousness in ourselves, and observation of the minds of others; and we are frequently able to apply a certain measure to these mental changes by their relation to things without.

* See Dr. Baly's translation of Müller's *Handbuch der Physiologie*, p. 680.

One particular topic rising out of this general view has not been so much considered, as its interesting nature, and relation to all the mental functions, might have rendered likely. This is, the variation in the faculty of the mind of holding one single image, or thought, continuously before it, as the subject of contemplation. The limit to this faculty in all men is certain and obvious, and in most cases narrower than is generally supposed. The persisting retention of the same idea manifestly exhausts the mind, and the effort persevered in beyond a given time, does often more speedily dissipate it. But nevertheless the power as to time is very different in different individuals; is susceptible of cultivation; and, if cultivated with care, not to produce exhaustion in the discipline, becomes a source of some of the highest excellencies of our moral and intellectual nature. It stands contrasted with that desultory and powerless state of mind which is unable to regulate its own workings, or to retain the thought fixedly on points most essential to the object of it.*

In all these instances we have the element of time entering, more or less directly, into our view of the mental functions engaged. Active diseases here, as in so many other cases, by disturbing the relation of these different functions, exalting some and depressing others, affords results more strongly marked than we can obtain in the state of health; and frequent examples, involving the same notion of time, will occur to all who are sedulous in watching these changes. I have seen within the last few hours a case of typhus mitior, in which the tendency has just come on to confusion and slight delirious rambling; where, though each question I put was rightly answered in the end, it seemed as if the mind had a long process to go through in attaining this. A case lately occurred to me, in a patient about sixty, where, without any actual paralysis, there had come on great enfeeblement of the sensorial functions, disordered perceptions, confusion of thoughts, and impaired voluntary power; but the conditions as to all these points, as often happens, varying much at different times. Here the patient himself expressed strongly the consciousness of time and labour being necessary for each voluntary act. He felt, to use his own words, " as if it were necessary to think for every finger in using it." A similar description I have often obtained from paralytic patients; indicating the slow and toilsome effort of volition they found needful to give motion to limbs so affected. This is obvious indeed to common observation. Time is seen to be required even to begin the act intended ; and so much labour to be necessary in pursuing it, that I have repeatedly noticed perspiration breaking out from the continued effort to raise a palsied arm to the level of the face ; and an exhaustion to follow, such as might ensue in health upon violent muscular exercise of the whole body.

* In Chapter XV. will be found some remarks which bear on this subject.

In another case, where there had been hemiplegia of two years' standing,—the memory of words, and power of articulation, being both impaired, but the intellect unaffected,—the singularity occurred of the frequent omission of one or more of the first syllables, in words of any length. On examination, aided by the patient himself, I found cause to believe that the mind here was occasionally conceiving words more rapidly than it could put the organs into motion to express them; and there existed an involuntary propension to remedy this difficulty by passing at once to the sounds terminating the words. Here then, also, if rightly interpreting the circumstances, time entered as an element into the action of the mind on the bodily organs. These paralytic disorders, indeed,—various in origin, progress, and modifications,—abound in curious instances, expressing the same general fact in different ways. I have many such in my recollection: but as they essentially resemble those just stated from recent observation, I need not detail them.

An estimate of the different duration of time required for the same operations of mind, under different conditions of the individual, would be interesting matter of inquiry; but exactness could scarcely be looked for, where the circumstances are so complicated. Instances like those just given, afford a sort of gross measure for one set of cases in which disease is concerned. And these, it must be added, are the cases showing more distinctly the origin of the diversity in physical causes. The parts ministering to the mental functions undergo change; and those especially which, through sensation and volition, connect the mind with the material world without. The more explicit instances furnished by disease or decay explain, by close analogy, the natural conditions of health, nor can we reasonably doubt that the varying quickness of perception and voluntary power are as much dependent on momentary changes in the brain and nerves, as are the states of sleep and waking; with which, indeed, they are in every way intimately connected. Under this general view there is no greater difficulty in the notion of time, than in that of intensity or vigour, as applied to describe the progress of mental operations; though perhaps less familiar to us in reasoning on the subject.

CHAPTER XXX.

ON PHRENOLOGY.

The evidence as to the system of phrenology of Gall, Spurzheim, and their followers, may be stated briefly thus:—

The phrenologists rightly regard it as probable, or even as proved, that there is some plurality of parts in the total structure of the brain, corresponding to, and having connexion with, the different intellectual and moral faculties. The partial and varying effects of accident, disease, or other less obvious change in the brain, in pro-ducing derangement of the mental functions, are the evidence of this assumption, and cannot be rejected as such. These effects are amongst the most remarkable which medical science affords in aid of our knowledge of man; and whether with or without reference to phrenology, a careful record ought to be kept of all which are well authenticated by trustworthy observers. They are precious materials for future comparison and inference.

The phrenologists rightly represent the old classifications of mental phenomena (which are chiefly expressions of function or capacity) as insufficient to denote the various propensities to thought, feeling, and action, observed in different individuals; manifestly original to a certain extent; and forming, in conjunction with certain acquired or modified habits, the particular character of each.

Thus far their doctrine has foundation in reason. But by no means equally so its other parts. The multiform division of these instinctive propensities, (as under this view they may fitly be called,) though doubtless right in some points, is arbitrary, inconsistent, or improbable in others; and even in some material respects very differently stated by phrenologists themselves. In the whole arrange-ment there is a strong flavour of human fiction;—a disregard, so to express it, of natural relation and sequence of parts. It is a sort of especial contradiction to the "*principe de la moindre action*," so generally prevailing throughout all parts of creation into which we are permitted to look; and it is yet further liable to this peculiar objection, that the limitation of the table of organs is not more rea-sonable than its extent. The principle of distinction adopted, is one which scarcely admits of boundary or exclusion.

Equally objectionable on other grounds is the remaining part of the system; viz., the attribution of these mental qualities or instincts to certain definite portions of the brain, discoverable from without; and discoverable on the presumption of the gross condition of quantity representing the intensity of quality, and the consequent vigour, or even compulsory nature, of the actions thereon depending. This relation of mere bulk of substance to the perfection or inten-sity of a faculty (for it cannot otherwise be stated) is, *primâ facie*, very improbable; nor is it attested by observation of the structure of the brain; either viewed in mass, or by the more minute dissec-tion and unfolding of parts, to which the authors of the system have themselves conducted us.*

* Admitting the great advance which has been made in the minute anatomy of the brain by these new modes of research, and appreciating the great merit of the observers, it is still difficult to see how the facts ascertained give support to their system of phrenology. The discovery of continuous and connecting fibres in the cerebral substance demonstrates, what must ever have been presumed, very complex relations of structure and function among the several parts of the

The facts of the general smallness and deficient development of the cerebrum in congenital idiotcy, and the ascertainment of the greater weight of the brain in certain persons of eminent intellect, may be admitted as their best reason on this point; but, duly examined, it will be found very insufficient as proof. It seems, indeed, that some phrenologists admit different intensity of action in the several organs, as qualifying the influence of size. Still the latter is the essential circumstance in the theory. It is that upon which the external demonstrations depend; and without which the o e principle of action presumed must be viewed in a new light.*

But the phrenologists put this part of their doctrine upon the evidence of fact; and the fairness, or even conclusiveness, of this appeal cannot be denied. If the facts tallied uniformly with their assumptions, or even in a certain large proportion of cases so as to make reasonable allowance for error or ambiguity, the improbability must be laid aside, of the mind being thus mechanically read from without, and the whole admitted as a new and wonderful truth.

Here then, by common admission, is a direct question of evidence, the amount and strictness of which are solely to be considered. And here, I think, it will be found, that the phrenologists are yet wanting in what is needful to establish their system; notwithstanding all the observation and ingenuity which have been bestowed on its proof.

Look at what they have in aid of their determinations, where the question concerns the relation between a certain outward form of cranium, and some faculty or quality of mind, alleged to be in correspondence with it. First, the equal chance of affirmative or negative as to each particular quality predicated. Secondly, the plea of a balance of some indications by others and opposing ones. Thirdly, the want of exact definition of many of these qualities or faculties; making it difficult to arrest for error, where there are

---

brain. But neither in the nature, nor distribution, of these nervous fibres, are there differences corresponding with the alleged locality or limits of the organs which the doctrine describes; and the periphery of the brain, in particular, may be said to be singularly devoid of any indications of such division. It is true that the circumvolutions are the parts of the organ which offer the greatest variations; but these are in no respect more consistent with the scheme proposed. Nor have the still more recent discoveries in this part of anatomy furnished, as far as I know, any evidence to this effect. See the writing of Tiedemann, Meckel, Wenzel, &c.

* The particular propensities of feeling and action, expressed in the divisions and organs of the phrenologists, must, in every intelligible sense of the term, be deemed instincts; and it has been sought to bring proof for the system, from corresponding relation of organs and habits in other animals. But, if not an objection, it would at least be a strange anomaly under this view, that certain insects, whose instincts are more complex, definite, and remarkable than any other which we can interpret by our own reason, should possess no cerebral organization but that of nervous ganglia, so little concentrated as barely to warrant the term of brain.

so many ways of retreat. And fourthly, the incidental discovery of character by other and more ordinary methods. I well know that the candid disciples of the system will not consciously avail themselves of all these methods. Nevertheless each one of them has more or less been made use of; and looking to the chances and facilities thus obtained, it may be affirmed that the number of true predictions in phrenology is less miraculous than it would be, were this number not to exist. This is a question purely of fact, and the statement just made may be disputed as such; but I think it will be found by those who look fairly into the matter, that the coincidences are not more frequent or remarkable than the assured average of chances would make them.

- In these few remarks I have chiefly sought to put the several points of the question into a clear light. It is obvious that these points are widely different in themselves, and differ much in their degree of probability. Respecting the evidence of that which is cardinal to the system, viz., the power of discovery of strong faculties and instincts by the external configuration of the cranium, the fairest test would be found, not in vague and ill defined moral propensities, respecting the site of many of which phrenologists themselves are far from agreed; but in a few simple and well marked faculties, such as those of numerical calculation, languages, or music; which have none others in obvious opposition to them; and the degree of perfection in which can be clearly defined. It is true that the phrenologists appeal to these in their evidence; and examples doubtless occur where such appeal has been made good: but the doctrine requires that it should more uniformly be so, than those will admit, who fairly look at any large number of instances in which the system has been put to proof under their own inspection.*

In the present state of our knowledge of the brain, and of its relation to the mental functions, an impartial view of phrenology requires, not that the doctrine should be put aside altogether, but that great abatement should be made of its pretensions as a system. To say the least, it is chargeable with what Lord Bacon has called " an over-early and peremptory reduction into acts and methods," and with the adoption of various conclusions, not warranted by any sufficient evidence. But on a subject thus obscure in all its parts, and where our actual knowledge is still limited to detached facts or presumptions, there is enough to justify the opinion being kept before us, as one of the outlines to which future observations may apply;—not fettered, as they now are, by the trammels of a premature arrangement.

* During some intercourse with Gall, and more frequently with Spurzheim, (both remarkable men, and deeply impressed with the truth of their opinions,) I had several occasions of noticing the failure of their judgment upon the particular faculties mentioned above, as well as in other cases where the peculiarity of external conformation, or of some quality of mind, made it almost needful that the doctrine should rightly indicate the relations upon which it professes to be based.

CHAPTER XXXI.

ON DISTURBED BALANCE OF CIRCULATION, AND METASTASIS OF DISEASE.

I PLACE these subjects together, not merely for mutual illustration, but because in some points they can scarcely be regarded apart, when looking to the phenomena of disease. It is another instance where much may be added to the extent and clearness of our views in pathology, by considering different disorders in relation to some common principle of morbid action. We thereby, even without aiming at new classification, gain knowledge of connexions, which escape notice, if confining ourselves to a single view, or to the limits of systematic nomenclature; and we obtain moreover various aids in practice, made more secure by resting on a wider basis.

Disorder or irregularity in the circulation of the blood, by whatsoever names in its different forms described, is such a principle of morbid action;—more universal perhaps, and more important in its effects than any other in the animal economy. Taking the expression, indeed, in its largest sense, it may be said to involve every possible form of disease. Scarcely one can be named, in which some unequal balance of blood, local or general, does not exist. From acute local inflammation of the most urgent kind, to chronic inflammation, plethora, or congestion, under the lightest forms; and again, to those momentary and ever-changing misdirections of blood which occur in some nervous disorders; we have a long series of morbid changes, in all of which this common fact is concerned, however various the causes of inequality, and however different, or even opposite, the state of the vascular system in the changes taking place.

It is further to be remarked, that all these morbid actions have connexion, more or less intimate, with corresponding changes in the healthy state; and that they become anormal chiefly by excess in amount or duration. The inequalities in circulation produced by mental emotion; by bodily exertion or posture; by digestion in its several stages; by exposure to heat or cold, or other atmospheric changes; represent in degree, or for a time, almost all such as are considered morbid in kind, and often pass into the latter without any obvious interval between. This manner of viewing the subject, through the relation of disordered actions to those of health, is here, as in all other cases, the best: whether we look to the theory of disease, or to its treatment in daily practice.

It is difficult, from the nature of the subject, to classify the various disturbances in the balance of circulation. The most general distinction might be that between inflammation, in the common sense of the term, and those irregularities, often much more extensive

and sudden, but where none of the characteristic marks of inflammation are present. Here, however, besides many exceptions and
doubtful cases, we come upon the wider question, whether there are
any distinctive characters of inflammation, certain enough to warrant their being thus classed apart. This doubt reasonably arises
as a result of all modern inquiry on the subject. Though it may be
difficult to go with one eminent pathologist so far as to remove the
term *inflammation* from medical use, yet it is certain that the gradation in all these states is such, as not to allow any fixed lines of
demarcation to be drawn, without error in fact, and frequent injury
in practice.* Still the pathological differences for each end of the
scale are so strongly marked, as fully to justify their separate consideration; and though the notion of metastasis, as commonly received, applies to both classes of phenomena, there is convenience
here also in keeping some such distinction in view.

So much has been written upon inflammation that it is not easy
to add either fact or opinion to those already before us. But the
other inequalities of circulation, though more considered of late
years, have not received the same minute attention. From the difference of the phenomena, research is here more difficult; and on
many points we are limited at present to facts drawn from other
parts of the animal economy. This very connexion, however, is
matter of great interest to pathology; and in all points of view
these unequal distributions of blood, which, without local inflammation, constitute so many forms of active disorder, deserve the diligent attention of the physician.

The most general manner of viewing the subject regards the
causes and conditions under which the blood is thus unequally transferred from one place to another, producing local excess or deficiency, as the case may be. It is clear that there is a natural
balance, or proportion, of blood to the several parts of the body
respectively; certain, and often great, deviations from which are
compatible with health, or even essential to the functions of life;

---

* All who have read on this subject, as well as studied it in actual practice,
will be conscious of its many perplexities ; and of the frequent impossibility of
diagnosis between inflammation and simple congestion, or the more curious
phenomena of turgescence. As an example of these difficulties we might specify
some of those curious instances, in which a state, having many of the received
characters of inflammation, is actually brought on by causes of depletion, such
as increase the proportion of serum to the coagulum of the blood ; and is relieved
by opposite treatment. Other anomalies might be named, familiar to every
practitioner. Some of these may best be explained by looking less than is
usually done to the mere vascular tissue of an inflamed part, and more to the
state of the fluid within the vessels, as primarily affected by the causes of inflammation, and determining the changes which ensue, both in the part itself,
and the system at large. An experimental memoir by Dr. Alison, read at the
meeting of the British Association at Dublin (see *Report of Sections*, p. 88), has
great value in relation to this topic.
  The opinion, advocated by Dr. Macartney, that inflammation can never be
rightly considered a reparative process, is another proof of the uncertainty which
still hangs over every part of this subject.

while yet greater deviations, or such as effect particular organs, or occur too suddenly, fall strictly within the name and character of disease. What are the physical causes producing these changes? Why is it, that even in healthy actions, and more remarkably in those of disease, mutual exchange of blood should take place, by sudden determination, between the skin and internal membranes? or why those more vague and various translations of blood which occur among different organs, without apparent unity of cause;— as the brain; the membranes lining the air-passages; the pleura and lungs; the peritoneum and membranes of the alimentary canal; the liver; the kidneys; the organs of generation; the mammæ; the synovial membranes? &c. That there are parts of the body more closely connected than others as respects these translations, and that there is some relation here both to similarity of texture and community of function, is certain from observation. But even could we derive any direct explanation from this, the facts would call upon us to go beyond it; and to show cause for those sudden changes in the balance and direction of the blood, where the structure and function of the parts successively affected are wholly different in kind.

Or it may be needful to enlarge the inquiry, to include the cases where, without actual increase or diminution in the quantity of blood in an organ, the rate of its motion is topically altered, so as to change for a time the condition of the part. It is not easy, indeed, to prove that such case exists. If it does (and perhaps the circulation through the brain furnishes the most probable instance), it comes within the scope of the subject, and receives illustration from the remarks which follow.

Four conditions at least may be taken into question, as respects the rationale of these changes. First, the variations in the heart's action;—secondly, the state of the capillaries of the parts to which the blood is for the time directed;—thirdly, the quality or quantity of the blood itself;—and fourthly, the influence of the nervous power upon the circulation. These questions in many points blend together; yet each is distinct enough to deserve separate consideration.

The first is by no means the most important, though on superficial view it may seem to be so. By whatever influence the motions of the heart are produced (and the question, as regards the nervous system, is scarcely yet decided), their immediate effect in propelling the blood towards the extreme vessels is one mechanical in kind; nor have we any certain proof that the arteries aid in this transmission by any power which they themselves possess. The action of the heart may be excessive or deficient in force; it may be disordered in frequency, regularity, or other characters of pulse; but still these inequalities affect more or less all parts of the vascular system; depending chiefly on the greater or less power of propelling blood into the minute vessels. The general inference remains the same, whatever opinion we adopt upon the questions still perplexing physiologists in respect to the circulation:—whether there be other motive power than that of the heart?—whether the arteries or capillaries have any vital contractile force aiding in this effect?—or whether the vital properties of the blood itself may assist or modify its passage through the extreme vessels? Under any of these views, it is equally certain that the agency of the heart, (to which, in the higher classes of animals, all other motive powers are subordinate,) must have the same general ratio to each part of the body, whatever the changes occurring in its own rate or vigour of action.*

As respects, again, the quality of the blood, and any influence the variations of the heart's action may have in altering this, though we cannot affirm it to be wholly unaffected, and might even suppose some changes to be made by the rate of motion, yet have we no certain evidence of such alteration; and the general presumption undoubtedly is that it reaches the extreme arteries little, if at all, altered in any essential character.

Nevertheless, the variations in the action of the heart cannot be wholly limited in their effect to changes in the general rate and diffusion of the blood. A different propulsion from the central organ must somewhat alter the proportion in which it reaches parts more or less remote; and even the same proportion of excess or deficiency will produce different effects according to the texture and function of particular organs; a point not sufficiently adverted to in the consideration of this subject. A given excess, for instance, as applied to the liver or kidneys, may have little influence on the system at large; while the same increased action through the brain, or even through some particular portion of this organ, may produce disturbances of circulation throughout other and various parts of the body. This, however, is a secondary effect, taking place through nervous agency. The action of the heart cannot alone, or in direct way, produce those singular translations of blood, respecting which we inquire; and we must go to other causes, beyond that of varying propulsion, for explanation of such changes in the body.

The second condition stated, viz., the action of the extreme vessels, and their relation respectively to the state of the blood and to the nervous system, is of much greater interest to the question before us. The subtle and delicate textures, glandular or otherwise, in which they terminate, fulfil (according to laws still very imperfectly known) all the more important changes in the animal economy. And to this part of the system (a view for which we are first clearly indebted to John Hunter), the physiologist and pathologist must equally and especially look for furtherance of knowledge in their several inquiries. After all the more exact researches of late years, we do but partially comprehend those minute and

* In descending through the scale of organized life, the functions of the capillary vessels in circulation become gradually of greater importance; till, arriving at vegetable life, we find them solely effective in this part of the economy of plants.

complex mechanisms by which, in spaces barely accessible to the nicest instruments, the various functions of absorption, secretion, and exudation, as well as the translation of blood from arteries to veins, are all simultaneously going on. What the immensity of creation is to the astronomer or geologist, such are these infinitely small dimensions of matter in space to the physiologist. Presuming, or knowing, that all organization, however minute, such as the many thousand lenses which compose an insect's eye, must be due to the action of distinct vessels, circulating, secreting, and absorbing, we have some vague measure of that exquisite minuteness of fabric and formative action, upon which life in its several parts essentially depends.

The discoveries of Dutrochet and others prove indeed that many of these changes may and do proceed, without the intervention of any continuous vascular structure, and that we need no longer look for the open mouths of vessels as essential to the functions by which one fluid is separated from another. It is still matter of dispute among physiologists whether the capillaries are really membranous tubes, or merely interspaces of tissue, through which the blood finds its passage. But though certain of these minute actions may be submitted to a common physical principle, it is obvious that we must admit essential differences of structure or nervous power, or both, to explain their actual diversities, and the relation of one common fluid to these separate functions. This is obviously true as regards the glandular texture; and even in the instance of the serous membranes, where the tissue appears so much more uniform and simple, the secretions from different membranes of this class vary in the proportion of water, animal and saline matters, they contain; and this more remarkably under the several conditions of health and disease.*

It is further manifest, and now generally recognised, that changes take place in these extreme vessels, or in the tissues of which they form the largest part, independent altogether of any previous alteration in the heart's action, and often connected with the latter only as an occasional cause of disturbance to it.† This is a point of great importance to the particular subject before us, and in truth to every part of medical science. The capillary vessels, as they are the

---

* Müller's admirable treatise on the Structure of Glands, as well as the later researches in his great work on Physiology, may be considered to have settled several principles in the general doctrine of secretion, particularly those which regard the relation of vascular structures to the effects they respectively produce.

It would be impossible to refer to all the questions that exist respecting the capillary system, and to the researches (through the microscope, injection, and other means) which have been directed to their solution by the most eminent physiologists of the day. They are indeed among the most important in physiology, as approaching nearest to those ultimate actions on which depend all the functions of life.

† The experiments of Dr. Philip, Le Gallois, and Serres, have shown that particular injuries of the brain and spinal marrow are capable of altering, or in some cases wholly arresting, the circulation through the capillary arteries.

seat and source of many of the great actions of life in healthy state, so have they like relation to disease in all its obvious forms. Here occur, as far as we can observe, the first morbid changes in fever and inflammation; and there is scarcely a symptom in the progress of such disorders, in which their functions, in one part or other, are not involved. The changes they undergo in all chronic diseases, either are originally, or become, an essential part of the malady. Vitiated states of the blood are testified in similar way; and through this part of the system morbid deposits and absorptions take place, and all the diversities of organic disease are more immediately produced.

The direct relation of the capillaries to the sensorium and nervous system is shown in various ways, which will afterwards be mentioned. At present we have only to notice this part of the circulation in its connexion with the sentient extremities of the nerves; the sensations derived from which are variously altered by the quantity and manner of transmission of blood through the extreme vessels. But beyond this, we must probably look to the capillaries as the first seat of those vital actions which are occasional to the system; as the enlargement of the uterus and its appendages during pregnancy; the swelling of the breasts and secretion of milk afterwards; and others which are too familiar to need recital. Any changes in the centre, or large branches of the vascular system, are undoubtedly subordinate to those which have their locality in the very organs thus determined to particular actions of life.*

Another important relation of the capillaries, requiring notice, is that to the external atmosphere, particularly to the fluctuations of heat and cold. I have spoken on this subject when treating of the influence of weather on the conditions of disease. It is manifestly through the capillaries of the surface that these external causes chiefly act on the body. Their actual effect in disturbing the circulation, and altering the balance between outward and inner parts, is shown in numerous cases, both in health and disease; to which, from their familiarity, it is merely necessary to allude as coming under this part of the subject.

Seeing, then, the numerous and remarkable functions of the capillaries throughout the body, it is certain that we must seek here the source, as well as evidence, of many of those disturbances in the balance of circulation which form the subject of this chapter. Altered or disordered action may be induced in the extreme vessels of any part by causes affecting the whole vascular system; but it often originates in them locally, and becomes thence a source of disturbance to the central organs; and this not merely where a particular function is to be performed, as in the cases just quoted, or in the more frequent and familiar cases where local irritation is applied;

* The singular case recorded by Dr. Houston, of an acardiac twin fœtus, shows that the capillaries may maintain in some degree, through their proper actions, the general movement of the circulation; one question, amongst others, which has created controversy on the subject.

but also from other conditions less cognisable within the part itself, altering the quantity and rate of blood circulating in it, and thereby changing, more or less in degree, its relations to the rest of the system.

Though discrimination of the cases is not always easy, yet multiplied instances might be given, and would be well worthy of collection, where changes take place in the capillary circulation of a part, having no connexion with the heart or general circulation, except in the effects they actually produce by reflected action upon them. Certain forms of metastasis, which I shall afterwards mention, furnish examples to this effect. One curious illustration, valuable in its generality, may be found in the fact (not much noted, though apparently unequivocal) that each stage of the simple febrile paroxysm may be represented locally in detached parts of the body, without obvious affection of the system at large. To a certain extent these partial effects happen even in the regular ague, especially when the paroxysms are slight. But the instances are more explicit, for our present purpose, of transient rigors, or flushes of heat, or sudden sweats, occurring on limited parts of the surface of the body, and disappearing where they have arisen.* I cannot state, on observation, that these circumstances do actually succeed each other in series; but in some cases it probably is so, and at all events the fact that they may happen singly, in this limited manner, is interesting in relation to a part of pathology, as important as it has hitherto been obscure.

Admitting, then, the general position that disturbances of the circulation may begin from the extreme vessels, and tend towards the centre, the question remains—one of the most subtle and difficult in physiology—to what agency these phenomena are due, which thus have local determination without apparent local cause; and which so frequently, rapidly, and unexpectedly, shift themselves from one place to another. In stating the third and fourth conditions of the inquiry, I have already referred to what seem the only intelligible sources of such effects; viz., differences in the blood brought to the part affected; or the influence of the nervous power in giving this direction. Any changes in the vessels themselves, either as regards elasticity or muscular power, must be considered

---

* The rigors and heat are here taken as proofs of the changes of capillary circulation in the part, and this inference is justified by all we at present know on the subject. If heat, especially, be not a consequence of increased influx of blood into the extreme vessels, it is at all events so uniform a concomitant that the connexion cannot admit of doubt. Topical changes of temperature, occurring suddenly from local irritation, make it evident that the immediate cause of this change is resident in the part. Still, unless it be shown that the local temperature, thus created, is above that of a part of the body, the vessels of which, in natural state, are equally full of blood as those of the irritated organ, it does not prove more than that increase of circulating blood brings increased temperature with it; and the general fact of proportion between the heat developed by an animal, and the quantity of its respiration, remains undiminished in evidence. The researches of ·Chossat, on the influence of the nervous system upon animal heat, have much interest here.

secondary to one or other of these causes. They cannot be conceived as initial actions, though they may modify such as have
begun.

The tendency, indeed, of recent inquiry has been to show that,
while the mechanical propulsion from the heart is the great cause
carrying the blood through its whole circuit, there are various and
ever-changing actions going on in the extreme vessels which check,
accelerate, or otherwise modify its movement, besides effecting
those other remarkable changes which belong to this part of the
system; and other observations seem to warrant the inference,
already noticed, that these actions are less due to the living solids,
to any direct contractions or relaxations of the vascular tissues,
than to vital changes in the blood itself, in passing through these
minute vessels. This view of the general relation of the solid and
fluid parts in the capillary system (though not necessarily involving
the assumption of a self-propelling power in the blood) is still the
subject of much controversy, the result of which is of equal interest
to physiology and pathology; bearing directly, it will be seen, on
the subject before us.*

We come, then, here to the third part of the inquiry, viz., the influence of changes in the quality or quantity of the blood on different
parts of the circulating and secreting system; a wide subject, on
which physiologists have hitherto obtained only insulated or imperfect facts. The difficulties, in fact, are great; involving on the one
side the most minute structure of solid parts, only partially known
to us in their intimate functions;—on the other, the numerous and
ever-changing conditions of a fluid, singularly complex as a chemical compound, possessed of vital properties which modify all its
others, incessantly altered by addition or subtraction of some of its
many ingredients, and liable to the graver and more permanent
alterations of disease. Incomplete, however, as our knowledge yet
is on these topics, we have proof enough to assure us that the
quality, as well as quantity of blood, must have effect, more or
less, on every part of the circulation. There is every reason to
consider the heart subject to this influence, in addition to that
derived directly from the nerves; and the modifications of its
action thence arising are clearly of great moment in the animal
economy.† The trunks of the arterial and venous systems may
not have other relation to the composition of the blood than as
regards its varying degrees of fluidity. The capillary and secreting
vessels are those where this influence reaches its maximum, and

* Magendie, Müller, Treviranus, Baumgärtner, Dutrochet, &c., may be cited
among the Continental physiologists who have chiefly engaged in this discussion. The two first-named strongly concur in negativing the idea of any spon-
taneous movement, or self-propelling power, in the blood.

† The observations which seem to show that certain variations in the sound of
the blood passing through the heart depend on differences of its composition,
have value as evidence here. Several instances have occurred to me where
there was cause to suspect this to be the case.

where the proofs are most numerous and distinct; especially, as might be inferred, under the actions of disease.

We have further reason for believing, though equally without knowledge of the proximate cause, that the vascular tissue of different organs is differently affected by given changes in the quality of the blood; a difference attested by changes in the functions of the several parts, and in the nervous sensibility appropriate to each. The ratio and order of these two effects are but little understood; and it is safer, perhaps, not to seek to distinguish them until more advanced in knowledge of these ultimate actions on the system at large. The attainment of such knowledge would probably show us the brain as the organ most remarkably affected by them. The alterations in the blood, of which we have evidence in the greater vessels, must be presumed to produce effects in the minute vascular tissue of this organ and the spinal marrow (especially, perhaps, in the cineritious part), of singular importance to the whole economy. Many problems in pathology, hitherto unsolved, may eventually be so, by looking to this source of morbid action.

Taking the simplest view of the subject, it stands thus:—That as the blood reaches the capillaries and secreting vessels of every organ and part of the body in the same state as to quality, whatever this be;—and as these several parts, from essential differences of tissue, vascular or otherwise, are capable of modifying differently the passage of the blood and the products therefrom in the healthy state;—so is it to be presumed that every change of quality in the blood will produce different effects according to these respective varieties of texture. One part may be little effected by alterations which will excite great disturbance in another. We can scarcely entertain any other view than this; looking at that delicate balance in the composition of healthy blood which, whether it be cause or effect of its proper vitality, has manifestly relations so important to every organ of the body.

This manner of viewing the subject illustrates the facts both of health and disease more consistently than any other. It recognises that appropriate vitality, vascular irritability, and nervous power of every part, which we cannot doubt to exist; and associates the peculiar functions of each with the changes going on in the system at large. Under disease especially, this regard to the specialty of organic structure is essential to a right interpretation of the phenomena.

It is uneecessary here to refer to the particular changes in the quality of the blood—whether altered proportion of its natural ingredients, or the addition of new elements—thus variously influencing the tissues to which it is sent. All we require is to show generally that alterations of quality must have effect on the circulation through particular parts or organs;·and in consequence may become a source of disorder to the general balance of circulation in the body. This is a topic on which it might be easy to dwell at great length, seeing the various knowledge acquired of late years respecting both the healthy constitution of blood and the changes it undergoes in disease; the latter sufficient in amount to justify the term of "lesions of the blood;" and the recognition of these, as including some of the most definite disorders which affect the human frame.

Without referring to ambiguous or disputed points in the physiology of the blood, we have evidence more than sufficient to assure us that the different degrees of its fluidity; the varying proportion of its serous and coagulable parts, and of the red globules; the several degrees of arterialization; the retention of the proper matters of the several secretions; or the admixture of foreign ingredients; must all have influence more or less on the movements through the vascular system. Looking to the principle of coagulation alone, its vital importance in every office of the blood, and the alterations it undergoes even in the living vessels, we have here a powerful cause of change pervading the circulation in every part, and producing effect on every solid tissue and fluid secretion throughout the body. It may be admitted as a general presumption, that each change in the quality of the blood must alter some of the secretions, and every alteration of secretion change more or less the quality of this fluid. The term "vital affinities" is one well warranted by the course and results of modern discovery.*

The views just stated regarding the influence of the quality of blood on its manner of circulation, apply to its variations in quantity also. These must mainly have effect, as in the former case, on the action of the heart, and on the movements through every part of the capillary system. The frequency and vigour of the heart's contractions clearly depend in part on the varying supply of blood to its cavities; and there may be fault either in the excess or deficiency of this; as is familiarly proved in the effects resulting respectively from undue plethora, or from excessive hemorrhage. In neither case are its actions rightly performed; and the influence of the disturbance, existing in every form and degree, is felt in some proportion throughout all parts of the body. Notwithstanding the frequent occasion for noticing them, and their great importance in the treatment of disease, these effects are still not sufficiently regarded in general practice. . Oppression of the heart by quantity of blood, beyond its power of ready propulsion, is sometimes mistaken for debility; and those singular disturbances to the nervous system which occasionally occur from great deficiency or sudden loss of blood, and which have reflected action in disturbing the heart, are

---

* Though not adopting the bold phrase of Bordeu, " *Le sang est de la chair coulante,*" we must admit that the further research is carried into the capillary circulation, the closer are the relations established between the solids and fluids of the body. No author has treated this subject more ably than Andral, in the first volume of his Anatomie Pathologique. I must refer also to the Lectures on the Blood and its Diseases, by M. Magendie, lately published ; which, aided by the experiments of M. Poiseuille, display the same boldness and originality as the other labours of this eminent physiologist. On the subject of the peculiar affinities of vital action we owe much to the researches of Tiedemann, Prout, and Raspail.

often wrongly interpreted, and made a motive for additional depletion. I have alluded to this subject in former chapters; but its importance may well warrant this further reference to it.

The varying pressure on their parietes may modify the passage
of the blood, even through the larger vessels; but the effect of
quantity is doubtless felt chiefly in the capillaries; and from the
same causes, already fully adverted to, which render this part of
the vascular system the seat of the most important changes taking
place in the circulation. We have various testimony of the fact in
the altered sensations, secretions, and other actions so produced;—
in the many forms of disorder, inflammatory, hemorrhagic, or
otherwise, well known as the effects of this cause;—and in the
irregular movements and sudden translations of blood, which are
prone to occur, both when the vessels are overcharged, and when
wanting of their proper fulness and distension.* The effects proceeding from the latter cause (the anæmia of some physiologists)
have, until lately, been less studied than they deserve to be. Their
influence upon the brain through the action of the heart and larger
vessels has just been noticed. It is probably, like that of quality of
the blood, most intimately felt in the capillary circulation of the
nervous centres, and thence becomes indirectly a source of disturbance and inequality to other parts of the system.

In considering the latter fact, which bears directly on the present
inquiry, we must still keep in mind the respective endowments of
each part (whether called vital or by any other name)—rendering them differently susceptible to all given causes of change;
liable to be acted upon in various order; and in many cases apt to
undergo sudden fluctuations in the blood circulating through them.
These expressions, though vague, do nevertheless characterize a
very important fact in the bodily economy. And they lead us immediately to the last division proposed in this inquiry; viz., the
influence of the nervous power in altering or disturbing the balance
of circulation.

This very curious topic may be considered in several lights; all,
it must be confessed, partaking of the imperfection of our present
knowledge; but, in their combination, authorizing conclusions of
much interest to this part of physiology. It is certain, from sufficient
evidence, that the irregularities of circulation, as well as its healthy
state, depend in various ways on the nervous system. The question
before us regards the nature and direction of this influence; and it
is embarrassed in many parts by the difficulty of distinguishing
what is cause, and what effect, where the actions and reactions
are so intimate, and exercised in modes so inaccessible to our
view.

The simplest and most familiar fact here is the influence of mental
emotions in disturbing the balance of circulation;—one nevertheless

---

* Many of these questions are ably treated in an Essay on Congestion, Inflammation, and Hemorrhage, by Professor Naumann of Bonn.

so striking in its manner of occurrence, as even to have produced theories which give a sort of locality to the passions in the organs thus affected. Dismissing all hypothesis, the result defined by ob-servation is, that these states of mind act immediately, and without any intervention of will, on different organs of the body ;—the action doubtless taking place through the nervous system, in some one or other of its parts ; but testified chiefly by changes in the vascular system and altered distribution of blood. These effects, whether of congestion or increased action, are varied by the nature of the emotion ; still more perhaps by difference of temperament. The heart is obviously the organ most affected ; and which has greatest influence in spreading the disturbance through the general circula-tion. But it is important to the argument to observe, that there are numerous local influences in the vascular system, sudden trans-lations of blood, and even well-marked changes in secretion, which cannot be thus explained ; but depend more immediately on the mental emotion forming the original cause of disturbance. It is needless to state examples of these facts, which are so familiar to common observation.

Besides the influence of mental emotions on the circulation, we have proof that it may be locally affected by the mere act of atten-tion of mind, voluntarily directed to a part. Here again we have reason to suppose that the effect may occur without any interven-tion of the heart's action ; but simply from the nervous influence, whatever it be, which associates each part of the body with the common sensorium ;—that *internuncial function*,—to use the phrase of a great physiologist,—which establishes and maintains the unity of every living being.

The latter consideration brings us to the view of another relation between the nervous system (still using this term in its largest sense) and the circulation of the blood ; illustrating some remarkable dis-turbances, real or apparent, in the latter function. This depends on the fact,—much more strongly marked in many other animals than in man,—that at different periods of life there is a varying degree of vital activity exercised by different organs ; directly at-tested to observation by the quantity and manner of circulation of the blood sent to each. It is simply the expression of a fact in the animal economy, of which the examples are numerous and familiar. The various phenomena of puberty are perhaps the most striking instances in man ; but one may be taken even from an earlier period of life, in that state of the brain during infancy and childhood, which seems connected with rapid development, and is indicated by great activity and mobility of the circulation through the organ. It cannot, indeed, be proved that any direct influence of the nervous system is the source of these actions ; which, strictly speaking, belong to the same causes as original organization and growth, and lie under similar obscurity. But neither can we affirm that any altered state or distribution of blood is primarily concerned in them ; and notwithstanding certain obvious analogies to vegetable life, it is safer perhaps to admit them in connexion with the nervous functions, than with any other. Their effects, when interrupted or otherwise disordered, in producing disturbance throughout the whole circulation, are well known in the history of disease.

Regarding the manner in which the nervous system acts on the circulation, independently of its more obvious influence through the heart, the main question is, whether the general distribution of nerves through the minute vascular structure of each organ or tissue will account for this, of which local neuralgia may be taken as the simplest case ;—or whether we must suppose also an especial power in the blood itself—what some have termed its innervation—to explain the vascular irritability common to the whole body, as well as that which exists, or is distributed, unequally to different parts. These are subjects where the intricacies of relation and invisible structure multiply around us ; and where, in the same proportion, language tends to encroach on the reality of facts. Yet there are many experiments sufficiently distinct to show that nervous influence is expressly directed to the circulation in one or other of these ways, and possibly in both. I have already noticed the observations which indicate that injuries of the brain and spinal nerves are capable of variously affecting, or even wholly arresting, the movement of blood through the capillary vessels, independently of the action of the heart. And other experiments are related, proving that section of the pneumogastric nerve has remarkable effect on the blood itself, in diminishing the proportion of fibrin, and destroying the power of coagulation.

Though there is some ambiguity in these, and all similar results, yet are they sufficient, in conjunction with more familiar observations, to justify the view of a direct nervous action on every part of the vascular system and its contents. In the latter case, where this action is immediate on the blood, there may be reason to suppose that the whole circulating fluid is equally and similarly affected. On the other hand, the nervous influence which belongs to the vascular tissues seems liable to every variety of local direction or limitation. If this distinction were well established, it might explain, by the concurrence or separation of the two agencies, many of the complex phenomena referred to in this inquiry. But it must be admitted that we are far short of any such certainty ; and that there is still a singular want of exact knowledge in all that concerns the relation between the nervous system and the circulation of the blood,—the two greatest functions of the living economy.

We have evidence, indeed, that both the cerebral and ganglionic nerves are engaged in this relation; but in what precise connexion with each other, or in what ratio to the several parts and functions of the vascular system, neither anatomy nor physiology have yet fully explained. The presumption undoubtedly is, from their obvious distribution on the trunks and branches of arteries, that the ganglionic nerves are those which chiefly give their appropriate irritability to the blood-vessels throughout the body. But here, as in all the relations of these nerves to other parts of the nervous system, we instantly lose every clue to further pursuit, and are obliged to limit ourselves to the expression of the simplest and most general facts.*

Pathology furnishes, as might be expected, many curious illustrations of this subject, though inadequate to the solution of the problems just stated. The most remarkable, undoubtedly, as being the most obvious in cause, are those derived from lesions of the brain and spinal nerves, and particularly from paralysis in its different forms. In the latter cases, we have often local changes in circulation, rendered very singular by the preciseness of their limitation to certain parts, in accordance with the distribution of particular nerves. This is well seen in certain slight and partial paralytic affections, where a portion of a limb, or even one or two fingers, may become almost bloodless, while the others retain their natural state.† I find among my notes many such instances of partial change in arterial circulation ;—some in which the effect was manifest even in the larger trunks of arteries leading to a part under this influence. An example has recently occurred to me of slight hemiplegia, evidently connected with cerebral disease, where the beat of the arteries on one side the head was wholly different in character from that on the other, as shown even in the carotid itself: and similar differences probably exist in many cases of this nature. The strong beatings, which sometimes occur in the course of particular arteries, are well known ; and though we may hesitate to describe them, with Laennec, as neuralgic spasms of the artery, yet is it difficult to attribute them to any other than nervous influence of some kind on the coats of the vessels so affected.

It is a question whether we can assign to the same cause, that rarer occurrence, where every part of the arterial system, to which we have access, is in a state of irritable action at the same time ; with a peculiar jar or vibrating beat, not unlike that attending some morbid states of the heart, yet here manifestly derived from another source, by which this organ also is simultaneously affected. There is a good deal of analogy between this condition, and what may be termed an hemorrhagic state of the arteries ; and there are some actual varieties of hemorrhage admitting of illustration from this source. It may possibly be produced by particular changes in the blood itself, thus acting on all parts of the vascular system ;—or from a state of the inner coats of the arteries, described by some authors, verging on inflammation. But I have seen one or two of these cases so singularly connected with cerebral and nervous irritation, as to make it probable at least that this formed the first step in the train of morbid actions.‡

* The late Dr. Fletcher, in his remarkable work on the Rudiments of Physiology, gave a more extended form to this doctrine of the ganglionic system, describing it as the source of all irritability in the body.

† I have also seen cases where the perspiration of a palsied limb was singularly altered in the quality of the matter perspired.

‡ In the most remarkable of these cases—a boy of four years old—the symptoms had existed ten days when I was called in, together with Sir Charles Clarke ;

I might take from another class of disorders,—such as hysteria, in the widest understanding of the name,—various illustrations of the influence of the nervous system in altering and disturbing the balance of circulation. But these are too familiar to require more than a reference to them, as part of the subject.

The preceding remarks, directed chiefly to those irregularities of circulation which are not inflammatory in the ordinary sense of the term, will show how wide is the topic, and how fruitful of questions still unresolved. Of the points severally discussed, the following may be stated as among the most important and best ascertained:—First, that the capillaries are, in numerous cases, perhaps in the majority, the first seats of these disordered actions, even where the causes reach them through the general circulation;—secondly, that the direction of such actions, as well as their degree, has relation to the particular endowments, nervous and vascular, of each part, and to the functions they severally perform ;—thirdly, that the quality and quantity of the blood in circulation, but particularly the former, have also much effect in determining the nature and extent of these disturbances;—and, fourthly, that there are further causes, producing or modifying them, in the influence of the sensorium and different parts of the nervous system; these causes operating, directly or indirectly, partially or generally, on the whole vascular system, exclusively even of the action of the heart.

It is unnecessary to point out further how integral a part these topics form of all pathology. I shall merely add a few remarks on the application of them, denoted in the title of the chapter, to the metastasis of disease;—a copious subject, abounding in curious

during which time he had been bled to the extent of nearly 30 ounces. We found the child delirious; the pulse from 120 to 130; hard, and with a tense vibrating thrill in all the arteries, especially those of the head, which I do not remember equally to have noticed in any other case ; and felt in the smallest artery to which touch could be applied. There was also a singular propensity to bite, apparently without passion, all those around him, even his mother and nurse ;—and further, a constant dread of falling, in degree far beyond that which arises from mere debility, and evidently depending on the state of the brain. The delirium speedily ceased ; but the fever, peculiar pulse, restlessness, and the other two symptoms just named, continued with little abatement for five or six days, and in slighter degree even for some weeks afterwards.—At this time, nearly six weeks from the earliest date of the illness, dropsical symptoms came on, and rapidly increased ; effusion taking place largely into the abomen, and by anasarcous swellings all over the extremities; with evidence also of some effusion in the cavity of the chest. All the preceding symptoms—and notably those of cerebral irritation and disordered action of the arteries—abated in the same ratio as these dropsical symptoms came on. The latter were thoroughly relieved by calomel, digitalis, cascarilla, and chalybeates ; and, at the expiration of about ten weeks, the child was restored to perfect health; without the occurrence of relapse, or the impairment of any organ or function of the body.

Some ambiguity may be supposed in this case from the effects of the large bleeding employed. But the narrative of the early symptoms gave reason to suppose that they had been essentially the same, before this depletion took place. Their sudden termination when dropsical effusions came on (here justly to be termed *arterial dropsy*), is a remarkable and illustrative part of the case.

results, and still, it must be owned, inadequately pursued in its various details. The instances of the occurrence, fully ascertained and described, are probably few in comparison with those which actually exist under forms less explicit and obvious. The term metastasis, indeed, in its largest sense, might apply in some part to almost every form of disease. Scarcely is there one in which certain of the symptoms do not undergo change of place ;—either from causes inherent in the nature of the malady, and therefore in regular series ;—or from fortuitous circumstances in its progress ; and that complex relation of parts and functions, which renders it scarcely possible that one organ should be morbidly affected, without disturbance to others also. The difference, however, as respects liability to translation, is great, even in diseases where only the latter causes are concerned. Some are prone to shift the seat of morbid action repeatedly, and on the slightest disturbance or provocation ;—others seldom and tardily ;—yet in each case, and in every particular disease, with a tendency to certain transferences, rather than others ; obviously arising from some inherent difference of circumstances, and often marked enough to require description as a character of the disease.

A general view of the subject involves mainly the two great functions, which alone pervade every part of the animal economy; viz., the circulation of the blood; and the nervous system, in its several parts, connexions, and sympathies. To these two agencies must we attribute all translations of morbid action from one part to another. Most of the foregoing remarks on the causes which produce disturbance in the circulation, will be found to furnish this inference; and those not least, which relate to the variations in the quality of the blood, either from internal changes, or the introduction of foreign matters into it. For in regarding the blood as an agent in the metastasis of disease, it is necessary to distinguish between the cases, where there is a mere transference of excess of quantity from one place to another, as in various instances of simple inflammation or congestion ;—and those more remarkable cases, where a morbid state of the blood, or a morbid matter present in it, become the subject, and apparently the effective cause, of such translation. Of the latter, the transferences of action in the contagious exanthemata, and some other eruptive diseases, afford striking examples; and among metastases of this kind we may reckon those also, less regular in form, which occur in gout, and in scrofulous or scorbutic habits, forming a character in these several disorders, of great importance both in pathology and practice.

The two conditions then, just stated, regarding the blood, and the direct influence of the nervous system, may be said to include all the instances which can fitly be termed translation of disease. The division, however, so made, though convenient both in reasoning and practice, is by no means easy to follow in all cases; and we must admit it as certain, that the several causes run closely and imperceptibly into each other. It may be, for example, that the simple redundance of blood, transferred from one part to another, is an effect of nervous influence thus directed;—a question already considered; and showing, as do so many others, how difficult it is, in these ultimate actions, to discover the true relation of cause and effect.—A similar doubt exists regarding the cause and manner of translation of morbid matters in the blood; and their relation to the inflammatory actions attending such change. These questions have also been discussed in several preceding chapters of this volume. They all include one consideration, never to be lost sight of; viz., that for every act of metastasis, however seemingly vague and irregular, there must be some definite cause; the discovery of which, whenever attainable, is important equally to the theory and treatment of disease.

In every general view of the subject of metastasis, regard must be had to the influence of similar texture of parts, whether continuous or otherwise, in determining these changes in the seat of morbid action. Though this similarity is obviously not indispensable, since some of the most remarkable metastases are independent of it, it doubtless is concerned in many cases of much interest in the history of disease;—particularly in the affections of mucous and serous membranes. The disorders of the air-passages, the alimentary canal, and the skin, afford many illustrations to this effect; indicating also the effect of continuity of surface and texture:—and they illustrate besides, in common with other organs, another very important fact respecting metastasis, viz., its frequent dependence on connexion of function between the parts which are the subject of such changes.

The latter circumstance might perhaps have been inferred, prior to all experience; but it is confirmed, as a fact in pathology, by instances exceedingly numerous, and often very remarkable. Besides those appertaining to the organs just named, we have many and striking examples in the urinary and generative systems, in the joints and muscular tissues, in the secreting organs, &c. And it may be to this principle we shall eventually refer certain cases,—as the singular metastases occasionally occurring in cynanche parotidæa,—which are wholly anomalous to our present knowledge, yet definite enough to prove a specific cause, the proper subject for future investigation.

The metastases,—whether in the form of inflammation, congestion, or other morbid action,—which are conjoined with, or depend upon, morbid states of the blood, are certainly amongst the most extraordinary phenomena of disease. Without repeating details, I may refer generally to what has been said in former chapters, regarding those translations in gout, scrofula, and other constitutional disorders, which, though they indicate simply various modes of development of the same cause of disease, come fairly under this denomination; and manifestly include many affections hitherto differently named, and ascribed to different causes. For, however varying in aspect or importance, we are not entitled to separate in principle those metastases which occur suddenly, from such as occupy a longer time in the transference of disordered action to another part. In each case the blood must be the medium of translation, and the difference of time is one merely of degree. This manner of regarding the subject is essential to the inquiry; and it will be found to confirm the inference, drawn from other sources, that the effects of a simple morbid matter, present in the blood, may show themselves in forms greatly more varied than is yet presumed in the theory of disease.

Another point worthy of more notice than it receives, is the state of the body during what may be called the act of metastasis;—that is, while the morbid matter, wholly or partially dislodged from one seat of its action, is in passage through the circulation to another part. It is certain, on observation of such cases, that during this time of transference, whether longer or shorter in duration, there is often a very notable disturbance of the heart, of the nervous system, and of various organs seemingly out of the ordinary course of the disease; which disappear, when the symptoms are again locally fixed. I find in my notes many curious examples of this fact; drawn not only from the familiar occurrences of gout, but from numerous other disorders,—erysipelas, psoriasis and other affections of the skin, certain strumous swellings, &c. The phenomena of the exanthematous fevers, and of all translations between the skin and internal membranes, afford instances to the same effect. The general fact might have been anticipated, seeing the certainty that every such passage of morbid matter (whether foreign to the blood, or an excess of some of its ingredients) must be through the circulation, and that its influence cannot be wholly dormant during this time. But I wish to draw attention to it, as one well meriting further observation, and leading to inferences beyond those which appear on first view of the subject.

Closely connected with the same general view of metastasis, are those cases, equally numerous as remarkable, where the translation forms what has been termed a critical termination of the malady; of which the abscesses occasionally occurring in fevers, and towards the close of many other disorders, are the most familiar example.* The change thus effected, by what is often an inconsiderable deposit of purulent matter in some part of the body, —remote, it may be, from those parts especially affected by the disease,—is, in truth, one of the most singular facts in pathology. For there are cases in which we cannot reasonably interpret it as a mere transfer of irritation; but must look to the actual nature and amount of the discharge, as that which gives relief to the system; thus furnishing another argument for the doctrine which derives many of these idiopathic fevers, and analogus diseases,

* The physicians of antiquity paid more attention to this subject of the crisis of disorders, whether by abscess or otherwise, than do those of our own time : and they are justified by its practical importance. I need not state proofs of what is so familiar in their writings, from the time of Hippocrates downwards.

from actual changes within the blood itself. And the same principle applies, on the other side, to those various cases, where the sudden suspension of an habitual discharge brings on symptoms in other and remote parts of the body; having no common aspect, yet manifestly to be referred to one specific morbid cause.

Other illustration of these views of metastasis may be drawn from the remarkable connexion between certain morbid actions of the kidney, and disordered states of the brain;—traceable in every degree, from the slight influences upon ordinary sleep, to the most serious affections of the latter organs; often occurring very suddenly; and manifestly depending, not on mere alteration of the quantity of urine, but chiefly perhaps on the imperfection of the secretion as respects the removal of particular ingredients of the blood, which are thereby injuriously retained in the system.* These cases have not yet been studied to their full extent; and the same remark may be applied to certain affections of mucous membranes —bronchitis, for example—which are frequently the subject of similar sudden translation;—involving in some cases, it may be, mere transference of blood, as where bronchitis supervenes upon hemorrhoids;—but in other instances, changes in its quality, produced by the new and altered secretions which takes place.†

I have alluded generally to the connexion by metastasis between the intestinal membranes and the skin;—one of the most important relations in the animal economy in state of health, and entering, more or less, into every part of the history of disease. Disorders of digestion, alterations of secretion, changes of temperature, the influence of acrid or poisonous substances, and numerous other cases, are attended by a reciprocity of action between these two surfaces, often marked enough to form a character for description, and in every instance deserving notice, both as pathological facts, and suggestions for practice. The rapidity of some of these translations, and varying rate of others, is a remarkable part of their history; of which multiplied examples might be given, were they not rendered needless by their familiarity.

As the title of this chapter includes the subject of metastasis chiefly in connexion with the circulation, I shall not do more than refer to that part of it which includes the more direct action of the nervous system in producing these changes. This is in itself a wide

* A note on this subject, which should have been inserted in the Chapter on Sleep, was accidentally omitted there. Some of the variations in the effect of wines and other fermented liquors, in producing intoxication, doubtless depend on this important relation between the functions of the kidneys and the brain.

† I have notes of some singular cases of this kind;—one, for example, in which there existed for many years a frequent and well marked alternation of headaches with hemorrhoids; each very severe in degree, and both almost altogether removed by the supervention of chronic bronchitis; which latter disorder has since continued, constantly and severely, for a long period of years. In the same case I have repeatedly seen a temporary translation for a few hours to the head, producing even delirium; which again was as suddenly relieved by the recurrence of a copious bronchial secretion.

and curious topic of research ;—expounding the character of a large class of diseases ; and embracing the whole subject of nervous sympathies, to whatsoever class of nerves they belong, and whether direct or reflex in kind. While thus slightly alluding to it, I may observe that a complete work on the metastasis of disease, in its most general acceptation, is still a desideratum in medical literature, and would possess great value. But to execute it rightly, all implicit adherence to names and systems must be laid aside. Some of the most important results are obtained from sources, and by observing relations, to which these methods of arrangements afford no clue ; and which must escape notice, if the latter are rigorously pursued. Various examples to this effect have been given in the present and preceding chapters ; and many others will be furnished by the experience of every observant physician. -

---

CHAPTER XXXII.

ON THE USE OF DIGITALIS.

AFTER all that has been written upon this medicine, there is reason to doubt whether its capabilities have yet been brought into full use. An agent which can thus alter the heart's action, and, under management, safely sustain this alteration for a considerable time, is a very important one in the hands of the practitioner ; affording means wherewith to control, more or less directly, all the actions of the system. It is, however, this singular sedative effect on the heart, and the occasional suddenness of the change so produced, which creates an apprehension as to its use, not warranted by what we learn from exact observation. Though employing the medicine somewhat largely in practice, I do not recollect a case in which I have seen any injurious consequences from this cause ;—none such, certainly, as were not speedily relieved by its discontinuance, and other means of easy adoption.

I am far from inculcating neglect of the symptom just mentioned. But while admitting that deviation below the average standard of the pulse is less frequent and considerable than excess above it, and that certain morbid states of the brain are sometimes thus indicated, I feel assured that alarm is too readily taken in the early effects of digitalis on the heart, even should intermittent action be one of these. Similar effects occur habitually from so many other causes affecting the body, without injury which can be especially referred to this symptom, that if there be justification on other grounds for sustaining the action, and care given to watching it, the practice may generally be pursued without any risk to countervail the good.

More attention too is required, than is also bestowed, in estimating the actual changes in the pulse. It is not enough to feel it once or in one posture only. The difference between recumbency and the upright posture will often totally alter its character; and it should be examined also after some cordial has been given, to ascertain the facility of bringing it back to its ordinary state. These and other precautions, by better determining the real amount of deviation produced, afford securities for the continued use of the medicine which are of great practical value.*

The manner of employing digitalis is undoubtedly of much consequence. I feel assured, on experience, that the combination with tonics and stimulants not only does not impair some of its specific effects, but even extends them by giving larger scope to its administration. This may be inadmissible when a direct sedative effect is required (though here, as in the case of Dr. Ferrier's original suggestion of digitalis and steel in phthisis, the line cannot always distinctly be drawn); but when the action of the kidneys is especially sought for, and in habits already debilitated by disease, such combinations are often of the greatest value. That with iron seems to me more beneficial in many cases than with bark ; nor producing any mischief or ambiguous effect from the seeming incongruity of the two agents. I have frequently given digitalis in the ordinary doses, for weeks together, in combination with the tinct. ferr. muriat., or the tinct. ferr. ammoniat., without finding cause to withdraw or intermit the medicine; and this in cases where the patients were far advanced in years, and the circulation become feeble from disease. It would be difficult to find any single combination more effective than this in old cases of general dropsy ; in œdematous swellings from debility ; or in the anasarca following scarlet fever, where, together with weakness, there is still left an excited and irritable state of the arterial system. The action of the foxglove, as a diuretic, seems even to be quickened and sustained by being conjoined with the steel; while the latter acts apparently as a safeguard against some of its peculiar effects.

It cannot be doubted that this medicine may often be given with safety and advantage, even where the action of the heart is already extremely irregular. The irregularity arises occasionally from causes which the digitalis is capable of lessening or removing; as from fluid actually effused. But, besides this less direct influence, it is probable that its immediate action on the heart,

---

* These suggestions regarding the pulse apply to many other cases, where we seek to know the effects of disease upon it ; and not, as here, the influence of the remedy. The value of its indications is often forfeited by the slight and careless manner in which they are taken. An inference may be formed at one moment, or under one posture, which the lapse of five minutes, and change of position, will altogether belie. It is true that this is less the case in fevers and inflammatory diseases : but there are many others where the view of the disorder and method of treatment may be wholly perverted, by trusting to a single observation. All recent inquiry into the pulse shows the need of attention to these points.

tending under certain circumstances to produce intermittent pulsation, may under other circumstances correct the irregularity already existing. And accordingly I have often found perfect equality of beat to ensue for a time upon its use, where the motions of the heart had been very unequal in their ordinary state.

The effect here is the same as that which frequently occurs from fever, or other cause of excitement to arterial action, in rendering regular a pulse habitually intermittent; but the fact is more remarkable in the instance of digitalis, from its peculiar influence on the heart under ordinary circumstances. We have reason, indeed, to suppose at least two different states of this organ, independently of structural disease, in which intermittent action may occur, from causes almost the converse of each other; and in this probably lies the explanation of the seeming anomaly in question. The point is a curious one in pathology, and meriting notice from the inferences it suggests.

I may further add on this subject, that I have often employed digitalis beneficially, in cases even where there was proof from auscultation, or otherwise, of the heart being actually diseased in structure. There is need here, however, not only of much watchfulness, but of discrimination as to the kind of disease. The enlarged and flaccid heart, though on first view it might seem the least favourable for the use of the medicine, is perhaps not so. At least, we have reason to believe that in the dropsical affections so often connected with this organic change, the action of digitalis, as a diuretic, is peculiarly of avail. Generally speaking, in all cases where there is obvious mechanical difficulty to the passage of the blood through the heart, so as on slight causes to give the patient apprehension of fatal stoppage, we are bound to be cautious, lest, in seeking to relieve quick and irritable pulsation, we should bring on some worse alternative.

The action of digitalis seems, indeed, peculiarly the subject of anomaly throughout; and I am partly led to these remarks, as pointing out the void there yet is in our knowledge of some of these very powerful physical agencies on the body. Scarcely even is the question wholly settled, whether it is directly or only indirectly sedative. The view of its action, as one of accumulation in the body, and sudden effect, is still uncertain;—or if thought to be determined in fact, liable at least to doubt in the practical inferences drawn from it. Another source of difficulty is the doubtful relation between the sedative and diuretic effects of the medicine; understanding by the former term, its peculiar influence on the heart and circulation. This connexion, though doubtless existing, and probably an integral part of its action, has not yet been rightly ascertained. In following the inquiry, there are certain points which occur in the outset, as essential to it; such as, more especially, the question, whether the action of digitalis, as a diuretic, is immediately upon the kidneys, or intermediately through changes it produces on the vital actions of the sanguiferous system? In answering this question (which may probably be done by affirming the latter opinion), we are called upon to refer to the fact, that it is chiefly in dropsy of the cavities of the chest, and anasarca, that its action as a remedy is of any avail. Pursuing this observation, it becomes likely that most of the doubtful or anomalous effects of the medicine will hereafter be found to resolve themselves into its influence, direct or indirect, on different parts of the vascular system; but much is yet required to substantiate this view, or to determine, if true, all its consequences.*

Until we thus, or through other means, acquire more exact knowledge of the mode of action of digitalis, we cannot look to obtain all those increased advantages in practice, which may be anticipated from its peculiar agency on the circulation. We must be content to proceed empirically, as we have hitherto done, in noting its effects in particular cases, and under given combinations. In proof of the present need of submitting all theory to practical observation, I may mention that though convinced of its value in combination with bark or preparations of iron, in dropsical cases, yet I am led by experience to acquiesce also in Dr. Withering's opinion, that its effects as a diuretic are often greater in states of feeble circulation and relaxed fibre, than where the habit is more vigorous and firm. Nor can I doubt, from observation, the truth of Dr. John Davy's remark, that patients weakened by disease often bear much larger doses than those in sounder health. Admitting the facts to be severally so, we must refer for explanation of the seeming contradiction, to the manner of action of digitalis on the vascular system, still so imperfectly known; and to analogy also in the case of mercury and some other medicines, where a certain state of the circulation is required to give specific direction to some of their effects.† We know too little, moreover, of the manner of action of iron and bark, to be able to affirm that they would prevent this state being attained; even though commonly using these medicines for purposes apparently of opposite kind.

The uncertainty of diuretic medicines in general is, indeed, a point where medical practice is greatly at fault. Scarcely can one be named on which we may uniformly rely; and the inequalities of action are rarely to be assigned to any known cause. As, however, they belong alike, or nearly so, to all these medicines, whether of mineral,

* Some experiments, made by injection of an infusion of digitalis into the arteries, seem to show the capillary circulation as directly affected; but it is very difficult in all these cases to determine which are really first in the series of effects. M. Magendie, by injecting tincture of digitalis into the jugular vein of a dog, reduced the beats of the heart from 120 to 84 in a minute, without, however, altering the arterial pressure, as indicated by the hæmodynamometer.

I have never seen an instance of ptyalism produced by digitalis; but the case recorded by Dr. Henry, and some earlier evidence of the same kind, make it probable that this is an occasional consequence of excess in its use.

† The experiments which prove that the facility with which poisons produce their effects by absorption, varies according to the quantity or dilution of the circulating blood, may be considered to bear directly upon this point.

vegetable, or animal kind, we must seek their origin not in the
substances themselves, but in the functions of the kidneys; liable
beyond all others to unceasing changes; and from causes and combinations so various, (interpreting, as they do, the state of every
other organ and function of the body,) that we may readily understand how medicines directed to them should partake in the same
uncertainty.

It is among the remedies of this class, perhaps more than any
other, that combinations have their greatest value.   Mercury, digitalis, squill, cantharides, diuretic salts, and the different vegetable
infusions having similar action, are severally capable of being aided
in this way, either by conjunction mutually, or with other agents.*
It must be admitted that the results so derived are purely empirical
in kind; not explicable when attained; and subject frequently to the
same failure as when the same medicines are given uncombined.
Nevertheless, these are the proper objects of diligent observation; and
the ability of the practitioner is in no way better shown than in
removing whatever may render his conclusions equivocal or obscure.

Intending these only as general remarks on the action and application of digitalis, I do not add to them by details of its employment in particular diseases.   I would merely repeat my persuasion,
that its use as a sedative to the circulation, in diseases of inflammation or excitement, might beneficially be much extended; superseding depletion in some cases, the use of narcotics in others.
Regarding its employment in pulmonary consumption, I am unable
to add anything to the ambiguous recommendation it has heretofore
received.   It clearly has no power over tubercular deposits; and
the only influence to be understood in such cases is that of abating
the rapidity of circulation, where greater than is natural; an effect
of less real moment than is generally supposed.   In this, as in many
other instances, the importance of a particular symptom as a test,
leads to a wrong estimate of its relations to the actual disease.   We
assume that we are proceeding towards cure, when merely diminishing one effect of a specific disorder upon the natural functions of
the body.

Respecting the several forms under which digitalis is used, there
is some reason to believe the infusion, rightly prepared, to be the
most certain and beneficial in its effects; and admitting of every
combination with other medicines which can in any case be re-

* In the instance of other diuretics, as well as digitalis, it would seem that
the direct conjunction with stimulants often adds to their efficacy. Ammonia,
for example, independently of its own occasional action upon the kidneys,
will often give other means more certain and speedy direction to this organ.
In another chapter (On the Uses of Diluents) I have mentioned the value of
these in their action on the kidneys, even in some dropsical cases; and it is well
worth while to keep in mind such possible aid to diuretic medicines, when
failing in their immediate and proper effect. It may be from disregard to this,
that various popular remedies have less effect in regular practice than under
older and more familiar methods of employment.

quired.   This, indeed, is an instance where, from the nature of the agent, it is singularly needful that the quality of its preparations should be equal and uniform.   It is certain that many of the inequalities and seeming anomalies in the effects of digitalis are owing to neglect of this important precaution.

CHAPTER XXXIII.

ON ANTIMONIAL MEDICINES.

I ANNEX this subject to the preceding, having chiefly in view what is still the insufficient use in English practice, of those medicines expressly sedative to the actions of the circulation.   I have noticed this in the instance of digitalis; and it is equally true as regards some of the antimonial preparations; and the tartarized antimony especially.   The opinions held in relation to the supposed sudorific effect of these medicines, has prevented due attention being given to their influence in allaying inordinate action; either of the brain, as in mania and delirium of different forms; or more generally in inflammation, or febrile states of the whole system.   In France, and still earlier and more extensively in some of the Italian schools, the use of emetic-tartar is well known to have been carried much further than in England, and under systematic views, as a contra-stimulant, which we scarcely yet fully recognise.   The appreciation of its powers is now, indeed, becoming more just and complete; but the progress is slow in relation to the assured benefits which may be derived from it in ordinary practice.*

In another chapter I have noticed the uncertain views which determine our employment of antimonials as sudorifics, and the probability that any such effect they have is due chiefly to their influence in abating the circulation and the febrile state.   To this may be added a reasonable doubt regarding the efficacy of some of the antimonial preparations most frequently in use.   My own experience suggests the conclusion which has occurred to others, that the antimonial powder of our Pharmacopœia is perfectly inert in any ordinary dose; and that the original James's powder has held a reputation barely justified by any method of its use; certainly not by the trifling quantities in which it is now given.   All the gain

---

* The writings, as well as practice, of Professor Tomassini of Bologna, may be cited in proof of the extent to which the use of tartar-emetic may be carried; and also for the best account of the doctrines of the new Italian school on this subject, to which the names of Rasori and Borda, as well as his own, have given reputation.   The work more recently published by M. Lapelletier, " De l'Emploi du Tartre Stibié à haute dose dans le traitement des Maladies," affords a complete history of all that is known on the subject.

we derive from these medicines as sudorifics or otherwise, is obtained far more largely, and with much greater certainty, by use of the emetic-tartar in similar cases : and this, in fact, is the preparation of antimony which, by proper management, may be made to supersede any other; and which, whether considering its power or variety of application, may fairly rank amongst the most valuable remedies we possess.

Of these applications, that which depends on its sedative effect is perhaps the most important. Without referring to any theories of this particular influence, or the mode in which it is exercised in the living body, it is enough to know that there is the power, directly or indirectly, of diminishing excess of action; and limiting thereby the degree, if not also the duration, of those conditions in which disorders of acute inflammation or inflammatory fever mainly consist.* As a febrifuge in the most distinct sense of the term, it may be doubted whether we possess any more direct or speedy in effect. It is impossible to have witnessed its effects, when adequately given, in acute pneumonia, or bronchitis, or croup, without recognising the same fact; and seeing that where it does not wholly supersede bleeding as a prior remedy, it at least abridges the demand for this; and comes in aid of it, by inducing the same state of the vascular system throughout the body. Its relation to mercury in these cases is that of most interest; the effect apparently the same, so as in many instances to make it doubtful which of the two remedies may best be relied upon for instant use; yet the mode of operation presumably very different.†

The evidence of Laennec, Louis, and other eminent French physicians, on many of these points, is more explicit than ours; as founded on larger use of the remedy, and more direct comparison of the cases of pneumonia so treated with those submitted to other means. I know not that its value has been equally attested in other forms of inflammation; but sufficiently so, and especially in affections of the brain, to show that the sedative action is not limited to one organ, but extends generally to the whole system.‡

---

* The reluctance shown by many to admit the phrase and idea of a direct sedative, may depend, in part, on too exclusive attention to the fact that augmented action is always followed by proportionate loss of power; becoming in this way the most frequent and familiar cause of sedative effect which is known to us. But the full admission of this general law by no means precludes the allowance of other actions upon the body, or certain of its functions, producing the effect at once, which indirectly results in the other case. Abstractedly considered, the notion of any part of vital action reduced below its average or natural state, is quite as intelligible as that of the same action raised above it.

† Dr. Stokes, in his work on Diseases of the Chest, remarks that the previous use of tartar-emetic in pneumonia seems to facilitate the further action of mercury in subduing the inflammation. He advises that in typhoid pneumonia the mercurial treatment should be pursued in preference to that by antimonials. What I have seen would lead me to concur in both these points of practice.

‡ The experiments of Sir B. Brodie, in the second of his valuable papers on the Action of Poisons (*Phil. Trans.* 1812, p. 205), render it probable that the brain chiefly is first acted upon by emetic-tartar so given, but with some evidence

Though the discussion as to the relative merits of the treatment by bleeding, and that by antimonials, in pneumonia, is not without use, yet it has perhaps placed the remedies too much in seeming opposition to each other. They come, in fact, in common aid towards the same object; and are often needed in conjunction;— the bleeding first, in such cases, for more instant and powerful effect, and possibly also as giving more power to the action of the tartar-emetic;—the latter as sustaining the effect of the depletion, and often preventing the need there might otherwise be of its repetition. When the inflammation is slight, its relief may frequently be trusted to the antimonial alone. This appears to be the view by which the relative employment of the two remedies may best be guided in practice.

I infer from my own observation, what is amply proved by that of others, that the sedative effects of antimony under this form are independent of all evacuation from the body. They may occur, where there has been neither vomiting nor purgative action; and where perspiration, if happening at all, comes rather in sequel and effect, than as cause of the changes produced. We must consider the vascular system, either directly, or through the influence of the nervous system, to be the part concerned in, and the subject of, these changes. Some ambiguity exists here, as to the nausea brought on by the use of the medicine; and the relation of such effect to its sedative agency. It is not always easy to separate these effects; which seem, indeed, to depend concurrently upon the same cause acting on the nervous system. But there is enough to show the sedative action to exist independently of this, in the fact that it occurs where the nauseating effect has either not taken place at all, or been removed.

It must be allowed that there are many singularities in the influence of this medicine as an emetic; and that we yet only partially understand the conditions which so variously modify this quality. The mode of administration is, doubtless, in part concerned; and particularly as regards the quantity of the fluid vehicle in which it it is given. The state of the stomach itself is another of the conditions. But there is also an influence derived from the general state of the body at the time; attested, as I think, in the case of fever; where, according to my experience, there is less effect from given doses in producing sickness, than when this state is absent. The same conclusion seems to be justified regarding its employment in inflammatory disorders. And further, it is manifest that a habit is acquired as to the medicine, lessening or wholly removing effects that have occurred on its first use; so that vomiting or nausea, very harassing in the outset, may cease to disturb the patient, even though the same doses are continued as before.

---

of direct action on the heart also. The suggestion of Magendie, that its fatal effects are due to an inflammatory state of the whole system, supervening upon absorption, does not seem warranted by any express fact; and is made less probable by the frequent absence of all inflammatory appearances on the coats of the stomach and intestines in such cases.

The influence, indeed, of dose and manner of employment, curious and important in all cases, well deserves notice here.   Our practice in England (limited, as I have said, by older views) seldom goes beyond such use of them in inflammatory disorders, as to sustain nausea for a time, and thereby repress the circulation; and even this intention is often made subordinate to the forcing of perspiration, as a means of relief.   It is certain that the full value of the medicine is not thus attained; and though we yet want proof of the efficacy or need of the large doses of emetic-tartar employed by some of the Continental physicians, it seems certain that those we use might beneficially be increased in relation to their sedative effect.*

The best test we have on this point is to be found in the objects for which we adopt the treatment; viz., the diminished action of the heart and arterial system, or the removal of some active irritation of the brain or other organ.   In looking to this test, as well as on other accounts, it is very generally expedient to give the medicine under its simplest form.   With a powerful agent of definite purpose in our hands, combination ought rather to be regarded as an exception than a rule of employment: enfeebling for the most part the principle of treatment, and perplexing its results.   I have elsewhere alluded to this maxim in practice; which, admitting all the needful qualifications, is still important enough to warrant a constant regard to it.

In the instance of emetic-tartar, its combination with opium is undoubtedly that which most merits notice.   This seems a fair example of a compound acquiring powers, which do not equally belong to either of its component parts.   Its value is attested by the observation of many physicians, particularly in cases of mania and cerebral irritation; and my own experience entirely concurs in this respect.   In cases more strictly inflammatory in kind, whether pneumonia, bronchitis, rheumatism, or inflammation of the membranes of the brain, the same combination is often useful; but under more reserve, both as to the period of the disorder, and the propriety of bleeding as a previous remedy.   The difference of opinion respecting the fitness of combining opium with the antimonial in such cases, arises probably from the different attention given to the latter points. Whether with or without emetic-tartar, it cannot safely be employed where bleeding is required.   But allowing for its unfitness in these instances, I still believe the harm done to be less, than were it given, under the like circumstances, not so combined.

Reverting to the use of this combination in affections of the brain, it is remarkable how speedy and assured the effect often is.   In the wild restlessness of delirium tremens this is sometimes very strikingly

* The doses of those French physicians, whose practice is best authority (one or two grains, so repeated as to extend from 5 to 20 grains in the twenty-four hours), may be assumed as affording every scope to the beneficial use of the medicine in different cases.   The maximum quantity here little exceeds what Rasori sometimes gave for a single dose.

seen. In fevers attended with much cerebral disturbance its employment has been attended. with similar good.* And in various forms of spasmodic disease I have experience of the same kind; giving evidence of benefits which are not so readily or completely obtained by the use of opium alone.

It is probable that other applications of the tartar-emetic in the cure of disease will hereafter be ascertained; depending, it may be, upon other modes of agency than that to which I have chiefly alluded.† For though employing the term *sedative*, thus far, in the most simple and practical sense in which we can understand it, it is obvious that much theory attaches to the subject; and that sedative action, so understood as merely opposed to stimulant, may occur not only from different agents, but in different ways as regards the organs first affected; and with varying influence on different parts of the system. The agency of the hydrocyanic acid (an important addition to this class of medicines, and perhaps the most explicit example of their effect) is evidently not the same as that of digitalis or tartarized antimony; and we have equal reason to suppose differences between the latter, seeing the diversity of their collateral effects. Though greatly instructed by modern inquiry in the action of poisons, yet is our knowledge likely to be much augmented in all that concerns their relation to the vital properties of the blood. And we have the assurance of great aid in the treatment of disease, by better determining the specific nature and application of those agents which are directly opposed to excess of action, either throughout the whole system, or in particular parts and functions of life.‡

* In a valuable paper by Dr. Graves (*London Med. Gazette for July* 8, 1837), this physician recommends the occasional use of emetic-tartar by enema; stating its effects to be the same as given by the mouth, and rightly commenting on the neglect of this means of administering various other remedies.

† In a late paper by Dr. Gemelle, (*Bulletin Général de Therapeutique, Mars,* 1838,) cases are given of the successful treatment of synovial affections of the joints by the internal use of tartar emetic.

‡ In alluding to the very powerful medicines of this class, and particularly to the prussic acid, it may be worth while to make one comment; needless, indeed, to all who are familiar with the principles of therapeutics; but requisite to be kept in view while these agents are still waiting, as it were, for recognition, and deprecated by many who see in them only the virulence of their concentrated forms. What we have mainly to regard, in estimating the medicinal value of any substance, or its just application to practice, is the well-defined nature of its action on some organ or function of the living economy. If this action be clearly ascertained, we have essentially a medicinal power in our hands. Every such agent, even the most simple, is capable of being misused by excess; and this excess, or the fitness of use, is determined, not by any comparison of the power of different agents, but simply by the amount of the effects appropriate to each. The prussic acid, diluted as befits the particular application given to it, is not, in any practical sense, a stronger medicine than others most familiar to us, nor more dangerous in use; and we have even some additional security in the more definite nature of its effects, and in the greater care bestowed on its administration.

CHAPTER XXXIV.

ON THE HYPOTHESIS OF INSECT LIFE AS A CAUSE OF DISEASE?

I PUT this title interrogatively, as expressing what is merely a speculation; and, in so far, distinct from all the other topics of this volume; yet sufficiently within the scope of possible truth to justify a few remarks upon it. In making these, the reasoning may conveniently be applied as an argument for the hypothesis; viewing it constantly, however, under the qualification just named.

The question is, what weight we may attach to the opinion that certain diseases, and especially some of epidemic and contagious kind, are derived from minute forms of animal life, existing in the atmosphere under particular circumstances; and capable, by application to the lining membranes, or other parts, of acting as a virus on the human body? This is by no means a new speculation; and it would seem to have been much more frequently started during the last century, than at the present time.* The greater exactness of modern inquiry rightly represses all opinions, which have not explicit facts for their support. Though the course of discovery has recently been approaching, in some points, nearer to the hypothesis in question, it still furnishes nothing beyond stronger presumptions and more numerous analogies; nor has any endeavour been made to collect or class these, with a view to more general results. Nevertheless the subject is one fairly open to inquiry; and the more reasonably so, as we possess no information regarding the causes of these maladies, which can supersede research, but rather have in our ignorance the motive for pursuing it through every new channel which science may disclose.

That there are conditions of animal life in the atmosphere, (however characterized), as minute, as numerous, and as variously diffused, as those of which the microscope informs us in water and other media, may be considered from analogy next to certain. Our actual knowledge carries us so far into these minute forms of existence, and by such uniform gradations, that we cannot suppose the series to stop, because evidence is no longer drawn from our own senses, or means of research. This would imply a sudden breach of continuity, such as we find in no other part of the scale

---

* Kircher is known as one of the earliest propounders of the opinion. Linnæus gave some sanction to it, by admitting into the Amœnitates Academicæ several memoirs on the subject. The most detailed is that by Nyander, entitled "Exanthemata Viva," in which small-pox, measles, the plague, dysentery, syphilis, and hooping-cough are all attributed to the agency of minute animals, chiefly Acari of different species. A second paper in the same work, on Lepra, applies the speculation also to this disease; and other memoirs, severally entitled "Mundus Invisibilis," "Miracula Insectorum," and "Noxa Insectorum," produce the hypothesis in a more general form.

of animal being. It is only of late that the wonderful eye of the microscope has clearly disclosed to us that vast domain of life to which the infusoria belong;—a new world of organized and active beings, which, but for the access thus afforded by the happy artifice of a single instrument, might have remained for ever as much hidden from our sense and knowledge as the invisible forms of insect life, of which the hypothesis before us presumes the existence.*

Whether we may hereafter reach more direct evidence on this subject is yet uncertain. Out of the direct dominion of the microscope these animals are removed, unless some such method as that suggested below be found attainable.† Other means, however, are conceivable, seeing the number and variety of resources furnished by modern science, and the unexpected quarters from which knowledge is often derived. I may name as an instance of this the paper of Dr. Wollaston (*Phil. Trans. for* 1820), "On Sounds inaudible by certain Ears;" showing the probable existence of whole domains of insect life, capable of exciting vibrations in the air, of which man's grosser hearing is wholly unconscious; but which, received by their finer organs as audible sounds, minister to purposes of enjoyment and activity among beings unperceived by any of the human senses.

Even admitting, however, that we may never reach actual proof of these more minute forms of life, be they insect or of other kind, the probability of their existence is little lessened by the failure; and if existing, the same analogy will lead us to other inferences, not less probable, as to those habits and instincts, in which they may be presumed to have affinity with the known insect genera. Such are, their frequent sudden generation, at irregular and often distant periods, under certain circumstances of season or locality, or under other conditions less obvious to apprehension:—secondly, the diffusion of swarms, so generated, and with rapidly repeated

* Even the unaided eye, however, gives us certain probable notices of these swarms of minute beings, which escape all individual examination. Reaumur and other naturalists have conjectured that the small floating clouds (*nubeculæ æthereæ*), like more opaque portions of the atmosphere, which, under summer temperature and in certain lights, are seen near the surface of the earth, are in fact insect swarms, depending for their fugitive existence on the conditions of the medium around them; but in this, as well as in their living habitudes, resembling the insect species more obvious to us.

† It has been supposed that the collection and condensation of dew, in situations where malaria or infectious miasmata abound, might afford a possible means of subjecting these material agents (for such they doubtless are) to chemical or microscopical research. If it were true, as presumed in the hypothesis before us, that minute insects are concerned in giving pestiferous quality to a portion of air, might not colouring matter, suitable to animal organization, be applied to the natural or artificial dew condensed from this air, so as to afford the chance of similar success to that which Ehrenberg has attained in his researches on the infusoria? The absence of any such observation, when he was himself seeking to discover infusoria in dew, does not disprove the possibility of this; as, from the difference in the cases presumed, the results, if ever thus obtained, would probably be only partial and occasional.

propagation, over wide tracts of country, and often following particular lines of movement. To which general inferences may be added another (resting on analogy, though of less explicit kind), viz., that certain of these animalcule species may act as poisons, or causes of disease, upon particular parts of the body exposed to their influence.

These inferences, supported by various reasons, and contradicted by no ascertained facts, give foundation to the question before us. Whatever is true as to the habits of insects obvious to our senses, is likely to be more especially so in those whose minuteness removes them further from observation. Their generation may be presumed more dependent on casualties of season and place;—their movements determined by causes of which we have less cognizance;—and their power of morbidly affecting the human body to be in some ratio to their multitude and minuteness. It cannot be deemed too mechanical an idea, that all conditions which give readier and more extensive access to the internal membranes, to any species capable of acting as a virus on these parts, may increase their influence as causes of disease. It occurs then, as the first point of inquiry, whether we have grounds for believing that animal life under this form can act as a noxious or poisonous influence on the human body. And here there are various facts which justify an affirmative answer; as showing that animal matter, applied to absorbing surfaces, may produce the most virulent symptoms of disorder, locally or generally, according to the nature of the virus, its intensity, or the relations of the texture first affected to other parts of the system.

The evidence on this subject varies in kind and conclusiveness. That which is most familiar and direct is our actual knowledge of numerous animal poisons; the product, as well of living secretions, as of changes taking place in animal matter after death. Respecting the former class, the most important to our present purpose, it is enough to refer generally to their many varieties in all parts of the animal kingdom, and particularly among the insects. From the dangerously active venom of the Argas Persicus and the tarantula, to the more harmless poisons of the bee, the wasp, the ant, and other insects which surround us, we have every gradation and variety of these secretions, which thus act noxiously on certain textures of the human body; and the instances would be much more numerous, if including those which affect other animals. In the cantharides we have a solitary example of their application to medicinal purposes.* The class of reptiles affords many well known

* In the narrative of the travels of Humboldt, Ehrenberg, and Rose, in Siberia, recently published, the last of these eminent naturalists describes a pestilence prevailing on the great steppe between the Irtish and the Ob, affecting very fatally both men and horses; the most obvious symptom that of suppurating tumours, chiefly on the exposed parts of the body. The opinion on the spot is, that the disease proceeds from the stings of insects; and there are various reasons for presuming it to be so. This is an instance before me at the moment; and

instances of such animal poisons, under the form of natural secretions, fulfilling purposes in the economy of the several animals possessing them. The virus in hydrophobia is an example of the poisonous production of disease. Recent observations have shown that the glanderous matter of the horse is capable of producing the same disorder in man; and it is probable that there are many more instances of this kind than we are yet acquainted with. Some of the secretions from diseased surfaces in the human body are known to acquire properties highly noxious, even to the frame within which they are generated; and we may perhaps attribute to the same cause the occasional poisonous quality of certain shell fish, which commonly are innocuous as articles of food. Or it may be that the latter are instances of a virus produced after death; as we have many examples of animal matter undergoing change of this kind during the process of decomposition, when life is extinct.

If it be urged that none of these instances (of which many more might be cited) apply expressly to the question, whether or not minute or invisible insect species may become causes of disease, the answer is, that the nature of the question supposes evidence of a different kind; and that we must seek for that of analogy and presumption where more direct cannot be had. Such evidence is found in the facts just stated, and in others still to be mentioned.

One argument, though also indirect, for the hypothesis before us, is founded on our increasing knowledge of the entozoa; and of the various morbid products, as well as diseased actions, which are due to the presumed propagation of these animals within the body. Without assuming what some have supposed, that tubercles and carcinomatous formations are thence derived, we have sufficient proof through recent discoveries, that these morbid actions from parasitic animals are much more numerous and varied than has heretofore been believed. It seems certain that future research will still further increase the number within our knowledge, and while indicating, by aid of the microscope, forms more minute than those yet discovered, will in this very minuteness suggest their more extensive agency as causes of disease.*

many similar, of greater or less authenticity, might be drawn from different sources both of ancient and modern date, attaching disease to the casual or periodical occurrence of this cause.

* Almost at the moment of transcribing this, I observe the notice of the discovery of minute worms (*Polystoma sanguicola* in the expectorated blood of phthisical cases (Andral, Delle Chiaje, and others had before discovered cephalocysts in the venous blood of man, and even of some of the invertebrate animals); and also of animalcules (*vibriones*) in syphilitic pus. The latter fact, however, appears from one of the papers already cited, in the Amœnitates Academicæ, to have been ascertained nearly a century ago. In other morbid secretions other animalcules have been seen; and, according to M. Donné, the author of some of these researches, with constant relation to the acid or alkaline nature of the discharge. The occasional presence of a minute worm (*Trichinia spiralis*), in the muscular substance, has been ascertained in this country; and still more recently another entozoon (the *Cysticercus cellulosa*) has been found by Dr. Knox and others in the same texture. That excellent observer, Mr. Owen, to whom we

The same remark will apply to the ectozoa, and to the spurious worms infesting the human body as well as many other animals. They afford further proof of the extent and variety of those connexions which subsist between different forms of living organization. It is a curious evidence of the progress of such research, that while only eleven species of intestinal worms are recorded in the 12th edition of the Systema Naturæ of Linnæus, nearly 1000 species are described by Rudolfi in his Entozoorum Synopsis, and others have since been discovered.

It is a remark of Ehrenberg, that, looking to the extreme fecundity of some of the entozoa, there is more cause for wonder at the limitation of their effects by the actions of the living bodies they inhabit, than at any morbid effects they appear actually to produce. The recent speculations of this eminent naturalist derive a sanction for their boldness from his remarkable discovery of the fossil infusoria, as well as from his researches among the entozoa, in their various species, and on different parts of the globe; in ascertaining the highly organized structure, astonishing minuteness, and fecundity of which, he has obtained arguments for the belief that they form a direct cause of many of the diseases affecting man.* The whole subject of parasitic animals and plants, and the mutual relations of each class, is indeed replete with curious matter of research; and now first pursued with an earnestness proportionate to its importance. It provides us with argument and analogy from every part of organic existence, in attestation of the fact, that the life of one being is in innumerable cases supported by the life of another; and that there are express relations of dependence of this kind established throughout creation, scarcely less definite and remarkable than those by which the functions of individual life are carried on.†

owe the best classification of the human entozoa, has been led by observation to suppose that the cataract of the eye is produced by a species of worm; a supposition at variance, however, with the results to which Sir D. Brewster has been led by his refined and beautiful researches on the crystalline lens in its healthy and diseased states. It is well known that minute animals (*filaria oculi*) have been seen in movement in the aqueous humour of the eye of the horse. Still more recently they have been observed in milk. Different animals, according to Gruithausen, exist in pus and mucus. Some of these statements need confirmation, and, above all, the identity of the animal in similar conditions of disease; but, if obtaining such proof, they manifestly become very important to all future inquiries in pathology.

* In connexion with his view (rendered doubtful by Müller), that the minute ova of parasitic animals may be taken up by the absorbents and deposited in particular textures of the body, he hazards the opinion that scrofula, in its various forms, may be thus produced;—a supposition not wholly new, nor incompatible with the fact of its being an hereditary disorder, but certainly requiring more evidence than has yet been given.

† It is a singular proof of the extent of this fact, that entomologists have ascertained more than forty genera of insects to be infested by parasitic worms (*filariæ*), and that it is often possible to determine the species of the insect by that of the parasite living upon it. I see a recent notice (1837) of a cryptogamic plant growing on the body of the common fly; the converse, (if indeed it be

In the foregoing remarks I have noticed only the more general reasons for supposing it possible that certain diseases to which man is subject, may be derived from animalcule life, existing in the atmosphere around us, and capable of acting noxiously on the human body. To carry the inquiry further, it is necessary to take some instance which may render more explicit its details, and connect together the analogies on which it is founded. Such instance is best sought for in the class of epidemic or contagious diseases; where, if evidence exists at all of the influence of this cause upon the human frame, it is most likely to be found. And amongst the number, there is none to which the hypothesis so well applies, as to the Asiatic or epidemic cholera; that strange pestilence of our own time, which, while affrighting every part of the world by its ravages, has seemed to put at naught all speculation as to its causes, or the laws which govern its course;—a disease, nevertheless, which by the mystery of its first appearance, its suddenness, inequality, and fatality, and the failure hitherto of every method of treatment, may well excite the inquiry of all who are zealous for the extension of medical science.

In taking this remarkable disorder for the instance required, I would merely affirm that it furnishes the best evidence in a case where we can attain none other than presumptive proofs. Presenting close analogies to other diseases of this class, its essential characters are so strongly marked, as to fit it well for being taken as a type of the rest. It must further be admitted that the ground is one singularly open for speculation. I have met with no opinion as to the causes and mode of propagation of the epidemic cholera, which can be considered to afford even-plausible explanation of the facts; and in putting to trial the capability of another hypothesis to solve the phenomena of the disease, we are but seeking, by comparison of difficulties, to attain the conclusion which is least liable to them. In truth, the manner in which the assured circumstances in its history annul all common theories as to its origin, has almost the force of an argument for any new opinion or line of research.

The outline of the problem to be solved may be stated thus. Here is a disease, which, appearing first in the Delta of the Ganges, has spread itself within the space of seventeen years round almost the whole habitable circumference of the globe; reaching Pekin on the one side, the Mississippi and Mexico on the other;—its general

correctly stated,) of the numerous cases in which animals live upon plants, and completing all the possible mutual relations of parasitic growth in animal and vegetable life. The discovery of monades within the bodies of certain of the entozoa is another circumstance not less worthy of notice. These facts are very interesting in themselves; and further remarkable as showing the exactness of modern observation, and the advance it has made into the most minute operations of nature. Ehrenberg has used a bold, but not unjustifiable figure, in speaking of the "*milky way* of the smallest organization," accessible to human research, like that of the heavens, only through artificial instruments; but yielding to these, in the one case as in the other, the most marvellous proofs of the infiniteness of creative power.

course traceable, step by step, over the whole of this wide distance, yet irregular in details both as to time and space ; the disorder frequently reaching more remote points long before it affected countries very near to the general line of its direction; yet never, even in these cases, without traces of every part of the intermediate course.* During the whole period since its first appearance, and in every place of its occurrence, the disease has been absolutely identical in kind; the only varieties those of degree. Wherever it has existed, a tendency is observed to its reappearance in successive years, though for the most part less extensively, and under other limits and conditions hitherto imperfectly known.

These are the points which it is essential to keep in mind in all reasoning as to the causes of cholera. Other peculiarities of the disease are scarcely less remarkable ; but these stand so completely at the threshold of the question, that no opinion can presumably be true, which does not include them, and furnish some explanation of their nature.

Holding these things in view, any hypothesis regarding cholera may best be prefaced by certain facts of negative kind ; the admission of which gives fairer space to the rest of the inquiry. Of these the first is, that no condition of physical change in the atmosphere are yet known to us—statical, chemical, or electrical—which afford even a probable solution of the phenomena of the disease. The Indian official reports furnish nothing that can be admitted as proof to this effect; nor has the more exact observation of Europe better warranted the opinion.† Among those who have written on the subject, there are some who have dwelt much on a presumed electrical state of the air as the exciting cause; but without any just or sufficient grounds for the hypothesis.‡ Admitting that there is much still to be learnt regarding this great natural agent, and its relations to the body, nothing certainly has yet been discovered be-

---

* The cholera had raged at New Orleans a year or two before it appeared in Sweden, and four years before it devastated Sicily and Naples. But it existed in ships making the voyage from Liverpool and Greenock to Quebec and New York ; and might be traced along the great line of river communication in the United States, as well as by the coast line from the Northern States to those of the Mexican Gulf.

† Some arguments drawn from the prevalence of storms, and seasons of drought or excessive rain, during the years directly preceding its first appearance in Bengal, even if they gave any sort of explanation for India, would in nowise explain the successive spread of the disease over other parts of the globe. Dr. Prout noticed a very small but constant excess in the average weight of the air, during part of the time when the cholera first prevailed in London ; but as there has been no repetition of this remark, it was probably a casual coincidence.

‡ It has been a favourite idea that negative electricity of the atmosphere might favour the production of cholera ; an opinion scarcely professing to have other basis than that the ordinary electricity of the air is positive. M. Peltier, from constant observations during 1835 and 1836, states that in 1835 the clouds were almost always in positive state; in 1836 generally neutral or negative. In neither of these years, except in a few insulated cases, did the disease appear either in France or England.

speaking its connexion with the disease in question; and the whole history of cholera is utterly at variance with such opinion. Staking the question on a single argument, is it possible that a state of electricity (compatibly with what we know of its laws) can exist in any one spot, capable of destroying life in a few hours in one person, while others in the same place are scarcely affected in their ordinary sensations? The supposition is highly improbable in itself, and stands in contradiction to every other physical law.

All the arguments used in a former chapter, to prove that the epidemic influenzas are in no way directly produced by atmospheric states or changes, apply with equal or greater force to the disease before us. No notion of an epidemic constitution (to acquiesce for a moment in a phrase which wraps ignorance in the garb of scientific language) can be of avail against the facts belonging to the history of the disorder—its course, manner and time of progress, and various aspects—as it has spread over the world during the twenty years succeeding the earliest cases at Jessore. Had I been writing a treatise on cholera, instead of a few remarks on a particular hypothesis, I might bring the most ample evidence for the truth of this negative assertion. The whole resolves itself into this:—that the disease, in its most distinct and virulent form, has existed in different places under every possible variety of atmospheric state; —and, conversely, that every such variation has existed in higher degree in the same places, without producing the disease.*

Nor have we the smallest reason, from knowledge or analogy, to assume that any gaseous, mineral or vegetable matter, diffused in the atmosphere, or exhaling from the earth, could create a disorder thus peculiar, or spread it in a manner so remarkable over the face of the globe. The notion of terrestrial or mineral exhalations,—a favourite one in all ages, and espoused by Sydenham,—is defective in proof in every case, and singularly inapplicable to the cause and circumstances of cholera. A natural morbid cause, or causes, (for which, in default of a better, we must admit the name of *malaria*,) may originate locally, and produce various local endemic or epidemic diseases; and of this we have sufficient evidence. But these very circumstances of limitation directly exclude any agent, so generated, as the source of a disease, to which it is impossible to assign boundary or limit.

Equally inapplicable, for the same reasons, is every theory founded on the temperament, habits, food, or other conditions of particular communities. The history of cholera, as followed through different countries and races of mankind, negatives at once all suppositions of this nature, nor need we follow them beyond the mere statement.

---

* I have myself at different periods been in five several places where the cholera was prevailing at the time, and have had sufficient proof of the different atmospheric circumstances under which it may subsist. Even with the disposition ever present to find especial causes for remarkable events, the records of former pestilences are equally wanting in admissible evidence as to any states of atmosphere or season likely to produce them.

Dismissing, then, as improbable or impossible these different views regarding the origin of cholera, we have to inquire what other opinion may best be held;—and particularly whether that hypothesis be tenable, which looks to animalcule life, diffused by the atmosphere or by man, as the source of the disease ;—a form of life not cognisable by our senses, or other direct means of research, but nevertheless subject to some similar laws of propagation and diffusion as species more obvious to us, and producing a virus which acts noxiously on the human body.

In pursuing this subject, we must take account severally of the more essential facts regarding cholera, to see how far they admit of such explanation ; premising, what will now be generally allowed, that the disease, though resembling the common cholera morbus in some of its symptoms, is actually distinct from it, as it is from every other disorder of which we have previous knowledge.*

The first condition is the obvious and assured one, that the cause of the disease must be a material poison ; definite in its nature, and specific in its effects.   We cannot reason on the subject without this admission ; nor, under the shelter of vague terms, apply to the phenomena any hypothesis which excludes it.   It is true that some of the suppositions already noticed admit a virus or specific cause; and use may be made of the analogies furnished by other disorders, avowedly infectious through matters generated within the body. But this is at best analogy of difficulty rather than elucidation ; and carries us little way towards solution of the circumstances which form the peculiar history of cholera.   It must be kept in mind that we have to deal here with a migrating malaria—a wandering cause of disease—capable, not merely of being diffused through the atmosphere, and conveyed along vast tracts or lines over the globe, affecting different places with a varying intensity which no known conditions of earth, atmosphere, or human habits, will explain ; but also possessing the power of reproducing itself, so as to spread the disorder by fresh creation of the virus which originally produced it.

This faculty of reproduction (admitting the term for what we can scarcely otherwise express) stands foremost among the conditions essential to a right theory of cholera.   Without it, there would seem a physical impossibility of explaining the phenomena of the disease ; and particularly its distribution and succession in different places and seasons.   A thorough study of these singular details of its history, keeping this principle in view, will not only confirm and illustrate the latter, but lead us to animal life, as the most probable source and subject of such reproduction.   Scarcely, indeed, is any

* This is a point where we may recognise the influence of names in opposition to the most obvious facts.   The Asiatic cholera, certainly unknown to us before, reached Europe from the spot where its origin is dated, by steps, every one of which is known and recorded.   The resemblances to another more familiar disorder is but what occurs in many other relations of disease, and does by no means prove identity of cause.

other conceivable in the present state of our knowledge. It is against all the analogy of nature to suppose this power to belong to inorganic matter; and the material of vegetable life is almost equally excluded by the obvious facts regarding the disease. We must look, then, for the source of this renewed production of the virus to some animal process: occurring either within the bodies of those affected, and acting therefore simply by infection; or produced by animal changes and propagation taking place without. In the hypothesis of production by certain animal species, minute beyond the reach of all sense, we have an explanation of the fresh creation and diffusion of the material cause; curiously conforming in many respects with our observations on the disease, and with what we know of the habits of insect life, under circumstances more open to research.

For analogy here, I might draw largely upon our knowledge of this part of the animal kingdom; but a few examples will suffice to explain the more obvious relations, and suggest the investigation of others.

One of the most striking facts in the history of cholera is the frequent suddenness of appearance and disappearance of the disease in given localities; while in other places of its occurrence, a more regular period of time is observed;—a few detached cases and slow progress at first; then a wide and fearful prevalence, and again a period of gradual decline;—with a ratio sometimes so exact between the mortality and the numbers attacked, as well as the period of the epidemic, as to have given a very precise form to some of the tables containing these facts.* The volumes written upon cholera, describing its progress through different countries, abound in curious examples of each kind; such as have endlessly perplexed the question as to the contagiousness of the disorder. Yet these conditions, seemingly incongruous, accord well with what we know of the habitudes of animal life, under the forms here presumed. The sudden appearance and rapid multiplication of insect swarms at certain times, and in situations favourable to their propagation, are facts familiar to naturalists. The diffusion of such swarms, sometimes by continuous flight for great distances, sometimes by tardy, broken, and divided progress, is equally familiar to observation, however scanty our knowledge of the animal instincts by which these movements are governed.† The same analogy extends

---

* A valuable report, founded on 9372 registered cases of cholera, as it occurred at Rome, was presented by Mr. Farr, at the Newcastle Meeting of the British Association. The principal results are, that the rate of mortality has its maximum on the first day of seizure, so that at the end of this day the chance of recovery in any number of cases exceeds that of death by one-sixth only. The ratio constantly and rapidly alters on succeeding days, so that on the third it does not exceed 10·5 per cent., on the fifth 5·6 per cent., &c. The mortality increases with the age at the rate of about 34 per cent. for every ten years.

† The Hessian fly, on its first appearance in America, afforded a singular example of this slow progressive movement. First observed in Long Island in

to the disappearance of these swarms ;—either suddenly, by further flight, or atmospheric changes on the spot,—or more gradually, by completion of their term of existence, want of food, or any physical causes tending to destroy their ova, or retard their development and the successive metamorphoses they undergo.

In many respects, indeed, the erratic and ambiguous course of cholera is well represented by the flight, settlement, and propagation of the insect swarms which inflict blight upon vegetable life. Their appearance at different and often distant periods, without obvious cause for such irregularity,—their direction to certain plants only,—their settlement upon these in clusters and detached localities,—the frequent suddenness of their change of place and final disappearance,—are all circumstances of curious analogy ; as also the curiously abrupt limitation of some of these swarms, showing itself in definite lines of direction, along which their work of destruction is carried on. These lines, though to our observation seemingly arbitrary, are doubtless connected with the instincts of life under this form, and with the relation of such instincts to the surrounding media. The cholera has been often defined in its course by similar lines of direction ; sometimes stretching over considerable tracts of land or sea ; more frequently obvious in particular localities ; but in neither case receiving explanation from any physical conditions of the globe, from currents of air, or local circumstances of soil and climate. Nor will human communication, though certainly concerned in part in the transmission of the disorder, resolve these singularities ; of which numerous examples might be cited, from the first appearance of cholera in India to its latest ravages in Europe. We have similar occurrences in the history of some other epidemics, but none so remarkable in degree.

Connected with these facts is the observation, seemingly well-attested, that the cholera sometimes spreads in face of a prevailing wind, and where no obvious human communication is present ;—a circumstance difficult, if indeed possible, to be explained, without recourse to animal life as the cause of the phenomenon. No mere inorganic matter could be so transferred, nor is vegetable life better provided with means for overcoming this obstacle.

Another analogy, as it may be considered, to the habits of insect life, is the apparent preference of direction along the course of waters, which has been noticed in the spread of the disease ;—one of the few facts regarding it which seem to have acquired anything like certainty, though not free from the contradictions and anomalies which press on every part of the subject. Again, the frequent occurrence of insulated cases of cholera, before the wider breaking out of the disorder in any given locality, though occasionally it may be attributed to infection, yet has peculiarities analo-

1776, it proceeded into the interior, at the rate of ten or fifteen miles in the year, destroying all the wheat in its progress. The appearance and spread of the *Blatta orientalis* in the northern parts of Europe is another fact of similar kind.

gous to the habits of the swarms of aphides, and other insects, infesting plants; and there are many instances for which it would be difficult to find any more plausible solution.

The reappearance of the disease in the same locality, at uncertain intervals, but generally during the hotter part of the year, is another fact bearing on the same hypothesis. The cases have usually been more detached than on the first ingress of the malady, and much less numerous, but often as fatal.* Difficult of solution on any hypothesis, these facts are less so perhaps on the supposition of an animal virus than on any other. It offers the contingencies of fresh swarms arising, or of the development of ova deposited in these places during the preceding incursions of the disease, and called more or less numerously into life by increased temperature or other causes.† The latter view accords better with the facts regarding cholera, and is reconcileable with all we know of insect life and reproduction. The ova may remain dormant for long and indefinite periods of time; yet, like the seeds of plants, retain the powers of life, and burst into active existence when circumstances occur to favour the change. One of the most singular facts in natural history is this sudden appearance of insect swarms, with all their instincts complete, in localities where they have not been seen for years before; either brought from unknown distance, or the produce of the ova of former seasons deposited on the spot, in preparation for this later development.‡

* Remarkable exceptions occur to this, as at Berlin; where the epidemic of 1837, notwithstanding it was six weeks shorter in duration than that of 1831, attacked a proportion of persons greater by one third, and with a somewhat higher rate of mortality; showing that the virus was more intense during the latter period.

† A valuable document on this subject is the paper by Dr. Budd and Mr. Busk, in the 21st vol. of the Med. Chirurg. Transactions, on twenty cases of Cholera, which occurred in October, 1837, on board the Hospital Ship at Greenwich. The circumstances of limitation to this vessel, in which the cholera had twice existed before, gave much proof of a local reproduction of the virus of the disease.

‡ Though such instances are familiar, even in our own country, I may briefly notice one, somewhat remarkable, and of recent occurrence. In October, 1836, a vast swarm of minute aphides (whether one of the numerous known species was not ascertained) passed over a wide district in Cheshire, Derbyshire, and the southern parts of Lancashire and Yorkshire. The air was so thickly filled with them, that the clothes and faces of persons walking out of doors were completely covered. When getting into the eyes they excited considerable inflammation. The height to which the column reached could not be known. From the best observations in one locality, its superficial extent must have been at least 12 miles in one direction by 5 miles in another; but the detached notices from other places make it certain that the continuous swarm was much more widely spread. No sufficient comparison appears to have been made of local observations to furnish proof as to the rate and direction of movement; but it is worthy of notice, that the town of Manchester was infested by these insects for two or three successive days. Wherever generated, or by whatsoever instinct carried on, there is cause to suppose that the swarm was in transit from one place to another, and possibly brought nearer to the earth by some peculiar state of atmosphere existing at the time.

And here we again approach to speculations, which, though founded on the most minute forms of existence, have yet a vastness in their obscurity, and in the results to which their solution would lead. I allude to the hypothesis of equivocal generation;—the question, whether animal or vegetable life (for the inquiry equally regards both) are in any case produced without the egg or seed of prior individuals of the same species? The result of modern research has been chiefly on the negative side of the question; and the old dogma of "*omne vivum ab ovo*" remains sanctioned to an extent, which could scarcely have been supposed within the scope of human observation. Nevertheless, we are still very far from certainty. Instances may be indefinitely multiplied to the effect just stated, and yet it may be possible that there are germs of life around us, awaiting development; or matter so constituted as to be capable of assuming new and various forms of living organization, according to the circumstances present to favour such change.*

Without entering on this controversy, we find in facts well ascertained, of the occasional length of time during which the ova of animal life retain their power of reproduction, much that bears on the hypothesis before us. There is reason to presume, that the simpler and more minute the form of organization, the greater is the faculty of thus retaining life in a dormant state: and if complete animal organization, such as that of the infusoria, or the vibriones of wheat, is capable of being restored to vital activity, after long apparent extinction, still more may animal ova be supposed retentive of the principle of life and reproduction. This consideration applies to one of the most curious questions respecting cholera;— how a poison should be thus locally generated, unknown before, but capable, by some means of reproduction, of being diffused over every part of the earth? Difficult though a solution is to every hypothesis, it seems almost impossible on any other than that of animal origin. This furnishes a reason why the disease, existing perchance at some anterior time, may have disappeared for ages; the seed of the pestilence, however, yet remaining, to be called into activity by future contingencies. Or, if we admit the doubtful assertion of some authors, that the same disorder has existed

---

* The generation of some of the viviparous infusoria seems inexplicable on any other view than this. The question is connected with the equally obscure one as to the immutability of species. In both, the greater familiarity of the idea of successive propagation by ova or seed disguises the fact that their propagation is quite as incomprehensible in itself, as the conversion of the same organic elements, under altered circumstances, into new forms. Notwithstanding this imperfection of our knowledge, the whole subject of organization, whether of animal or vegetable life, affords a signal testimony to the progress of modern science;—realizing on the one hand some of the poetical imaginations of antiquity;—on the other, by mathematical exactness of observation directed to the most minute forms of matter, laying a basis for discovery, of which the boldest speculator can scarcely yet see the full extent.

The Memoir of MM. Beauperthuy and Roseville, on microscopic animalculæ as a cause of putrefaction, is one of the most curious of the recent inquiries bearing on this subject.

repeatedly in India, though never with equal virulence, no view will so well explain the diversity, as that which admits on the one side all the instincts of animalcule life; on the other, the varying casualties of place, season, and human communities.   Swarms may be evolved in a given locality, and perish, before migration or communication to man have given cause to wider extension of the disease.

The whole subject of this presumed migration will occur as a difficulty in the hypothesis, seeing that we have no evidence of any of similar extent in the animal kingdom ; and that the manner and duration of insect life are in many respects opposed to one, which involves such variety of country and climate; most of the species known to us appearing to be submitted to geographical distribution, like plants, and the other classes of the animal kingdom.   What may be said in reply (even admitting the restriction to insect life, properly so termed) is, that we are singularly ignorant of all that relates to animal migrations in general ;—that our knowledge becomes less as we descend to the more minute forms of life ;—that the facts known respecting the occurrence of insect swarms meet some of these objections ;—that the ova themselves may be widely disseminated ;—and that the rapidity of propagation and change, incident generally to this part of creation, if introducing some difficulties, provides the means of obviating others.

Pursuing the hypothesis (still tentatively upon all these points), we reach the question as to the infectious nature of cholera, and may gain from hence some further argument in removal of the objections just stated.   If this point, so warmly contested, be answered in the affirmative, man becomes an agent in the diffusion ; and the transit over continents and oceans, otherwise impossible, is brought within comprehension, and the analogies of other disease.   Much of this controversy might, as I think, have been obviated by a regard to the principles mentioned in a former chapter.   It seems certain that the virus of cholera, whatsoever its nature, may be spread in different ways.   That the atmosphere, though not in any of its states the cause of the disease, forms one medium for diffusing it, and this over great distances, is clearly to be inferred from numerous facts in its history.   From the same evidence, and particularly from the details of its introduction into new localities, and passage across seas, it is impossible not to admit that its transference is frequently effected by human means ; and it may perhaps be affirmed, without involving the question in more doubtful phrases, that man, the peculiar recipient of this cause of disease, is also the principal agent in its diffusion.   On a question of this nature, it is always well to select a few proofs unequivocal and complete, wherewithal to meet the many ambiguous or anomalous cases which are certain to occur: and it would be easy to state several such in the history of cholera, scarcely admitting of other interpretation than that just given.*

* One, which I think includes every condition of perfect evidence, is the transportation of cholera from the infected towns of Liverpool, Dublin, and Greenock,

Allowing this, some of the apparent contradictions which have embarrassed the question as to contagion may be solved by referring to the habitudes of that class of animal life which the hypothesis assumes; and particularly to the circumstances which favour the propagation, diffuse the ova, direct the flight, fix the resting places, or modify the virus, of the swarms thus supposed. We can understand in this sense the respective relations of man and the atmosphere to the spread of the disease. The human body may be a means of concentrating the morbid cause; and conveying it, possibly in a state more prone to inflict the disorder, to distant and detached localities. The atmosphere, the medium in every case of communication from one body to another, may itself, independently of man, carry the miasma over wide distances; and by its changes in temperature, humidity, and electrical state, produce many of the modifications observed. And in the separate or concurrent agency of these causes of communication a plausible solution is found of some of the more singular anomalies of the disease.

That man should be so peculiarly the subject of cholera is a difficulty which belongs to all hypotheses, but least perhaps to that of an animal origin. It is difficult to conceive any other physical cause thus far exclusive in its effects; while, in support of this view, we have various analogies in insect-life, and in the habits of parasitic animals already noticed. Though man, however, is chiefly obnoxious to this virus, whatever it be, we have proof that he is not exclusively so; and it is worthy of note, that the most distinct evidence relates to its effects on birds; and to the rare appearance of certain species of birds in the localities where cholera is prevailing at the time.* The cause assigned in the hypothesis under review is at least as probable as any other in explanation of this curious fact.

The question, connected with the preceding, why the miasma of the cholera should destroy some persons, and leave others in the close vicinity little if at all affected, applies equally to other disor-

---

to Quebec; in vessels having emigrants on board, among whom the disease existed during the whole passage across the Atlantic. The details of this occurrence, including the place, time, and manner in which the cholera first showed itself in Quebec, are such as to leave no point of ambiguity. The circumstances which attend the transmission of the disorder over land are not often so explicit in their conclusions.

The Treatise on Pestilential Cholera, by Dr. Copland, published in 1832, contains an excellent statement of the argument regarding contagion, as of all besides relating to the disease. In adopting the opinion of its infectious nature, he has ably and justly dwelt on the inadequacy of the experiments by inoculation, and certain other modes of exposure, to negative this opinion.

* This fact of the effect upon birds is fully confirmed in a late report of the Medical Faculty of Vienna, upon whom the inquiry as to the influence of cholera upon other animals, was expressly enjoined. A similar fact has been noticed in the history of other pestilences of older date, and attributed vaguely to atmospheric changes affecting this class of animals. The report just named is the most complete document we possess on the subject, and contains many very curious facts.

ders of contagious and epidemic kind, and presents similar difficulties to every hypothesis; yet greater perhaps to the notion of an inorganic agent, than to a supposition which includes all the conditions of animal life; and particularly that form of life which is so rapid and abundant in reproduction, undergoes such remarkable changes, and is submitted to instincts of which we have so little cognisance. No view, as far as can be seen, better applies to the various degrees of the disorder;—from the slight and ill-defined uneasiness about the epigastrium and bowels, subsiding without further issue,—to the powerful and virulent disease, producing instant collapse, and destroying life within a few hours of the earliest seizure.

These considerations bring us more directly to the pathology of the disease, and the relation of the various alleged causes to its actual symptoms. The weak part of medical science lies here, where morbid agents from without come into contact with living actions in the body: and, fairly examining into this subject in all its relations, we shall find how little real knowledge has been gained from the earliest date of medical history to the present day. Singular though the symptoms of cholera are, in their suddenness and fatality, they offer no difficulty which does not equally belong to other kindred diseases. We may even go a step further, and affirm that the notion of an animal virus, applied to absorbing surfaces, and engendering the disorder by entering into the circulation, is that which on the whole best accords with the character of the disease, and with the analogies most obvious to other morbid affections. We have many proofs of the power and virulence of different poisons of this class, and of the remarkable changes they produce on the nervous system and the blood. The action of the morbid cause in cholera seems to have most kindred with these; the change which takes place with such rapidity in the properties of the blood being, as I think, the great feature in the disease; the basis probably of all the other symptoms. The extreme depression of animal heat throughout the body;—the peculiar secretions so largely poured out from the inner surface of the intestines;—the suppression of the natural secretions;—the severe spasmodic actions;—the various effects on the nervous system;—and the typhoid and other symptoms which occur in sequel to the acute stage of the disease;—are all more readily and consistently explained, by looking to this altered state of the blood, as the effect first resulting from the influence of the morbid cause.* Some of these symptoms indeed scarcely show themselves where the cholera exists in so virulent a form as to ter-

* I would apply the same remark to the diseased or disorganized state of the inner coat of the blood-vessels, observed in many of the dissections after death from cholera, and particularly described by Dr. Mackintosh.
The recent experiments of Dr. Namias, of Venice, show that inoculation with the blood from cholera patients under collapse will often destroy other animals, as rabbits, within a few days, and by changes which render their blood again destructive to others of the same species.
32*

minate life in a few hours; proving thereby that they are not essential to the character of the disorder, nor to its event.

It is conceivable indeed, and we have no direct proof to the contrary, that the original impulse of the virus of cholera may be upon
some part of the nervous system; but I consider the supposition
much more probable which makes the influence on the blood the
first in the series of changes; and it is undoubtedly that which has
most obvious and general relation to the other symptoms of the disease. If the magnitude of the effect here seems out of proportion to
the cause, we have but to look to the certain influence of other morbid agents on the blood;—whether the imperceptible virus of many
contagious diseases;—the minute quantity of certain other animal
poisons producing death;—or the action of different salts in preventing the coagulation of this fluid. Inability to explain the rationale of such changes applies alike to every view of the subject;
and cannot therefore be admitted as an exclusive objection to one
alone.

As respects the prevention and treatment of cholera, little need
here be said. Neither the hypothesis of which we are treating, nor
any other alleged cause, can be considered as affording even plausible suggestions to this effect. The requisitions in common to each
are, the discovery of means to prevent the access of the cause;—
or a specific capable of obviating the virus when received—or remedies adequate to sustaining the body under its effects;—objects,
it must be confessed, hitherto wholly unattained. The singular
uniformity in the proportion of deaths, in every place of the occurrence of cholera over the globe, not only affords proof that no valid
means of cure have been discovered for the disease, when fully developed; but shows, moreover, how inert even the most drastic
remedies become, when directed against this extraordinary poison.
Methods of treatment the most opposite, yet equally insisted upon
by their respective advocates, and many of them such that their
use would be dangerous in other cases, lose here all their distinctive
effects, and are found alike inefficient and harmless. I doubt not
that in some habits, and especially when the morbid cause is present
in slight degree (a contingency ever to be kept in mind), good may
be done by all means which tend to moderate the symptoms, restore
right secretions, and sustain the powers of life. But until the proportion of mortality is distinctly abated under some given plan of
treatment, and the effect well attested by comparison with other
places where different methods, or no methods at all, have been pursued, the conclusion will remain, that no real antidote has yet
been discovered; and that the cases interpreted as cures, derive
this character from causes which we neither recognise, nor can
command.

If the disease should still continue in the world, and a remedy, justly
so called, be happily discovered hereafter, it will probably be of the
nature of a specific antidote to the action of the virus on the blood.
I hazard this opinion, looking to the singular importance of this ac-

tion in the pathology of cholera; to the promise which animal chemistry gives of new methods of altering the state of the blood ; and
to the actual results obtained by means expressly applied to the
object in question.   I allude to the treatment by saline injections
into the veins; which, though not yet thoroughly established by experience, has nevertheless in many cases been found to possess singular power in checking the progress of collapse; and approaches
nearer, perhaps, to a successful issue than any other method yet
employed.   Still it is only an approach ; and the problem yet
remains to be overcome, either by accident, or the better fortune
of future experiment.   Casualty may perchance serve us better
here than reason; but we are bound to follow the latter as far as
we can.

The best contingency, next to that of a specific remedy, seems to
be the discovery of means capable of sustaining or restoring the
nervous power of the vital organs, so rapidly and deeply affected by
the disease.   Any agent equal to fulfil such purpose must presumably be both simple and powerful :—whether electricity, in any form
of its action, may be capable of this, is a question not yet fully answered. Speaking generally of the treatment of cholera, I certainly
do not believe that an efficient means of cure will ever be attained
by dealing with the symptoms in detail.   The magnitude of the disease, and intensity of its cause, are beyond this means of reaching
them; and it is probably only in the milder cases that any such result can thus be obtained.   After all, is it just to speak of our ignorance of a remedy for cholera as a peculiarity of this disorder ?
Have we any more certain or specific cure for other contagious or
epidemic diseases, unless dignifying with this name that mitigation
of symptoms, and prevention of particular mischiefs, which alone
come within the rule of safe practice in most of these cases? The
instance is one among many, where long familiarity with certain
disorders, or their milder character, disguise the connexion they
have with other diseases, less known and of greater virulence. The
preventive remedy discovered for small-pox is an eminent, though
partial, exception to the remark ; and an indication, at the same
time, of what may yet be possible in other diseases where a specific
virus is present ;—the cause of malady to the individual, and the
means of its dissemination to others.   Whatever the nature of the
virus of cholera, the contingency of discovery is the same here as
elsewhere: and if, like the small-pox, it is to be considered a new
form of disease, engendered in the world, and destined to remain
as a wandering pestilence there, the attainment of this object is
manifestly most important to human welfare.

These remarks, however, have no peculiar application to the
hypothesis before us.   This has now been discussed in as much detail as a speculation merits to be in which direct proof is altogether
wanting; and which a main argument is the inadequacy of all other
hypotheses to explain the facts.   I have not noticed the further objection which may be urged against it, that, if well-founded, its

application would not be limited to cholera, but must of necessity extend to certain other contagious or epidemic diseases, (and especially to the epidemic influenzas,) of which the essential conditions are so far the same, as to warrant the belief of a similar, though not identical, cause.   The justness of the inference can in no way be denied; nor the extent to which it would carry speculation in advance of actual knowledge.   This in truth is the wider question, serving as title to the present chapter ;—how far, and in what manner, living animal matter may become a source of disease; and the case of cholera was taken merely as furnishing the most various and singular illustration.

The general question is one still open to research ;—sanctioned in its object by our ignorance of other causes for these genera of disease ;—affording some curious presumptions where certainty may be unattainable ;—and involving a topic than which none is more remarkable, viz., the origin and progress of those disorders, which, if not newly generated, have first appeared in our parts of the world within the period of modern record ; and become endemic, where there is no authentic trace left by history of their prior existence.

CHAPTER XXXV.

ON THE PRESENT STATE OF INQUIRY INTO THE NERVOUS SYSTEM.

D'ALEMBERT has well designated the space which lies between geometry and metaphysics, " L'abîme des incertitudes et le théâtre des découvertes."   A remarkable part of this wide intellectual domain is that occupied by the science of the nervous functions, forming, in the present state of our knowledge, a sort of neutral ground between the sciences which deal with matter in its various forms, and those which have relation to the functions of animal life and mental existence.   It is this vicinity to the region of metaphysics which has given to the subject its peculiar ambiguities.   Language here labours vainly to follow the suggestions of thought or consciousness ; and the discussion has been endlessly perplexed by the effort of philosophers of all ages to give phraseology to their doctrines, without any covenanted understanding of the ideas they involve.

The deep interest now felt in this branch of physiology, and the active and refined inquiry directed to it, may warrant some observations on the subject, even though not adding to the facts already known.   It is one of the cases in science where a nearer approach to truth is sometimes gained by recasting the order of facts, and using them in new combination. In the following remarks I shall merely touch upon some parts of this wide topic; putting much interrogatively, as best befits what is still so uncertain or obscure.*

Language, indeed, must not alone be charged with the difficulties which belong to the inquiry. Our progress is at every moment stopt;—on the one side, by the intricate and subtle organization it is needful to decipher;—on the other, by those more insuperable bounds which, in the very constitution of the human mind, seem placed to prevent too close a contemplation of its own workings; or even of the manner of relation to the material instruments through which it acts. It may be that some men, by higher capacity of reason, whether invested in language or not;—or by greater power of concentration, if this term better express the act of mind;—do really approach nearer than others to the comprehension of these great functions of our nature. But every such difference is trifling in relation to the undiscovered and impassable space that lies beyond; and the highest attainment is that which can best define the boundary of research, and labour for truth and knowledge within it.

A question, illustrating these remarks, and which stands indeed foremost in the inquiry, is that regarding the nature, various forms, and functions of the nervous power. Whatever opprobrium has been thrown, justly or unjustly, upon this phrase, it is certain that we cannot dispense with some term equivalent to it, in reasoning on the phenomena of animal life. At every step we are obliged to admit the conception of the fact thus expressed; and however inadequate our present means to determine its nature, and relations to the mental and physical parts of our being, we can no more deny reality to such a power, than we can to the effects of which it is the obvious source. Other terms,—energy, agency, element and principle,—have on the same grounds been applied to denote it; all readily lending themselves to any relation with physical agents which may hereafter be ascertained; but liable in common to the objection of designating as one principle or element, that which we know not to be really such. For the inquiry brings us directly to the most essential of the questions regarding the nervous power, viz., its unity:—whether it be one and the same agent, producing diversity of effect from the manner of its transmission, or from the various fabric and vitality of the parts on which it acts;—or whether there are two or more powers, coming under this common appellation as acting through nervous structure, but really different in nature, and thereby producing different results.

This question, to which I shall afterwards revert, becomes more definite as we proceed to specify the several functions appertaining to the nervous system, and especially those of the nerves of sensa-

---

* Those who desire to learn the actual state of knowledge in this complicated inquiry, will do well to refer to a series of most able articles in the British and Foreign Medical Review; embracing its relations to all other branches of physiology, as well as to the higher and more general principles of inductive science.

tion and voluntary power.   Here the obvious machinery is nearly or altogether the same :—it is every where blended for the purposes of mutual action and relation :—yet are the functions themselves so utterly unlike to our comprehension, that we can in no way conceive the same physical agent, however modified, to be capable of fulfilling both.   The opinion, early admitted by many physiologists, that the difference is simply that of the action being centripetal in the sensitive nerves, centrifugal in the motor, merely translates the difficulty into another form ; and is less tenable since the distinctness of these two classes of nervous fibres has been fully demonstrated.

The inquiry extends, and under equal obscurity, to the nervous influence of organic life ; if this term be permitted for the power by which numerous muscles are moved, and the several offices of circulation, absorption, and secretion performed, without any direct intervention of the two great functions just named ; though in such various and close relation to them, that it seems equally impossible to dissever the two agencies as to understand their dependence on a single source of power.—And further, in connexion with these organic functions, we are required to recognise the direct influence upon them of all mental emotions, even of the simple act of attention of mind ;—testified in every part of life ;—during sleep and dreams, as well as in waking state ;—connected with some of the most remarkable sympathies of our nature ;—and depending, we must suppose, upon relations of nervous structure for all that concerns its distribution to the several organs of the body.

Nor can we with certainty stop here, when seeking to analyze those different functions of animal life which are performed through the nervous system, in the general understanding of the term.   The question occurs, suggested by unceasing consciousness and observation, whether there is not some proper and independent energy, of which, however it be designated, the brain is the immediate source and seat ; by which the higher animal functions are maintained and brought into relation with others, and unity given to every part of the individual being ;—a principle various in power in different individuals, and forming what has been termed the temperament of each ;—varying also in the same individual at different times, and by its excess or deficiency in the living organization becoming a source of disorder to the functions both of body and mind.   Description applied to this sensorial agency-might, in truth, extend throughout all the phenomena of health and disease ; from the exuberant excitement of high bodily and mental vigour to the sudden collapse which threatens, or occasionally produces, instant death.   And its terms might be borrowed, as well from the language of familiar use, as from that which has been current at all times in the schools of philosophy.

It will be manifest that we are treading in this place on the extreme boundary of human knowledge.   The close proximity on one side to the mental functions,—on the other to the doctrine of a vital principle, in the numerous shapes which this has assumed,—places the question under an obscurity we can scarcely hope to remove. It may be that the principle inquired into is not really a separate and single element of power, but merely a quality or degree of the other actions by which mind is connected with material organization :—that we are not entitled to express more by it than a greater or less sensibility ; a higher or lower degree of the voluntary power ; or the varying strength of impressions made on the body by mental emotions. This indeed is one part of that question, metaphysical more than physiological in its nature, which has perplexed reasoning men in every age, and been fruitful of dispute in proportion to its obscurity. We have powers before us for contemplation, which we cannot identify as the properties of any physical agents, nor interpret by any analogy beyond their own action; and which, while giving unity to many separate organs and functions, seem to be derived from, and supported by, the combination of these functions themselves. On the other side we find them indissolubly blended with the great separate unity of the mind and will; a relation which, from the very conditions of the inquiry, must ever remain a sealed question to the present comprehension of man.*

On many of these points it is expedient for the highest interests of science, that inquiry should not, by any artifices of language, be pressed beyond this boundary. Though insusceptible of strict definition, it is certain and obvious as a general limit, and becomes mose so as our knowledge increases in exactness. The precaution suggested by one of the wisest of the ancients, Το γινωσκειν τινων δει ζητειν αποδειξιν, και τινων ου δει, is applicable to every age of philosophy. Within this boundary, indeed, there is space enough for the utmost zeal of research; and it is enlarged, rather than narrowed, by the abandonment of all abstractions which are not absolutely requisite to classify the phenomena observed.

These remarks directly apply to the question of a vital principle ;—a term which, as expressing an agency independent of organization, and itself capable of organizing and giving life, has found its way into every part of physiology and general philosophy; and which, even where rejected by men of acute understanding, is still often seen to lurk in their writings, under some less palpable form of expression. In reasoning, for example, on the active principle of animal organization—that which operates in the original evolution and unceasing maintenance of the animal frame—some modern physiologists have almost given separate existence to this, as the *primum movens* of the system; therein approaching to the theory of Stahl and early writers ; and still more explicitly to the doctrine of a vital principle in one or other of its forms.† Upon this latter

* These remarks apply to the notion held by certain writers of the existence of another sense, needful to establish a community of feeling and consciousness in all parts of the body ; the *Gemeingefühl* or *Selbstgefühl* of some German physiologists.

† In describing the principle of organization (the *nisus formativus* of earlier

subject I do not enter further, having nothing to add to what has been so ably written upon it of late years. To suppose the existence of a principle of life, independent of the organs and functions of living bodies, and superadded to give activity to them, is, in the present state of our knowledge, to substitute a bare phrase for the reality of facts. We gain from it no explanation of the vital actions and affinities, the relations of which are the proper objects of study; nor even of the phenomena of generation, and of propagation by simple division in some of the lower animals, which seem most to authorize the conclusion;—but rather impose injurious limits on all other parts of the inquiry which are fairly open to human research. We interpose a separate agent, (for in no other sense can the doctrine of a vital principle be understood,) when all that is warranted to our understanding is the assumption of existing and active laws.

I have dwelt longer on these topics, as illustrating some of the difficulties of the subject, and the manner in which they affect the course of research into the nervous system. Recurring now to the question, what other attributes of life depend directly on this part of the animal economy, the large and singular class of actions, termed instinctive, comes into view;—sufficiently separate from those already mentioned to warrant the inquiry whether there is any especial organization for them, or any nervous function with this appropriate destination. As anatomy affords no direct answer, we must seek it by defining, as far as can be done, the nature of the actions we so denominate. If limiting our view of instinct to those express motions which invariably follow the excitement of certain sensations, independently of volition or any conscious act of mind, it is clear that there is an especial structure fitted for this function as part of the great system of organic life; and the doctrine of reflex actions by the nerves affords illustration of many of the particular phenomena. And further, as respects the instinctive motions which take place through voluntary organs, we have presumption that the nervous structure is the same for both, in the fact, that any given series of muscular actions, become thoroughly habitual by repetition, approaches to the class of instincts, as far as the will is concerned; or at least cannot be discriminated by any insight we have into these mysterious relations of life.*

writers), the German physiologists have availed themselves of the richness and redundance of their language to give a more copious and distinct expression of these powers than any we have ventured to adopt. No other modern language could furnish such phrases as "die bewustloss wirkende zweckmassige Thatigteit,"—"die nach vernunftigen Gesetzen wirkende organizirende Kraft," &c., which we find in the writings of Müller, and which appear to give more of individuality and independence to this power than is usually recognised at the present day. His discussion of the question of identity, or other relation, of the mental principle (das psychische princip) to that of life, is a striking specimen of the acuteness of this eminent physiologist.

* It must be mentioned, however, that Sir C. Bell has sought in certain instances to distinguish the nerves of instinctive motion from those of voluntary power.

But it is obvious that we must not limit the meaning of instinct to mere motions only. The term carries us beyond, to those long trains of acts, of which such movements, whether strictly automatic, or involving any exercise of volition, are but the machinery; —acts involving, as far as we can see, no operation of thought or consciousness of the object to be attained, yet more precise and uniform than any results of animal intelligence;—far more remarkable, moreover, in other animals than man; multiplying in number and extent as we descend in the scale of being; and at the lowest part becoming identical with existence itself, and closely associated with corresponding functions of vegetable life.

In the subjoined note will be found some remarks on this interesting subject.* Its relation to the topic before us is comprised in

* It would be difficult to add anything new to what has been written on instinct, and yet the main questions continue unresolved. Bayle has justly termed the actions of beasts "un des plus profonds abîmes, sur quoi notre raison peut s'exercer;" and, in fact, the relation of these actions to the higher reason and more limited instincts of man, while illustrating some points, does in others make still wider this great chasm in human knowledge. No certain connexion has yet been ascertained between the two classes of phenomena, though so blended together that it is often as difficult to dissever them in detail, as to refer their separate workings to any common principle.

Definition has been busy with the subject, and under a wide range of description. We have proof of this in the singular difference of analogy by which Laplace and Cuvier have severally described animal instincts. The "affinité animale analogue à celle qui rapproche les molécules des cristaux" is an expression of the former, less happy than the "somnambulisme" of Cuvier,—the determination of actions by innate sensations or images ever present on the sensorium. But it will be obvious how far these and other analogies fall short of any true theory of instincts ; nor can we safely carry the expression of our knowledge beyond particular facts, which it is impossible to contravene ; and certain relations, less definite, yet marked enough to furnish a basis for inquiry.

The main fact, to which all others are subordinate, is the essential difference between instinctive actions and those of reason. Though ingenious men have sought to undermine this opinion,—some by raising instinct to the character of reason ; others by submitting the latter faculty to a metaphysical necessity, intelligible only as an instinct,—yet are the examples so decisive of separate origin to these two classes of actions, that no subtlety of argument is of avail against them. The hereditary nature of instincts ; their instant perfection, prior to all experience or memory ; and the preciseness of their objects, extent, and limitation for each species, are the more general facts on which the opinion is founded. The particular examples illustrating it are endless, and their variety such, that the conclusion to which they concur becomes irresistible.

Pursuing the subject, the questions which follow are, on the one side, the relation of these two great functions of instinct and reason ; on the opposite, the connexion of animal instincts with those of vegetable life. The former has naturally most engaged the attention of philosophers ; and we find the names of Bacon, Newton, Descartes, and Locke annexed to the subject, in sequel to those of antiquity ; and followed by many eminent writers of modern times. The last in order, but high in ability, is Lord Brougham, who, in his Dialogues on Instinct, espouses on this point the opinion proposed by Sir Isaac Newton in his 31st Query ; viz., that the Deity himself is virtually the acting and moving principle in animal instincts ;—seeking, as Newton had done before, to separate this doctrine, and the ubiquity of the Deity, from that grosser Pantheism into which

the question, whether there is any organization as far connected with these trains of action, as the cerebral part of the nervous system is with the processes of thought and feeling? or whether

so many philosophers of every age have fallen while dealing with these abstruse subjects.

Unless, indeed, we merge both reason and instinct in this common chaos, it is difficult to avoid the general conception just stated. The instinctive action has an express object of which the animal has no prior cognisance; to attain which its living organization goes through certain movements and changes, definite, identical, and constant in each one of the species. Here all proper reason or volition of the individual is excluded; and the Creator of the organization becomes, in every sense intelligible to us, himself the motive power. At this point the argument is at an end, or passes into a mere tissue of words without meaning or result.

Recognising, then, this essential distinction between reason and instinct, we find in the various conjunction of the two in the same being some of the most remarkable phenomena of animal life. To pursue the subject in detail would require a volume rather than a note. If, with Cuvier, we term instinct the *supplement* of intelligence, we may proceed in the same view, and affirm that the two faculties exist throughout in inverse ratio to each other; the completeness of instinct in reference to the life of the individual being greater as the intelligence becomes less. In man instincts form the *minimum* in relation to reason. They multiply, or become more constant, as we descend in the scale; and a point doubtless exists (though indeterminable) in the series, where they govern all the actions of life; the appearance of exception to the law depending probably on our imperfect knowledge of its operation in particular cases.

In this view there is an admission of the similarity in kind of the intelligence of other animals to that of man; a subject on which, well considered, no doubt can exist. The expression of Cuvier,—"leur intelligence exécute des opérations du même genre," must be allowed in the fullest sense; and the only questions left regard the proportion of the several faculties as compared with man; their relative amount in different animals; and their relation to the particular instincts of each. The first of these is the one in which we are most concerned. Though unable to enter upon it here, I may briefly state that memory (the lowest of the intellectual faculties) is that in which there appears the largest participation of other animals with man; while we have no proof that they possess in any degree that higher faculty of determining by will the course or change of thoughts;— the especial prerogative of the human being, and that on the right governance of which the superiority of one man to another mainly depends.

After all that has been written on the difference between reason and instinct, it is difficult, even in the case of man, where the scope of the latter is so limited, to define where it ends, and where reason begins. The question runs speedily into metaphysics, and is lost there. How, in fact, can we avoid considering as instincts many of those marked natural propensities of thought, feeling, and action, which designate individual character? Like instincts, they are innate; —they strongly modify, often control, the whole course of life;—in some cases they are felt as opposed to the reason of the individual, yet dominant over it;— in extreme cases they become a sort of madness, by opposition to the reason of the species.

In considering this curious question of the relation of human instincts to those of lower animals, it seems to me that a valuable distinction may be derived from the latter source; viz., their respective development in species and individuals. In the lower animals, instincts are chiefly those of the species; directed especially to physical objects; uniform and permanent; and with little of intellectual faculty to modify or control them. In man, instincts are more those of the individual; less numerous and definite in relation to the physical conditions of life; more varied and extensive in regard to his moral nature; yet subject as such to the control of his intellectual powers. Domestication in animals, like education in

nervous structure is merely concerned as furnishing instrumental power for carrying them on? Notwithstanding some observations which seem to show that certain instincts are altered or impaired by injuries to the brain and spinal marrow, we have no evidence on the subject free from ambiguity. Perhaps the most plausible is that furnished by the remarkable changes which the nerves of insects undergo, in their changes from the *larva* to the *pupa* state, and again to that of the *imago*: but here there is an obvious source of doubt in the actual diversity of life in these states, limiting the inference to the change of function taking place, and not having any necessary relation to those trains of action in which we understand instinct to consist. There is much obscurity in this subject, and great difficulty in establishing valid distinctions, and finding terms to express them. Instinctive actions are so closely blended with those of voluntary kind—the excitements and immediate instruments the same—that, while recognising the essential differences, we are perpetually at fault when seeking to follow them into different parts of the economy of life.

There yet remains what may be considered one of the great offices of the nervous system, viz., the establishment of connexions of feeling and motion among the several parts of the living being, —a function partly comprised in those already described, and indicated especially in the influence of mental emotions on the body; but testified further in the numerous and complex sympathies which depend upon particular nervous connexions; some of them known to us by actual observation or experiment; others undetected, but of certain existence. The most remarkable among these sympathies (and bearing closely on the question of the unity of the nervous power) are those which depend on the relation of nerves of different endowments;—the excitement of motion in one part by sensation in another;—or, conversely, of sensation by motions;— and again, the connexion of both with the peculiar nervous functions of organic life. A very important step has been made in this part of physiology by the explicit determination of those sympathetic or reflex actions, between the sentient and motor nerves, which occur directly through the medulla spinalis, without intervention of the brain. These discoveries of relation, even though not yet expounded by anatomical observations, do greatly extend and better define our knowledge of the whole organism of nervous life; and are of singular value to every part of pathology, as well as in explanation of the natural functions of the body. They esta-

man, has a certain effect in subduing some of their instincts; but this effect is partial and scanty in degree. In man, on the other hand, all the higher principles of mental cultivation are deeply involved in the question. The actions of his early infancy are instinctive, and closely resemble those which form the highest attainment of many other animals. It seems the proper destination of reason, as given him by his Creator, to subject these actions to the power of will;—to acquire mastery over the instinctive propensities of his nature;—to cultivate some, to moderate or subdue others, to give due proportion and direction to all.

blish more clearly than before a simply automatic part of the nervous system, with which the sensations and volitions of the mind are only indirectly concerned;—which has within itself the instruments of excitement and consequent motion, producing actions which are probably prior to all others in date—and to which the cerebral and intellectual functions are superadded gradually, blending with and modifying, but never superseding them. The connexion of these automatic sensations and motions with some of the phenomena of instinct has already been stated. Their relation to nervous structure, and to the voluntary actions, will be mentioned afterwards; all points of great interest, and meriting more explicit notice than this slight outline will afford.*

The foregoing remarks merely, indeed, recite the general problems of the nervous system;—the several points to be solved either by anatomy, or by observation of the phenomena of life, where solution is possible; and those which rational physiology will relinquish as beyond the scope of present attainment. The statement of what has been recently done in furtherance of the inquiry by the two means just mentioned, would make a volume in itself; and I can only briefly notice those particular results which seem to present conclusions of greatest importance. The sources of information on this subject are now indeed so numerous that more is not required.

The application of anatomy to the brain and nerves is twofold: first, that which relates to the intimate structure of the nervous substance in its several parts: secondly, that which regards the distinction, distribution, and connexion of different portions of the nervous system. The latter direction of research is at present the most important to physiology; and will probably always remain so, seeing the difficulty of drawing any plausible inference even from the most minute and refined examination of nervous structure. This examination, begun by Ehrenberg with the aid of the microscope, and ably pursued by other physiologists, has, it is true, disclosed many curious facts; some of them unsuspected, and all which may possibly aid hereafter in explaining the phenomena and relations of the nervous system.† Such are the tubular structures of the filaments composing the medullary substance of the brain and nerves;—the cylindrical form of these tubes, with the tendency in certain parts to assume a varicose appearance;—the existence in them of a viscous matter or medulla, more fluid in the brain than in the nerves, and becoming granular by coagulation;—the absence of anastomosis or union between these tubular filaments;—the

* In an earlier part of this volume I have stated my impression of what we owe of discovery in this part of physiology to the sagacity and zeal of Dr. Marshall Hall, and of the great value of the application he has made of his views, both to the theory and treatment of disease.

† Treviranus, Müller, Remak, Valentin, and Burdach are those who have most successfully followed Ehrenberg in this inquiry; and the general accordance of results is sufficient to give assurance of their truth, amidst some discrepancies of detail.

seeming identity of structure in the sentient and motor nerves;—and the peculiar granular matter diffused through the vascular texture of the cineritious substance, as well in the ganglia as the brain, and distinguishing the organization of this part.

These results, however, though interesting, afford no clue to the movements and combinations in which nervous action intimately consists; nor can it be shown that the parts thus described are really the elements of nervous structure. Even the assured distinction of office between the cineritious and medullary substance remains undetermined by such researches; and all other views, directed to varieties of function, are embarrassed by a degree of structural uniformity, which offers neither inference nor explanation. If these and similar facts ever become the basis of more exact knowledge, such result is perhaps more likely to arise from the growth of science without, than from any internal evidence they can themselves afford.

Passing to that more general anatomy which regards the distribution and connexion of the parts of the nervous system, we find it almost as difficult to classify, as to enumerate, the facts derived from the industry and refinement of modern research. The obscurity of functions is here also a main cause of perplexity. For in no branch of medical science is the connexion closer between dissection and experimental physiology; the latter being almost essential to the exposition of parts, which are thus interblended and bound together; and the aspect of which so little explains their endowments, that experiment is required to interpret relations seemingly the most obvious to the eye. Our knowledge of the symmetrical nerves of the spine might be termed barren, until the great discovery of Sir C. Bell of the separate functions of the anterior and posterior roots, not merely expounded these particular offices of parts, but indicated further the mode of research as applied to other analogous structures. The later investigation of the course and functions of the cerebral nerves, in which Magendie and Mayo have borne so eminent a part, furnishes an example to the same effect; where, though much is still left undetermined, the method of inquiry affords the best security for its ultimate attainment. This also is the subject where, from similar causes, comparative anatomy and physiology are of greatest avail; illustrating by the successive addition of parts and endowments the mutual connexion of all; though, it must be owned, adding also difficulties to the research, by showing conditions where action, such as is commonly deemed voluntary, takes place after the removal of that part of structure to which this function is presumed to belong.*

The circumstance last stated brings us to what is one of the

* I have only just received Mr. Carpenter's volume (*Principles of General and Comparative Physiology*), but have looked sufficiently into this excellent work, to see in it the best exposition we possess of all that is furnished by comparative anatomy to our knowledge of the nervous system, as well as to the more general principles of life and organization.

greatest attainments in the physiology of the nervous system; viz., the more express definition of the structure and offices of the cerebro-spinal axis; in its relation on the one side to involuntary or instinctive actions; on the other, to the sensations and volitions which connect the mind with the material organization around it. Recent inquiry here has removed errors obscuring all former views on the subject, and the minute dissections which have shown, not only the distinction of different parts of the spinal cord, but also a continuous structure of separate nervous filaments extending severally from them, through the medulla oblongata, to parts within the brain, indicate though they cannot explain) those combinations of mental and automatic or instinctive acts, which may well be reckoned among the most singular phenomena of animal life.

But, though this portion of structure is better defined than heretofore, much remains to be done for its complete demonstration. Even the manner of division of the spinal cord is not fully determined; some ambiguities are left as to the functions of sensation connected with the posterior column; and the appropriation of office to the middle or lateral columns is still uncertain. The questions of origin or termination in particular parts of the brain are also unsettled, even as to the manner of expressing these facts; and much is to be learnt as to the commissures or decussations between the portions of the cord itself. Further, it remains to be proved, whether there is any especial structure corresponding to the reflex actions performed through the cord, and independent of all connexion with the brain;—a true spinal system, on the excitor and motor nerves of which depend the mechanical parts of respiration, the ingestion and egestion of food, and the actions generally of the orifices and sphincters throughout the body. This, however, is a point of such importance to all our views of the functions of organic life, that it probably cannot long remain uncertain.*

Among the circumstances recently ascertained respecting the sentient and motor nerves, those perhaps which bear most importantly on future knowledge are, the situation of ganglia on the posterior terminations of the spinal nerves;—the convergence under the same sheath of nerves fulfilling these separate functions,—the individuality of every nervous filament, as far as we can observe, from its peripheral extremity to the centre;—and the manner of termination of nerves, either singly, or in a net-work, or by connecting loops between the fibres, as in the muscles generally throughout the body. These and other facts, now authorizing few conclusions, will doubtless hereafter form a part of that more certain and connected knowledge, to the attainment of which all such observations do more or less directly contribute.

The apparatus of the sympathetic nerve and its ganglia, that which chiefly ministers to organic life, may justly be named the

* The able Treatise of Mr. Grainger, in vindication of the opinions of Dr. Marshall Hall, is well known; but I am not aware that his anatomical argument for a distinct system of spinal nerves is yet fully substantiated by observation.

terra incognita of the nervous system. Its anatomy has the support of a very partial and obscure physiology; and its relations must be put interrogatively, even for the organs and functions which appear to have closest dependence on them, of which the action of the heart is a conspicuous instance. The manner of connexion of this system with the cerebro-spinal, presents a long series of unresolved questions; and the experiments of Dr. W. Philip and others, while deciding certain points, have added to the number remaining for solution. The nature and offices of the ganglia—whether generating, or merely modifying and directing the passage of power from the greater nervous centres—are known to us but by presumption; and this too vague to be recorded as matter of science. The connexion of the sympathetic nerves with the vascular system, and with the general irritability of the body, are other points of equal interest to physiology, but not less obscure in every circumstance of proof.

Our present state of knowledge regarding the brain involves similar questions; multipled in number and difficulty by that closer involution of parts which has suggested to some physiologists its description as a group of ganglia; and by the nearer approach to the mental functions, if a phrase involving the notion of space be admissible for what we cannot conceive to have any common or congruous quality with it. When we get beyond the apparent connexions and terminations (the latter term itself ambiguous) of the fasciculi of the sensory and motor nerves, the anatomy of the brain becomes little more than a description of appearances, variously arranged by different observers; and physiology is limited to insulated facts, derived for the most part either from pathology, or from comparative anatomy and experiments on living animals. All these classes of facts have been greatly extended in number and minuteness, and many remarkable presumptions derived from them; but examining fairly into the subject, it will be seen how few are the conclusions which can be recorded as final and complete. Pathological observations, however great their ultimate value, have hitherto, by their discordance, rather perplexed than illustrated the inquiry; and the results of actual experiments so partially concur with these, and with each other, that almost every inference requires to be verified by future research.

I have had occasion in former chapters to allude to this topic; and to state certain of the more remarkable deficiencies of our knowledge, as well as those points where we have better authority for connecting certain parts of structure with given faculties or functions. Without entering into details beyond my present object, I may again name, as a striking example of the former, our ignorance of the respective offices of the cineritious and medullary portions, whether of the brain itself, or other ganglia. Their diversity is attested by many essential differences of structure and distribution; but from none of these sources do we obtain evidence of the nature of their endowments, or relation to each other; and all opinions hitherto entertained on this subject must be considered

merely speculative. The most plausible perhaps is that which regards the medullary or fibrous portion as conducting and combining the powers which originate in the cineritious part; but the
vagueness of this expression shows how far it is removed from certainty. The same may be said regarding the functions of the
cerebellum ; which, notwithstanding dissections of singular minuteness, and much experimental observation, are still known to us only
in certain partial phenomena of motion ;—possibly not the most important of the attributes of this organ.*

The term of medulla oblongata is perhaps an unfortunate one, as
defining, by a single name, parts separate and of various character;
and two of them, the motor and sensory columns, apparently only
in passage to portions of the brain and cerebellum beyond. Ex-
cepting what we know of the functions of these columns, and of the
connexion of the corpora olivaria through the pneumogastric
nerves with the proper respiratory motions, I doubt whether anything certain can be affirmed of this part of the cerebral structure.
The experiments of Flourens and others, which appear to indicate
it as the peculiar seat of sensation and volition, even though we
may be unable to interpret them otherwise, are yet liable to the
doubts which attach in some degree to all observations of this nature.

Though we cannot strictly attribute more to the commissures,
however named, than the connexion of different parts of the brain,
and particularly of the opposite sides of this complex organ; yet
are these connexions of singular interest, both in health and disease ;
and warranting the closest regard to the structure which maintains
them. In a former chapter (On the Brain as a Double Organ), I
have referred to this subject; to the inferences suggested by the
view of unity of result, connected with doubleness of structure ; and
to the possible or certain effects arising from difference of the two
sides, however produced, or from morbid changes in the parts thus
connecting them. I need not revert to the topic, further than in
stating the importance of more minute attention to these portions
of structure, than is generally given in morbid dissections of the
brain.

Omitting necessarily in this sketch what has been attained by
modern anatomy in relation to the proper cerebral nerves, and the
questions which still remain to be solved as to their particular endowments and connexions, I may refer to another point of great
import in the physiology of the brain; viz., the functions of the
cerebral hemispheres ;—parts which, from their magnitude, peculiarities of structure, and progressive development from the lower

* In illustration of the doubts belonging to this subject, I may mention one or
two cases of which I have notes ; where, though the want of proper direction of
the movements of the body was a conspicuous symptom, examination after death
showed no obvious change in the cerebellum. It must be admitted, however,
that our ordinary dissections of disease of the brain, though much improved, are
still by no means minute enough for the conclusions it is so important to obtain
from them.

vertebral animals up to man, are manifestly of singular importance to some of the higher faculties of our being. That the exact nature of the relation should be yet unknown might have been mentioned as another proof of the imperfection of this part of physiology, and of the difficulties besetting it. The results of lesion or disease; the congenital deficiencies of this structure in idiots; and the direct experiments of Flourens and other observers, have seemed to some physiologists to warrant the phrase of " the seat of intellectual functions," as applied to this portion of the brain. A better expression, because more consistent with our knowledge, is, that the organization of these parts so ministers to certain mental faculties, that any deficiency or injury of structure impairs in some proportionate degree the functions thus connected. For reasons already given, it is as important as difficult, in this inquiry, to restrict language to the simple denotation of facts. And the complex nature of the faculties themselves,—needfully separated by definition, yet portions of a unity to our consciousness—tends further to embarrass all conclusions from the several sources of information just named.

If any particular inference be justified here, it is probably that which regards the cerebral hemispheres as serving especially to the functions of memory and association, in the simplest understanding of these terms. Pathological facts and dissections (of which I find two or three striking examples among my notes) afford many arguments for this belief. As far as we can attach definite notions to points thus abstruse, it would seem that memory, distinguished from the mental act of recollection, must have closer connexion with material structure than any other intellectual faculty. Its fluctuations in the ordinary course of life are more various and extensive;—its direction and objects are often curiously partial, and liable to the most sudden and singular changes;—it is more readily affected by disease or other physical accidents;—and its final decay is antecedent to, and often independent of, that of the higher powers of the understanding. The mind deals with memory, almost consciously, as something that is *without* itself, and over which it has only limited control: while at the same time this faculty is so preëminent in man, and fills so great a part of life, that we might naturally expect some large and conspicuous part of structure to be attached to its functions.

From this train of reasoning it would be easy to pass into those speculations, regarding the connexion of the higher mental faculties with material organization, which have been the subject of controversies in every age of philosophy. But I refrain from this topic, not merely as one exhausted in argument, but believing the relation to be wholly inapproachable by human reason in its present state. I will merely remark, in correction of a prevailing misapprehension on the subject, that the further we proceed in unravelling the brain as a system of nervous fibres, condensed into one complex organ for the establishment of their several relations and functions, the more in fact do we detach the mind itself from all

matèrial organization. By showing the general similarity of cerebral structure to those other parts of the nervous system which
conduct sensations and volitions, and minister to sympathetic
actions—functions all subordinate to the mental principle—we dis-
lodge the latter, if it may be so expressed, from any local tenement.
And while allowing the influence of every part of the brain upon it,
and of some parts more than others, we still more directly annul
any assumption that these material functions are in themselves acts
or conditions of the sentient principle.

I allude to this particularly, as it is a common error, both of those
who indulge in, and those who deprecate and dread such speculations, to suppose that, in proving these particular relations, we tend
to identify the operations of matter with those of mind. Were
research a hundredfold more minute and certain in its results, the
separation of the two would remain to all comprehension exactly
what it is at the present moment. But in truth, both anatomy and
physiology, as we have seen, are still engaged in settling points of
structure far below those of the ultimate organization of the brain.
Many of the appearances on ordinary dissection are probably
owing, not to the true nervous matter, which is small in quantity,
but to the membranous covering which every where accompany
and invest it.* Even those microscopic observations which show a
tubular structure of the medullary substance leave all uncertain as
to the peculiar matter existing within. Chemistry gives no indications on which to found a single inference; and the conclusions
from pathology are rendered vague and insufficient by dealing only
with the grosser parts of structure and connexion. These difficulties, inevitable in occurrence, are yet capable of being overcome
up to a certain point; but such as attach directly to the relation
between organized structure and mind are insuperable in their
nature; and we may best serve science by leaving them aside from
the direction of our pursuit.

The question regarding the existence and properties of a physical
agent, operating through the brain and nerves, is one wholly separate
from these metaphysical speculations; and may be entertained
(whatever the ultimate success of the research) as reasonably as
any other inquiry in science. It has, in truth, been much and variously discussed;—sometimes vaguely, as a crude hypothesis;—by
other and more eminent authors, experimentally, and with a definite
theory in view. Allusion has been made to the question in the first
part of this chapter; and I now again refer to it, after having intermediately noticed the several functions belonging to the nervous
system, and what has been done by anatomy and physiology in
relation to the subject. Though such agent be in nowise cognisa-

---

* In a memoir read before the British Association at Cambridge (*Report of
Third Meeting*, p. 449), Dr. Macartney has well illustrated these facts; adding
a conjecture that even the lowest animals may have some portion of nervous or
sentient matter diffused through their structure, not aggregated into cords or
masses as in those higher in the animal scale.

ble by our senses or direct observation, yet is its existence, and diffused action throughout the system, proved almost in the same sense as that of the circulation of the blood. The remarkable arrangement of nerves in the body, whether single or collected into central masses, might be received in evidence of their serving to this conveyance, even had we not the more explicit proof of functions impaired or destroyed, by injury to the conducting nerves, or to the nervous centres in which they terminate. The demonstration, thus simple and precise, of an agent transmitted through space, and by means of a definite structure, does not admit of any reasonable doubt. It is enforced, moreover, by looking to other phenomena, illustrating its properties and laws of action; the latter being as legitimately the object of research as are the laws of light, heat, and electricity, to which in many points they offer such singular analogy.

The observations which bear upon this subject, by illustrating nervous action, in state both of health and of disease, are too numerous for recital. Omitting all details, I shall merely advert to the more general inferences they afford; some of them ambiguous, but others determinate enough to be received as part of our knowledge of the nervous system; and so far connected as to serve in many ways for mutual illustration. Here, however, we must again refer to the difficulty stated in the outset; the question, namely, whether we can reason upon a single agent, where the functions performed differ thus widely in their nature? We are still unprovided with any answer on this point. That which is obvious to no sense, and defined only by certain observed effects, is beyond the reach of such discrimination; and we must be satisfied with conclusions of more general kind. What we may justly infer, looking to the common aspect of nervous structure, and to the connexion of nerves of different classes with each other and with common centres, is its being an element of the same nature; capable of similar relations of quantity or intensity; of translation to different organs along the course of nerves; and of suspension by like causes of injury or disturbance. Whether the hypothesis of electricity, to be mentioned hereafter, might afford some explanation in the various modes of excitement, action, and conduction which belong to this element, is an inquiry too vague to warrant more than a mere statement. Still, it is through this class of analogies that the unity of the nervous power may best be maintained; and with stronger presumptions than any we can derive from supposed differences of texture in the nerves themselves.

Another question, among the many connected with the agent of nervous power, has been the mode of its transit through the nerves; whether by passage of a current, according to the ordinary understanding of electrical transmission; or by movements within the nerves, having more kindred with those which enter into the undulatory theory of light. This question (connected with the preceding, and equally difficult of solution) requires notice here in its bearing upon all that regards the other properties or conditions of nervous agency. It might seem on the latter view, for instance, that we cannot rightly speak of its quantity, excess, or deficiency; terms which the phenomena almost impose upon us, to express the notions they suggest. Reasoning strictly, however, and with close appeal to the analogy of these other great agents, the inquiry may be prosecuted in a similar way, under either of the views just mentioned. In electrical science, and in those of light and heat, the phenomena admit of double interpretation, to an extent which could scarcely be deemed possible, without knowledge of the fact. In each of these cases, however, certain of the higher conditions of inquiry are better satisfied on one hypothesis than another; and the same may eventually happen in our researches regarding the nervous power. Meanwhile the knowledge we possess accords best with the notion of an agent transmitted progressively along the course of the nerves, to fulfil its functions in the several parts to which they conduct. And this application is most explicit in regard to those of sensation and voluntary power, where experiment is easiest, and observation least ambiguous in its results; and from which all inferences must chiefly be derived.

Of the several properties or conditions we can assign to the nervous power, that of quantity is perhaps the most determinate. The terms of excess and deficiency, exhaustion and repair, familiar in common use, seem to be warranted in fact, as well as for the familiar expression of certain bodily states or feelings; and we can scarcely explain a single phenomenon of the sensorial and organic functions, without the virtual admission of this idea. Though unable to assign with certainty the structure or living action, by which nervous power is generated, (a condition which must be admitted as almost essential to the argument,) yet does this deficiency in nowise alter the inference.* It is certain from observation, that the production takes place chiefly in the central organs, and that constant supply from them to the conducting nerves is necessary to maintain the power of the latter, and all the peculiar actions, single or sympathetic, of animal life. Even as regards the functions of the ganglionic system of nerves, though apparently endowed with some nervous power independent of that of the cerebro-spinal system, yet

---

* Of the several opinions propounded on this subject, that perhaps is the most plausible which regards the cineritious portion of the nervous substance as the seat of this action. The complex and highly vascular structure of this part, as determined by the microscope, and by the beautiful injections of Dr. Arnold of Zurich, is strikingly contrasted with the straight cylindrical fibres chiefly composing the medullary portion; and this difference, while indicating different offices, suggests the latter as the conducting medium to that power which is generated in the former. If this were so, it would follow that the element in question is produced throughout various parts of the nervous system, and not from one central source; a supposition which, in some points, better accords with the phenomena. If we should ever proceed beyond bare presumption on this question, it will probably be, not through any anatomy, however refined; but from physiological reasoning, or observation of the injuries of disease.

is this in various ways subordinate to the latter, and requiring a certain amount of communication to sustain its actions unimpaired. However obscure these relations, they all involve, in one part or other, the notion of quantity; not so definitely as in the case of the voluntary power, but still admitting no other interpretation of facts.

Of quantity, considered in this general sense, the best exponents are simple excess and deficiency, in as far as they are obvious; and we have in fact various proof of the existence of these respective states in all the functions of life. The great difficulty here is the one before alluded to, of distinguishing between sensorial energy—that influence derived from the higher animal functions and communicated to every part of the body—and the agency, whatever its nature, by which impressions or influence are actually conveyed along the nerves. I have noticed what may fairly be deemed our incompetency to deal with all the abstractions of this question. Though the notion of identity cannot be maintained, and some authors have separated them even as widely as matter and spirit; yet is it difficult to adapt language to the separate description of their properties and effects.*   As respects especially the conditions just named, of excess or deficiency, there seems a common application to both; nor can we reason upon the phenomena without incurring this admission, even as respects the mental faculties, strictly so termed.

Limiting ourselves, however, to the simplest expression of facts, it is certain that there are constant variations in the amount of that power by which the mind and higher animal functions are maintained in activity, and associated with the bodily organs and the world without. These variations occur among different individuals, forming in part what may be called the temperament of each; but they are yet more manifest in the same individual at different times. The deficiency is that which we most familiarly recognise; expressed, on the one hand, by the simple sense of exhaustion or fatigue of these functions, of which the cessation of action is the appropriate repair;—on the other hand, by that more sudden collapse or loss of power of which we have frequent consciousness in life; sometimes without obvious cause; much more remarkably under the various accidents of disease. Acute pain, and generally any excess of sensation, is a cause of such exhaustion:—the violent or protracted exercise of the voluntary power in muscular action has similar and more obvious effect:—and the same is produced by intent thinking, or by deep and painful emotions, continually pressing upon the mind. Exhaustion from any one of these causes (and we might perhaps add to them a less definite influence from the nervous system of organic life) has some common effect upon all; not strictly to be measured by degree, but enough to show clearly

* Much is owing in this part of physiology, as in many others, to the researches of Dr. Wilson Philip; who has, more clearly than most other authors, defined the separation of the sensorial and nervous power, independently of his views regarding the nature of the latter.

a common character in the power which is the subject of these fluctuations.*

Though excess in its amount is less familiarly recognised than deficiency, yet is this attested by various phenomena; probably by many which are not usually thus interpreted. Admitting, indeed, its generation by a living action, this deviation from the medium state must be presumed to occur, either by excess of such action, or by default of expenditure upon the several functions to which it ministers.† Many familiar examples might be cited, where the augmentation, slight in degree, is testified only by effects compatible with health;—increased sensibility, and greater energy of the active powers, but under entire control of the will. These effects pass by regular gradation into the more extreme cases which constitute disease; and I cannot doubt that various morbid states, not recognised in this light, are really due to the excess of that which is the element of nervous power.‡ In a former chapter (On Morbid Actions of Intermittent kind) I have spoken on this subject; adducing instances in epilepsy and other spasmodic disorders, where the notions of accumulation, excess, and sudden expenditure, seem needfully to be involved; and interesting, moreover, as examples of this power, so altered, passing in great part out of voluntary control. Without repeating these, a further question may be added (also alluded to before), whether certain forms of mental derangement may not be owing to, or modified by, this excess? In mania especially, some of the symptoms might well receive this explanation;—the excited sensibility and irrepressible vehemence of action; the protracted muscular exertions without proportionate fatigue; and the endurance of long-continued wakefulness without suffering.

This inquiry as to the influence of quantity of the nervous power merits more attention, as a part of pathology, than it has generally received. Whether in any intelligible sense, we can speak of its *intensity* also, as a property distinct from the former, is very doubtful. The analogy to another imponderable agent, like electricity, must not seduce us too far into inferences, to which language often

---

* The subject of pain as a cause of exhaustion of nervous power, is one of very great practical interest to the physician. It is certain that the degrees of pain are not to be estimated by any obvious similarity of lesion, or exciting cause. The *sentient state* of the individual is also concerned; varying in different persons, and at different times in the same person. Whether the variation depends on the sentient extremities of the nerves, or on the ganglia at the root of the sensitive columns, it may be difficult to determine. The recent researches, which have done so much to verify and extend the discovery of Sir C. Bell, show that the latter have close relation to the nature and perfection of this function; and a particular observation of Mr. Newport might lead to the inference that the size of the ganglia, and the proportion of cineritious matter they contain, are the circumstances chiefly concerned.

† Though, on some of the points here discussed, we approach the ground occupied by the Brunonian doctrines, yet nothing can be found to warrant the particular opinions which have borne this name.

‡ Among these gradations, many cases occur where there seems a necessity for disposing of the excess of the nervous energy;—when slight in amount, by common exertions of muscular power;—in morbid cases, by violent and irregular muscular acts which suddenly expend or give an outlet to the force.

lends a false appearance of reality, injurious in many ways to the better interests of science.

There is more foundation for admitting time as an element in the actions of the nervous power. In a preceding chapter I have considered this in reference to the mental functions; and recognising, in the present case, an agency conveyed through nerves to and from the central organs of this system, we must allow it as possible that there may be inequalities in the rate of motion, at different times or in different nerves. No observation, however, free from ambiguity, has yet been obtained on the subject; nor does analogy justify the expectation that any such estimate will ever be within our reach.

In considering the general attributes of the nervous power, a question still occurs, of singular interest to all our views of the economy of life, viz., whether this element, so generated within the living body, and distributed to all parts of it, in relation to their several functions, is capable of any mode of diffusion beyond this limit, and of producing effects on other living organization without? We cannot assert this to be impossible; and one or two high authorities have affirmed its probability. But a fair regard to the proofs alleged will show these to be ambiguous in many essential points; and a presumption against the principle is derived from the absence of all certain evidence; where, if true, it might be looked for, familiarly and unequivocally, in every part of life.*

From this topic we readily pass to a question, which has furnished material for discussion to the most eminent physiologist, and is still awaiting the possible solution of future research, viz., the nature of the agent fulfilling these great functions of animal life. Is it one that can be supposed identical with any of those surrounding us in nature, or must we admit at once that it has no type elsewhere in creation? This question is brought more within our scope, by being limited in effect to electrical agency; physiologists having adopted this as rendering the only plausible account of the phenomena. Nor can it excite surprise that they should have been so prone to assume this great element as the moving principle in the nervous system; seeing the vastness, or almost universality, of its operation throughout nature; and the actual proofs of its intimate and various relations to this part of the animal economy. Followed through new modes of development, and tested by more certain and delicate instruments, it has been found in some cases evolved and concentrated by vital actions:—in others, exciting, modifying, or even apparently supplying, the place of these actions in the body;—while, regarded in its relation to chemical action, and to the whole

* These alleged proofs are chiefly furnished by the Mesmerists; to whose views this principle is necessary as a basis; though, in point of fact, they carry the scope of their belief infinitely beyond, and to conclusions wholly incongruous with it;—making the transmitted energy produce powers in the recipient, which are in no sort possessed by the person communicating it, and which nothing but miraculous interposition could explain.

doctrine of affinities and polarities, it has the aspect of connecting together the phenomena of animal and organic life more completely and naturally than any other principle we can assume.

It would be impossible to pursue, into details, the controversy which still exists on this subject. Collecting generally all that has been done by experiment, and the reasoning applied to its results, we must admit that no certain or unequivocal proof of identity with the nervous power has been attained; but much cause shown, and foundation laid, for further research. The main argument against it is, that electricity, under the form of the voltaic current, can continue its excitement to muscular action, through a nerve divided or injured in such manner that the proper nervous influence is wholly arrested in its course. This argument, strong in the precision of the fact, cannot well be obviated but by assuming a different form of electricity from any yet known, as that generated and acting in the animal frame;—an assumption not warranted by other evidence, though rendered plausible by the various and remarkable modifications of this agency, familiar to us in the electricity of the machine, of the voltaic pile, of the magnet, of thermo-electric combinations, and of electrical fishes. The latter phenomenon, which appears on first view an argument for the opinion, loses its weight as such, by the ascertainment of the extensive and peculiar apparatus of nerves and cells existing in these animals, and providing for an electrical function essentially distinct from any attribute of the nervous power, and closely resembling those effects of accumulation and tension which we obtain by various artificial apparatus.

The production of muscular contractions by electrical excitement to the nerves of sensation, as well as of motion;—the similar action of other stimuli, mechanical or chemical, where we have no certain proof that electricity is involved;—and further, the absence of effect on the most delicate electrometer from contact with the nerves of muscles, in which strong contractions are taking place at the time:—are circumstances difficult of explanation by the theory in question; and obviously requiring some manner of electrical excitement and action, different from any yet known, to entitle us to admit this as the cause of the phenomena.* The generation of animal electricity, independently of external relations, is most readily understood as the effect of those vital actions (perhaps comprising all which take place in the body) where, by chemical change or otherwise, matter is abstracted from, or added to, organs in the discharge of their several functions. But as the doctrine in question

---

* The experiments and reasoning of Prevost, Dumas, and Edwards, in favour of the electrical theory of nervous power, and the argument of Müller against it, may be mentioned as embodying nearly all that can be said in relation to the sentient and motor nerves. The valuable researches of Dr. W. Philip, in support of the same doctrine, have been directed to certain of the vital functions; and, were there not still some ambiguity and want of uniformity in the results, his remarkable experiment of restoring by a voltaic current the action of digestion, suspended by section of the par vagum, might go far towards deciding this point of the question.

supposes these actions themselves to be the effect of electricity in its state of nervous power, we are admitting the difficult view of operation in a circle; and must rather presume some more direct mode of generation (of which, it may be, the electrical animals afford the type) and the existence of properties or relations, as to intensity, distribution, and manner of influence, of which we have no cognisance in its other states.* It is a reasonable question whether identity can be admitted, where the circumstances are, to our present knowledge, thus distinct.   If hereafter we should prove the affirmative, it will probably be in the same sense, and as part of the same train of discovery, by which all these great imponderable agents of the natural world are gradually submitted to a common principle, the highest and ultimate object of human science. Meanwhile it may safely be affirmed, that if any one of the powers of inanimate nature, as we now distinguish them, be concerned in the functions of the nervous system, electricity is indisputably that which best fulfils all the conditions required.   This seems to be the utmost point to which any conclusion can yet justifiably proceed.

In the preceding remarks on the course and state of modern inquiry into the nervous system, I have only partially noticed many topics, inseparable from the subject, and of the highest interest in physiology.   Such are, the especial relations of the powers acting through this system to the vital powers of organic life;—that greatest of all the known links in creation;—connecting together, into common functions and effects, principles wholly distinct to our present conception; and, in the different proportion of those which operate through and are represented by the nervous system, constituting all the forms and gradations of animal life.   The vital properties of the blood, and those inherent in the muscular fibre (the just definition of which we owe to two illustrious physiologists,) are the great foundation of organic existence, as distinguished from inorganic matter; and the modes in which these properties are severally excited to action, by the powers of the sensorium and nervous system, form in effect the chief problems of physiological science.   Every influence of the nervous system on the matter composing the animal frame must, as far as we can understand, be applied through, or upon, these two media.   And to the same relations there is most reason to look for what concerns the phenomena of generation and reproduction; admitting always that we approach but the threshold of this mystery, and that the action of organization, in giving similar vital properties to inorganic matter, must presumably be for ever hidden from our knowledge.

I have alluded to many of these questions in preceding parts of this volume; and in the last chapter especially, to the influence of the nervous system on the circulation of the blood.   Its various re-

* Regarding the torpedo and gymnotus, it is yet wholly uncertain whether the large nervous ganglia, appropriate to their extraordinary power, act directly in generating electricity, or only in giving energy to the extensive organs by which it is accumulated and directed.

lations to muscular action have been a fruitful subject of research to physiologists; accompanied with greater facilities for observation than in the case of the blood; and involving two great topics, each of singular interest in the economy of life;—first, the relation of the nervous power to the proper vital contractility of the muscular fibre; secondly, the connexion of the voluntary and involuntary motions throughout the body. The former inquiries (founded on the distinction which Haller has not too strongly designated a *lex æterna*) have still left many points undetermined; such, for instance, as the proportion which the nervous and contractile powers respectively bear in all the various phenomena of muscular action, exhaustion, and intermission. These two powers are independent; originate in different sources; and may apparently exist at the same time in very different ratio to each other. The agent of stimulus through the nerves may be deficient, or exhausted by one set of actions; while the contractility of other muscular parts remains unimpaired. Or, as we have reason to suppose that the nervous power is unequally generated at different times, it may occasionally be in excess above the muscular contractile power, which we know to be sometimes enfeebled generally throughout the body, by default of nutrition or other cause. The various combination of these circumstances (multiplied further by the distinction of voluntary and involuntary motions) is presumably a source of many singular results and anomalies, both in health and disease, which are not generally thus regarded; and I believe that more explicit attention to them under this view might solve many difficulties which still embarrass the subject.

The relation of voluntary muscular actions to those of involuntary kind presents questions as numerous, and equally complex in their nature. There are no more interesting topics of inquiry than the functions (such as respiration, deglutition, and the action of all the sphincters) in which both are concerned; and where, though commonly in concurrence, they are often found in opposition to, or impeding each other. And a remarkable result of such inquiries is the evidence they furnish as to the limited and secondary nature of voluntary motions. Not only do these come last, and by aid of repeated effort and education; but they also soonest pass away under the influence of habit; especially in the case of the conjunction just described. The exercise which gives them highest perfection for use, does, in certain degree, remove them from that consciousness which seems essential to any just definition of the will; and the most distinct acts of volition are those in which muscles are brought into modes of exercise altogether new. Of the combined and complex movements which form the habits of life (for the action of a single muscle is comparatively rare) more cannot be affirmed, than that we will certain acts, which particular muscular combinations, wholly unknown to us in their details, are able to fulfil. It is a main business of physiology, in its present state of progress, to distinguish and better define these results; and what has already been done is an augury of conclusions more general than any yet obtained, and of certainty more complete in all stages of the research.

In closing this chapter (a mere outline of the inquiry), I may again remark that the topic is that to which all separate researches in physiology converge; blending themselves in this common centre,—on the one hand, with the higher doctrines of life, reproduction, and mental existence;—on the other, with those great general powers or laws of inanimate nature which are ever in action within and around us. Physiological science, on the matter in question, seems at this moment to be on the verge of some greater discovery; resembling in this respect the actual state of other physical sciences —those of light, heat, electricity, chemical forces, and perchance gravitation—which the course of modern inquiry is ever tending to reduce to certain common laws. It is a question of deep interest, already referred to, whether the relation here is not closer than that of mere analogy; and whether future research may not associate some of the functions of the nervous system with the more general elements of force and action in the physical world. Vital laws, and what we term physical laws, stand precisely in the same relation to our knowledge. They are continually approximating as this knowledge advances; and may not impossibly in the end be submitted, even in human comprehension, to some common principle, embracing the whole series of phenomena, however remote and dissimilar they now appear.

All science tends to prove the unity of creation, through the evidence it affords of mutual and universal relation of parts. The expression of an eminent philosopher, " L'univers, pour qui sauroit l'embrasser d'un seul point de vue, ne seroit qu'un fait unique, et une grande vérité," though in one sense it may seem a vague imagination, yet, in a larger scope of view, involves the great result and term of all philosophy. The " single fact" and " great truth," is that of one Almighty Cause ;—a conclusion to which we are irresistibly carried forwards from every side ; surmounting in this inference those intermediate gradations of existence or power, which are too dimly seen to be rightly apprehended by the faculties of man in his present state of being.

THE END.

Standard Works

ON

ANATOMY, MEDICINE, SURGERY,

AND

THE COLLATERAL SCIENCES.

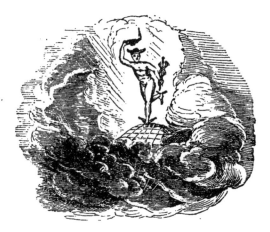

PUBLISHED BY

ED. BARRINGTON & GEO. D. HASWELL,

293 MARKET STREET, PHILADELPHIA.

NEW WORKS.

LISTON'S ELEMENTS.

ELEMENTS OF SURGERY, IN THREE PARTS. By Robert Liston, Fellow of the Royal College of Surgeons in London and Edinburgh, Surgeon to the Royal Infirmary, Senior Surgeon to the Royal Dispensary for the City and County of Edinburgh, Professor of Surgery in the London University, &c. &c. Third American, from the Second London Edition, with upwards of one hundred and sixty illustrative engravings. Edited by
SAMUEL D. GROSS, M.D.,
Professor of Surgery, Louisville Medical Institute. Author of Elements of Pathological Anatomy, etc., etc. 1 vol. 8vo.

"We are here presented with a republication of Mr. Liston's admirable and much praised work on Surgery, which has been subject to the alembic of a critical and learned friend, Dr. Gross. He has added "copious notes and additions," such as the progress of surgery in the United States demands in order to meet the wants of the surgeon. Professor Gross has also given an entire article on Strabismus, and another on Club Feet, which were wholly omitted in the English copies. They may be regarded important, inasmuch as they give a completeness to an otherwise unfinished treatise. The execution of the book is good; the paper firm, and well secured in the binding. The plates are uniformly well executed, and the impressions distinct."—*Boston Med. and Surg. Jour.*

"In another essential feature this edition is greatly improved. With the principles is taught also with it the practice of surgery; and both morbid structure and operations are doubly described; first by the author and editor, and next by the graver of the artist."—*Bull. Med. Scien.*

"Mr. Liston's reputation as a clear, accurate, and scientific surgical writer, is so widely known and admitted, that formal panegyric is quite unnecessary Dr. Gross has discharged his duties as editor, with all the sound sense, accurate discrimination, and experienced judgment, which all who knew him expected. The additions and notes, are indeed profitable and interesting; and our only regret is, that they are not still more numerous than they are. The volume is inscribed to Professor Parker, of the College of Physicians and Surgeons in this city,—the beauty of its typography, and 'getting up,' will be readily taken for granted by all who know the publishers,—and the illustrative engravings are executed in a style very creditable to American art."—*N. Y. Lancet.*

PUERPERAL FEVER.

THE HISTORY, PATHOLOGY, AND TREATMENT OF PUER-
PERAL FEVER AND CRURAL PHLEBITIS. By Drs.
GORDON, HEY, ARMSTRONG, and LEE; with an INTRODUCTORY
ESSAY by CHARLES D. MEIGS, M.D., Professor of Obstetrics and
the Diseases of Women and Children in the Jefferson Medical
College, Philadelphia. 1 vol. 8vo.

"We have peculiar satisfaction, in announcing the publication of this very judiciously
arranged series of treatises, on one of the most important and interesting diseases, which
demand the attention of the physician." "Dr. Meigs' Introductory Essay is concise and judicious, and will be read with profit. He speaks in the highest terms of commendation of Dr.
Gordon's invaluable treatise — a treatise which cannot be too generally diffused and studied.
Altogether this volume presents the most acceptable and useful compend of the doctrines
and practice of the best authorities, with regard to 'Puerperal Fever,' with which we have
ever met."—*N. Y. Lancet.*

DIGESTION.

DERANGEMENTS, PRIMARY and REFLEX, of the ORGANS of
DIGESTION. By ROBERT DICK, M.D., author of "A Treatise on
Diet and Regimen." 1 vol. 8vo.

"It is the fullest, most comprehensive, and decidedly the best account of derangements of
the digestive organs that we have encountered. While it embraces all that is important or
interesting to be found in the writings of other authors, it contains much original information, which the physician will find of great practical usefulness."—*Western and Southern
Medical Recorder.*
"We recommend this volume most warmly to the attention of our readers."—*London
Lancet,* No. 937.
"This volume may, in fact, be denominated with no small degree of propriety, an ency-
clopedia of dyspeptic disorders, and we unhesitatingly commend it, as the most useful and
comprehensive treatise on this class of diseases, with which we are acquainted.—*N. Y.Lancet.*
"We have perused this work with pleasure and instruction. It is decidedly the best
compilation in the English language on the extensive class of disorders and diseases
comprehended under the term dyspepsia, united with a very large proportion of original
matter, both in the form of able comments on other writers, and practical information
derived from the author's own experience."—*Johnson's Medico-Chirurg.* for Jan. 1842.

LIVER AND SPLEEN.

DISEASES OF THE LIVER AND BILIARY PASSAGES;
by WILLIAM THOMSON, one of the Physicians of the Royal Infirmary of Edinburgh; and CLINICAL ILLUSTRATIONS OF
THE LIVER AND SPLEEN, by WILLIAM TWINING; Surgeon
of General Hospital of Calcutta, &c., &c., 1 vol. 8vo.

"The present work we regard as remarkably well calculated to remove several of the
objections and difficulties now referred to. It is distinguished throughout by a much greater
degree of precision in the pathological history of the different morbid states of the liver than
any work hitherto published on that subject. It contains not only the most ample and
complete accounts of the various dynamic disorders and organic changes incident to the
organ hitherto given, but these states are described and distinguished in a much clearer
and more methodical manner than any other treatise yet before the public. In accordance
with this we observed, also, in the therapeutic principles and precepts established by the
author, a much more rational development and application of therapeutic measures than it
has yet been our fortune to witness."—*Edinburgh Med. and Sur. Journal.* October, 1841.

"The work before us is an excellent compilation of the subject of hepatic affections,
functional and structural; and, as such, it is infinitely more valuable to practitioners and
students, than any original essay, however ably executed. We cannot do better, therefore,
than strongly recommend the work as the best in the English language, on the important
subjects of which it treats.—*Medico-Chirurg. Rev. October,* 1841.

"These two works, when united, form, we may safely say, one of the most valuable and
attractive volumes on this important class of diseases which have been issued from the
press. We may, *en passant,* remark, that the volume is got up in a very superior style."—
N. Y. Lancet, March 26, 1842.

CLINICAL REMARKS ON SOME CASES OF LIVER ABSCESS
PRESENTING EXTERNALLY. By JOHN G. MALCOLMSON, M.D.
Surgeon Hon. E. I. C. Service, Fellow of the Royal Asiatic Society, and
the Geological Society, London, 1 vol. 8vo.

MATERIA MEDICA:

A PRACTICAL DICTIONARY OF MATERIA MEDICA, *including the Composition, Preparation and Uses of Medicines ; and a large number of Extemporaneous Formulæ : together with important Toxicological Observations; on the Basis of Brande's Dictionary of Materia Medica and Practical Pharmacy ;* by JOHN BELL, M.D., Lecturer on Materia Medica and Therapeutics, &c. &c. 1 vol. 8vo.

"Mr. Brande's is an excellent work, and with the retrenchments, additions, and alterations of Dr. Bell, may be regarded as one of the most valuable works on the Materia Medica, we now possess. It has an important advantage over many of the treatises on this subject, in giving a large number of prescriptions for the administration of the principal articles. This renders it especially valuable to the young practitioner." —*Balt. Jour.*

A THERAPEUTIC ARRANGEMENT and SYLLABUS of MATERIA MEDICA. By JAMES JOHNSTONE, M.D., Fellow of the College of Physicians, and Physician to the General Hospital, Birmingham.

"This book cannot but be particularly useful to those who intend to lecture or write upon the Materia Medica; as well as to the students for whose particular use it is prepared."—*Brit. and For. Med. Rev.*

ÆTIOLOGY.

ARETÆUS ON THE CAUSES AND SIGNS OF ACUTE and CHRONIC DISEASE. From the Greek, by T. F. Reynolds, M.B., F.L.S., &c., &c. 1 vol. 8vo.

"The correct detail of symptoms, the nervous style, the graphic delineation of disease, displayed in this author's work, the poetic and quaint fancies scattered throughout, give a certain value and interest, that may fairly excuse an attempt to reinvest part of them in a vernacular garb."

"We certainly have no hesitation in recommending this curious volume to the notice of our readers. Its price is a mere trifle."—*New York Lancet.*

SEMEIOLOGY.

OUTLINES OF PATHOLOGICAL SEMEIOLOGY. Translated from the German of PROFESSOR SCHILL. With copious notes by D. SPILLMAN, M.D., A.M., &c., &c. 1 vol. 8vo.

"The signs of disease exhibited by the principal tissues and organs, are treated of in a succient and comprehensive manner, by Dr. Schill, and as a work of daily reference to assist in distinguishing diseases it cannot be too highly commended."—*Balt. Jour.*

"An elegant and accurate translation of a very ingenious and instructive work. We do not know any other source from which we can so easily and profitably obtain all that is really useful in the semeiology of the ancients; and the erudite translator and editor has so very creditably supplied the deficiencies of the author's *abrige* of the labors of modern workers, in this most important department of modern science, that we can in good conscience commend the book as one of unequivocal merit."—*New York Lancet.*

VENEREAL.

HUNTER'S TREATISE ON THE VENEREAL DISEASE. With Notes by Dr. BABINGTON. With Plates. 1 vol. 8vo.

"Under the hands of Mr. Babington, who has performed his task as editor in a very exemplary manner, the work has assumed quite a new value, and may now be as advantageously placed in the library of the student as in that of the experienced surgeon."—*Brit. & For. Med. Rev.*

"The notes, in illustration of the text, contain a summary of our present knowledge on the subject; the manner in which these notes are constructed is at once clever and perspicuous; and the modes of treatment prescribed, spring from a right apprehension of the disease. We would recommend to the reader the note on the primary venereal sore; the note itself is an essay in every word of which we fully concur."—*Med. Gaz.*

A PRACTICAL TREATISE ON VENEREAL DISORDERS, AND MORE ESPECIALLY ON THE HISTORY AND TREATMENT OF CHANCRE. By PHILIPPE RICORD, M.D., Surgeon to the Venerea Hospital at Paris. 1 vol. 8vo.

GRAVES & GERHARD.

CLINICAL LECTURES; by Robert J. Graves, M.D., M.R.S.A., Professor of the Institutes of Medicine in the School of Physic, Trinity College, Dublin, with additional Lectures and Notes, by W. W. Gerhard, M.D., Lect. on Clin. Med. to the Univ. of Penn.' Physician to the Philadelphia Hospital, Blockley, etc. 1 vol. 8vo.

"In the volume before us, a series of clinical lectures by Dr. Gerhard is given, and forms a most appropriate and acceptable addition to those of Dr. Graves. Between these two distinguished physicians we can trace many points of resemblance. We find in both the same professional zeal,—the same powers of close and correct observation,—the same discriminating tact,—the same disregard of idle theory,—and the same decision in the application of right principles. No student or practitioner should be without this volume. *It is in itself a library of practical medicine."—N. Y. Lancet.*

"No man in the profession has done more for clinical instruction in this country than Professor Gerhard. The lectures of Professor Graves have been long before the public, and the fact of a second edition being called for, is proof that their value is understood. Our space will not allow us to give a detailed notice of them, we can only commend them heartily to our readers. To the student and young practitioner they are truly invaluable; especially would we recommend them to students pursuing their studies in the country, and who have no opportunity of seeing hospital practice. Reading, we all know, is but a poor substitute for clinical observation, still where the latter cannot be obtained, the STUDY, not the mere reading, BUT THE STUDY of these lectures of Graves and Gerhard, is the best substitute we know of—to country students, then, in particular, we would earnestly recommend this book. Of the lectures which Professor Gerhard has added, we will only say, that they are worthy to be associated with those of Graves; as Americans, we are proud of the association, proud to see one of the first, if not the very first, of the European Clinical Teachers followed "*passibus aegiis*" by our countryman."—N. Y. Med. Gaz.

"This volume contains a fund of practical matter, useful and interesting to the practitioner and student. There are few works which will better repay a perusal."—Am. Jour. of the Med. Sciences.

DISEASES OF CHILDREN.

A TREATISE ON THE DISEASES OF CHILDREN; WITH DIRECTIONS FOR THE MANAGEMENT OF INFANTS; by the late Michael Underwood, M.D. From the ninth English edition, with Notes, by S. Merriman, M.D., and Marshall Hall, M.D., F.R.S., etc.; with Notes, by John Bell, M.D., etc., of Philadelphia, 1 vol. 8vo.

TETANUS.

A TREATISE ON TETANUS, being the ESSAY for which the Jacksonian Prize was awarded by the Royal College of Surgeons in London. By Thomas Blizard Curling, Assistant Surgeon to the London Hospital, &c.

"This book should be in the library of every surgeon and physician. It is a valuable work of reference. It does not pretend to originality, for originality on such a subject was not wanted. But a compendium of facts *was* wanted, and such a compendium is this volume. We cannot part from Mr. Curling without thanking him for the information we have received in reading his work, and for the matter it has enabled us to offer to our readers."—Medico-Chir. Rev.

EYES.

A MANUAL OF THE DISEASES OF THE EYE. By S. Littell, Jr., M.D., one of the Surgeons of the Will's Hospital for the blind and lame, &c., &c.

"We confidently recommend the work of Dr. Littell to the senior, as well as to the junior, members of the profession. It is replete with information; yet so terse in style, and compressed in bulk, as at once to entice and repay perusal. It is no small triumph to the author to be able to say that he has introduced almost all that is valuable, and everything absolutely necessary to the student within the compass of 200 pages, and we would deliberately recommend our young friends to read this work."—Br. & For. Med. Rev.

GUMS.

THE GUMS; with late Discoveries on their Structure, Growth, Connections, Diseases, and Sympathies. By George Waite, Member of the London Royal College of Physicians. 1 vol. 8vo.

CHEST.

LECTURES on the PHYSIOLOGY and DISEASES of the CHEST, including the Principles of Physical and General Diagnosis, illustrated chiefly by a rational Exposition of their Physical Signs: with new researches on the sounds of the heart. By CHARLES J. B. WILLIAMS, M.D.; Third edition, 1 vol. 8vo.

"Evidently written by a man thoroughly acquainted with his subject."—*Lancet.*
"We strongly recommend this work to the attention of auscultators."—*Med. Chir. Rev.*
"I gladly avail myself of this opportunity of stronglyrecommending this very valuable work."—*Dr. Forbes's Translation of Laennec.*
"Of all the works on this subject, we are inclined much to prefer that of Dr. Williams."—*Med. Gaz.*

LECTURES ON THE DIAGNOSIS, PATHOLOGY, AND TREATMENT OF THE DISEASES OF THE CHEST. By W. W. GERHARD, M.D., Lecturer on Clinical Medicine in the University of Pennsylvania, etc., etc. 1 vol. 8vo.

"A series of clinical lectures—concise, lucid, and eminently instructive. We have no more able expositor of diseases of the chest than Dr. Gerhard, and any work of his on these important subjects is certain of grateful acceptance by his professional brethren."—*New York Lancet.*
"To our readers, therefore, we recommend the book of Dr. Gerhard as the fullest and most judicious manual, in relation to the diseases of the chest, which they can procure."—*Western and Southern Recorder,* June, 1842.
"These lectures constitute a useful and practical digest of the existing knowledge of the diseases of the chest (lungs, and heart)."—*Bulletin of Medical Science.*

A PRACTICAL TREATISE on the PRINCIPAL DISEASES of the LUNGS. CONSIDERED ESPECIALLY IN RELATION TO THE PARTICULAR TISSUES AFFECTED, ILLUSTRATING THE DIFFERENT KINDS OF COUGH. By G. Hume Weatherhead, M.D., Member of the Royal College of Physicians, Lecturer on the Principles and Practice of Medicine, and on Materia Medica and Therapeutics, &c. &c. 1vol. 8vo.

PRACTICAL OBSERVATIONS on DISEASES of the HEART, LUNGS, STOMACH, LIVER, &c., OCCASIONED by SPINAL IRRITATION: AND ON THE NERVOUS SYSTEM IN GENERAL, AS A SOURCE OF ORGANIC DISEASE. Illustrated by Cases. By John Marshall, M.D. 1 vol. 8vo.

CUTANEOUS DISEASES.

A PRACTICAL TREATISE ON DISEASES OF THE SKIN, arranged with a view to their Constitutional Causes and Local Character, &c. By SAMUEL PLUMBE, late Senior Surgeon to the Royal Metropolitan Infirmary for Children, &c. Illustrated with Splendid Coloured Copperplate and Lithographic Engravings. 1 vol. 8vo.

PLUMBE *on Diseases of the Skin.*—"This excellent Treatise upon an order of diseases't the pathology of which is, in general, as obscure as the treatment is empirical, has jusr been republished, edited by Dr. John Bell, of this city. We hail with pleasure the appeaof ance of any new work calculated to elucidate the intricate and ill-understood subject he skin-diseases. The late Dr. Mackintosh, in his Practice of Physic, recommends it as the 'best pathological and practical treatise on this class of diseases, which is to be found in any language.'"—*Phil. Med. Exam., Jan.* 17, 1838.
"This work is one of the most excellent on the Diseases of the Skin in the English language."—*West. Jour. of Med. and Phys. Sciences, Jan.* 1838.

BANDAGES AND BANDAGING.

THE SURGEON'S PRACTICAL GUIDE IN DRESSING, and in the Methodic APPLICATION of BANDAGES. Illustrated by ONE HUNDRED ENGRAVINGS. By THOMAS CUTLER, M.D., late Staff Surgeon in the Belgian Army.

"The Author seems to have spared no pains in procuring correct descriptions of all the surgical apparatus, at present employed in bandaging and dressing, both at home and abroad. He has given numerous illustrations, in the form of well executed woodcuts, and has altogether produced what we conceive to be a very useful, and by no means an expensive publication."—*Medical Gazette.*

CLINICAL MEDICINE.

MEDICAL CLINIC; or, Reports of Medical CASES: By G. ANDRAL, Professor of the Faculty of Medicine of Paris, etc. Condensed and Translated, with Observations extracted from the Writings of the most distinguished MedicalAuthors: By D. SFILLAN, M.D., etc., etc.; containing *Diseases of the Encephulon, &c.*, with Extracts from OLLIVIER's Work on *Diseases of the Spinal Cord* and its Membranes. 1 vol. 8vo.

LECTURES on Subjects connected with CLINICAL MEDICINE By P. M. Latham, M.D. Fellow of the Royal College of Physicians and Physician to St. Bartholomew's Hospital.

" We strongly recommend them [Latham's Lectures] to our readers; particularly to pupils attending the practice of our hospitals."—*Lond. Med. Gaz.*

TEETH.

A TREATISE ON THE TEETH. BY JOHN HUNTER. With Notes by THOMAS BELL, F.R.S. With Plates. 1 vol. 8vo.

" The treatise on the teeth is edited by Mr. Bell, a gentleman accomplished in his art. Mr. Bell has studied his subject with the greatest minuteness and care; and in appropriate notes at the foot of the page corrects the author with the air of a gentleman, and the accuracy of a man of science. The matter contained in these short notes forms an ample scholium to the text; and without aiming at the slightest display of learning, they at the same time exhibit a ready knowledge on every point, and an extensive information both of comparative anatomy and pathology.—*Med. Gazette.*

BLOOD, INFLAMMATION, ETC.

TREATISE ON THE BLOOD, INFLAMMATION, AND GUN-SHOT WOUNDS. BY JOHN HUNTER, F.R S. With Notes, by JAMES F. PALMER, Senior Surgeon to the St. George's and St. James's Dispensary, &c., &c. 1 vol. 8vo.

LECTURES ON BLOOD-LETTING. BY HENRY CLUTTERBUCK, M.D. 1 vol. 8vo.

HISTORICAL NOTICES ON THE OCCURRENCE OF INFLAMMATORY AFFECTIONS OF THE INTERNAL ORGANS AFTER EXTERNAL INJURIES AND SURGICAL OPERATIONS. By WILLIAM THOMPSON, M.D., &c. &c. 1 vol. 8vo.

A TREATISE ON INFLAMMATION. By JAMES MACARTNEY, F.R.S., F.L.S., &c., &c. Member of the Royal College of Surgeons, London, &c., &c. 1 vol. 8vo.

LECTURES ON THE BLOOD, AND ON THE CHANGES WHICH IT UNDERGOES DURING DISEASE. By F. MAGENDIE, M-D. 1 vol. 8vo.

MIDWIFERY.

A PRACTICAL TREATISE on MIDWIFERY; Containing the Results of Sixteen Thousand Six Hundred and Fifty-four Births, occurring in the Dublin Lying-in Hospital. By ROBERT COLLINS, M.D., Late Master of the Institution. 1 vol. 8vo.

" The author of this work has employed the numerical method of M. Louis; and by accurate tables of classification, enables his readers to perceive, at a glance, the consequences of the diversified conditions, in which he saw his patients. A vast amount of information is thus obtained, which is invaluable to those who duly appreciate precision in the examination of cases."—*Balt. Chron.*

A PRACTICAL COMPENDIUM OF MIDWIFERY; being the Course of Lectures on Midwifery and on the Diseases of Women and Infants delivered at the St. Bartholomew's Hospital by the late ROBERT GOOCH, M.D. Prepared for Publication by GEORGE SKINNER, Member of the Royal College of Surgeons, London,

LECTURES on the MORBID ANATOMY, NATURE, and TREAT-
MENT of ACUTE and CHRONIC DISEASES. By the late JOHN
ARMSTRONG, M.D.; Author of "Practical Illustrations of Typhous and
Scarlet Fever," &c. Edited by JOSEPH RIX, Member of the Royal Col-
lege. of Surgeons. 1 vol. 8vo.

The *British and Foreign Medical Review* says of this work:

"We admire, in almost every page, the precise and cautious practical directions; the
striking allusions to instructive cases; the urgent recommendations of the pupil to
be careful, to be diligent in observation, to avoid hurry and heedlessness, to be attentive to the poor. Nothing can be more excellent than the rules laid down for all the
parts of the delicate management of fever patients: nothing more judicious than the
general instructions arising out of the lecturer's perfect knowledge of mankind. . . . . .
His prudent admonitions respecting the employment of some of the heroic remedies, as
mercury, arsenic, and colchicum, attest his powers of observation and his practical
merits." "The pious office of preserving and publishing his Lectures has been performed
by Mr. Rix, with singular ability."

INSANITY.

A TREATISE on INSANITY and other DISEASES AFFECTING the
MIND. By James Cowles Prichard, F.R.S. M.D. Corresponding Member
of the Institute of France, &c. 1 vol. 8vo.

"The author is entitled to great respect for his opinions, not only because he is well
known as a man of extensive erudition, but also on account of his practical acquaintance with the subject on which he writes. The work, we may safely say, is the best,
as well as the latest, on mental derangement, in the English language."—*Medico-Chir.
Rev.*

A TREATISE ON MENTAL DISEASES. BY M. ESQUIROL.

APHORISMS on the TREATMENT and MANAGEMENT of the
INSANE: with considerations on Public and Private Lunatic
Asylums, pointing out the errors in the present system. By J. G.
MILLINGEN, M.D., late Medical Superintendent of Lunatic Asylum,
Hanwell, Middlesex, &c. 1 vol. 8vo.

"Dr. Millingen, in one small pocket volume, has compressed more real solid matter
than could be gleaned out of any dozen of octavos on the same subject. We recommend
his vade mecum as the best thing of the kind we ever perused."—*Dr. Johnson's Review.*

PHYSICAL AGENTS.

ON THE INFLUENCE of PHYSICAL AGENTS on LIFE. By W. F.
EDWARDS, M.D., F.R.S., etc. Translated from the French, by Drs.
Hodgkin and Fisher. To which are added, some Observations on ELEC-
TRICITY, and Notes to the work. I vol. 8vo.

"This is a work of standard authority in Medicine; and, in a physiological point of
view, is pre-eminently the most valuable publication of the present century; the experimental investigation instituted by the author, having done much towards solving many
problems hitherto but partially understood. The work was originally presented in parts
to the Royal Academy of Science of Paris, and so highly did they estimate the labours
of the author, and so fully appreciate the services by him thus rendered to science and
to humanity, that they awarded him, though a foreigner, the prize founded for the
promotion of experimental physiology.

ANIMAL ŒCONOMY.

OBSERVATIONS ON CERTAIN PARTS OF THE ANIMAL ŒCO-
NOMY, Inclusive of several papers from the Philosophical Transactions,
&c. By JOHN HUNTER, F.R.S., &c., &c. With Notes by RICHARD OWEN,
F.R.S. 1 vol. 8vo.

SURGERY.

LECTURES OF SIR ASTLEY COOPER on the PRINCIPLES and PRACTICE of SURGERY, with additional Notes and Cases. By FREDERICK TYRRELL, ESQ., Surgeon to St. Thomas's Hospital, and to the London Ophthalmic Infirmary. 1 vol. 8vo.

LECTURES ON THE PRINCIPLES OF SURGERY. By JOHN HUNTER, F.R.S. With Notes by JAMES F. PALMER, Senior Surgeon to the St George's and St. James' Dispensaries, &c. &c. With Plates. 1 vol. 8vo.

"We have perused these lectures with no ordinary feelings of satisfaction. They embody an immense amount of important facts, directed with no common skill to the illustration and improvement of medical science generally, and of the surgical department in particular. Indeed we have no hesitation in saying, that, whatever be the position of the reader in the profession, he will not relinquish the perusal of these lectures without the consciousness of having usefully employed the time which he may have bestowed upon them. For they constitute, in the fullest sense of the term, a philosophical disquisition on the science of Surgery; and hence, embracing the great principles on which the whole art of healing rests, their interest will be felt by all who regard Medicine as a true branch of science, and who delight to witness the gradual development of principles in the right interpretation of the phenomena of nature."

"We cannot bring our notice of the present volume to a close without offering our testimony to the admirable manner in which the editor and annotator has fulfilled his part of the undertaking. The advancements and improvements that have been effected, up to our own day, not only in practical surgery, but in all the collateral departments, are constantly brought before the reader's attention in clear and concise terms."— *Brit. & For. Med. Rev.*

JOHN HUNTER'S WORKS.

THE COMPLETE WORKS OF JOHN HUNTER, F.R.S., 4 vols 8vo., comprising his Lectures on the Principles of Surgery; A Treatise on the Teeth; Treatise on the Venereal Diseases; Treatise on Inflammation and Gun-Shot Wounds; Observations on Certain Parts of the Animal Œconomy; and a full and comprehensive Memoir. Each of the Works is edited by men of celebrity in the Medical Science, and the whole under the superintendence of JAS. F. PALMER, of the St. George's and St. James's Dispensary. This is the only complete edition of the works of the distinguished physiologist ever published in this country.

"One distinctive feature of the present edition of Hunter's works has been already mentioned, viz: in the addition of illustrative notes, which are not thrown in at hazard, but are written by men who are already eminent for their skill and attainments on the particular subjects which they have thus illustrated. By this means, whilst we have the views entire of John Hunter in the text, we are enabled by reference to the accompanying notes, to see wherein the author is borne out by the positive knowledge of the present day, or to what extent his views require modification and correction. The names of the gentlemen who have in this manner assisted Mr. Palmer, are guarantees of the successful performance of their task."—*Med. Gaz.*

PATHOLOGY.

OUTLINES OF GENERAL PATHOLOGY. By GEORGE FRECKLETON, M.D., Fellow of the Royal College of Physicians.

RHEUMATISM,

BOUILLAUD ON ACUTE ARTICULAR RHEUMATISM IN GENERAL. *Translated from the French*, by JAMES KITCHEN, M.D., Philada.

HYSTERIA.

AN ESSAY ON HYSTERIA, being an analysis of its irregular and aggravated forms; including Hysterical Hemorrhage and Hysterical Ischuria. With numerous Illustrative and Curious Cases. By THOMAS LAYCOCK, House Surgeon to the York County Hospital. 1 vol. 8vo.

UTERUS.

LECTURES on the FUNCTIONS and DISEASES of the WOMB, by CHARLES WALLER, M.D., Bartholomew's Hospital.

ON DISEASES of the UTERUS and its APPENDAGES, by M. LISFRANC, La Pitie Hospital.

ON DISEASES of the PUERPERAL STATE, by J. T. INGLEBY, Edinburgh. 1 vol. 8vo.

" We can very cordially recommend them as affording a concise and practical exposition of the pathology and treatment of a most important class of diseases, and which cannot be too attentively studied."—*N. Y. Lancet.*

" The present volume contains a short and succinct practical account of the principal morbid states either of the functions or the structure of the womb, the best methods of distinguishing them, and the means which experience has shown to be the most effectual in removing them. The reader will find that he obtains, in a small compass, a distinct view of the nature and treatment of each disorder."—*Edinb. Med. and Surg. Journ.*

CONSTIPATION.

A TREATISE on the CAUSES and CONSEQUENCES of HABITUAL CONSTIPATION. By JOHN BURNE, M.D., Fellow of the Royal College of Physicians, Physician to the Westminster Hospital, &c. 1 vol. 8vo.

" For some interesting cases illustrative of this work, the author is indebted to Dr. Williams, Dr. Stroud, Dr. Callaway, Mr. Morgan, Mr. Taunton, Dr. Roots, Sir Astley Cooper, Sir Benjamin Brodie, Mr. Tupper, Mr. Baller, Dr. Paris, Mr. Dendy, Dr. Hen. U. Thomson," &c.—*Preface.*

URINARY DISEASES.

URINARY DISEASES AND THEIR TREATMENT. By ROBERT WILLIS, M.D., Physician to the Royal Infirmary for Children, &c. &c.

" We do not know that a more competent author than Dr. Willis could have been found to undertake the task ; possessing, as it is evident from his work that he does possess, an accurate acquaintance with the subject in all its details, considerable personal experience in the diseases of which he treats, capacity for lucid arrangement, and a style of communication commendable in every respect."

" Our notice of Dr. Willis's work must here terminate. It is one which we have read and trust again to read with profit. The history of discovery is successfully given; cases curious and important; illustrative of the various subjects have been selected from many new sources, as well as detailed from the author's own experience, chemical analyses, not too elaborate, have been afforded, which will be most convenient to those who wish to investigate the qualities of the urine in disease; the importance of attending to this secretion in order to a proper understanding of disease is strongly insisted upon ; in short, a book has been composed, which was much required, and which we can conscientiously and confidently recommend as likely to be useful to all classes of practitioners.—*Brit. & For. Med. Rev.*

MEDICAL EXPERIENCE.

CURIOSITIES OF MEDICAL EXPERIENCE. By J. G. MILLINGEN, Surgeon to the Forces, Member of the Medical Society of the Ancient Faculty of Paris, etc., etc.

" *Curiosities of Medical Experience.* By J. G. MILLINGEN, Surgeon to the Forces, etc. The Author or Compiler derived the idea which prompted him to write this work from D'Israeli's 'Curiosities of Literature;' and, in our view, he has made a book equally curious in its way with that one. The heads of his chapters are numerous and varied ; and all his subjects are treated in an agreeable and comprehensible style to the general reader, The drift of the Author, too, is decidedly useful. We shall endeavour to give some extracts from this work."—*Nat. Gaz.*

EPIDEMICS OF THE MIDDLE AGES.

EPIDEMICS of the MIDDLE AGES.   From the German of I. F. C. Hecker, M.D., &c. &c.   Translated by R. G. Babington, M.D. F.R.S.—

No. I.—THE BLACK DEATH IN THE 14th CENTURY.

" Hecker's account of the ' Black Death,' which ravaged so large a portion of the globe in the fourteenth century, may be mentioned as a work worthy of our notice, both as containing many interesting details of this tremendous pestilence, and as exhibiting a curious specimen of medical hypothesis."—*Cyclopedia of Practical Medicine—History of Medicine by Dr. Bostock.*

No. II.—THE DANCING MANIA.

" Medical History has long been in need of the chapter which this book supplies; and the deficiency could not have been remedied at a better season.   On the whole, this volume ought to be popular; to the profession it must prove highly acceptable, as conveying so much information, touching an important subject which had almost been suffered to be buried in oblivion, and we think that to Dr. Babington especial thanks are due for having naturalised so interesting a production.   The style of the translation, we may add, is free from foreign idioms: it reads like an English original."—*Lond. Med. Gaz.*

RETENTION OF URINE.

AMUSSAT'S LECTURES on the RETENTION of URINE, CAUSED by STRICTURES of the URETHRA, and on the Diseases of the Prostate, translated from the French by James P. Jervey, M.D.

DENGUE.

ON DENGUE; ITS HISTORY, PATHOLOGY, AND TREATMENT By S. Henry Dickson, M.D., Professor of the Institutes and Practice of Medicine in the Medical College of S.C.

MEDICAL EXAMINATIONS.

HINTS ON THE MEDICAL EXAMINATION OF RECRUITS FOR THE ARMY; and on the Discharge of Soldiers from the Service on Surgeon's Certificate : Adapted to the Service of the United States.   By Thomas Henderson, M.D., Assistant Surgeon U. S. Army, &c., &c.

PHYSIOLOGY AND HYGIENE.

ESSAYS ON PHYSIOLOGY AND HYGIENE ; viz:

I. Reid's Experimental Investigation into the Functions of the Eighth Pair of Nerves.

II. Ehrenberg's Microscopical Observations on the Brain and Nerves, (with numerous engravings.)

III. On the Combination of Motor and Sensitive Nervous Activity ; by Professor Stromeyer, Hanover.

IV. Vegetable Physiology.

V. Experiments on the Brain, Spinal Marrow, and Nerves. By Prof. Mayer, of Bonn (with woodcuts).

VI. Public Hygiene.

VII. Progress of the Anatomy and Physiology of the Nervous System, during 1836. Ry Professor Muller.

VIII. Vital Statistics. 1 vol. 8vo.

MEDICAL AND TOPOGRAPHICAL OBSERVATIONS.

OBSERVATIONS on the PRINCIPAL MEDICAL INSTITUTIONS and PRACTICE of FRANCE, ITALY and GERMANY: with Notices of the Universities, and Cases from Hospital Practice: With an Appendix on ANIMAL MAGNETISM and HOMŒOPATHY. By EDWIN LEE, Member of the Royal College of Surgeons, &c. 1 vol. 8vo.

"Mr. Lee has judiciously selected some clinical cases, illustrating the practice pursued at the different hospitals, and he has wound up the volume with an amusing account of animal magnetism and homœopathy—those precious effusions of German idealty, for which we refer to the work itself."—*Meuico-Chirurg. Rev.*

MEDICAL AND TOPOGRAPHICAL OBSERVATIONS UPON THE MEDITERRANEAN AND UPON PORTUGAL, SPAIN, AND OTHER COUNTRIES. By G. R. B. HORNER, M.D., Surgeon U. S. Navy, and Honorary Member of the Philadelphia Medical Society. With Engravings. 1 vol. 8vo.

"An uncommonly interesting book is presented to those who have any disposition to know the things medical in Portugal, Spain, and other countries," and "will doubtless be read, also, with marked satisfaction by all who have a taste for travels."—*Bost. Med. and Surg. Jour.*

ON DEW.

AN ESSAY ON DEW, and several Appearances connected with it by WILLIAM CHARLES WELLS, M.D., F.R.S., etc.

ANATOMICAL EXAMINATIONS.

EXAMINATIONS in ANATOMY and PHYSIOLOGY; being a complete series of Questions and Answers; designed and intended as preparatory to Examinations at the different Medical Schools throughout the United States. To which are annexed, Tables of the Bones, Muscles, and Arteries. By THOMAS SYDENHAM BRYANT, M.D., Surgeon U. S. Army.

NOTES AND REFLECTIONS.

MEDICAL NOTES AND REFLECTIONS. By HENRY HOLLAND, M.D.; F.R.S., Fellow of the Royal College of Physicians, and Physician Extraordinary to the Queen.

RANUNCULACEÆ.

HE MEDICAL PROPERTIES of the NATURAL ORDER RANUNCULACEÆ, &c., &c. By A. TURNBULL, M.D.

DR. P. S. PHYSICK.

PROF. HORNER'S NECROLOGICAL NOTICE OF DR. P. S. PHYSICK; Delivered before the American Philosophical Society May 4, 1838.

JOHN HUNTER.

THE LIFE OF JOHN HUNTER, F.R.S. By DREWRY OTTLEY. 1 small vol. 8vo.

"In the summing up of Mr. Hunter's character, Mr. Ottley exhibits equal judgment and candour."—*Brit. & For. Med. Rev.*

DALE'S ESSAY.

ESSAY UPON THE QUESTION, IS MEDICAL SCIENCE FAVORABLE TO SCEPTICISM? By JAMES W. DALE, M.D., of Newcastle, Delaware. Pamphlet.

Lightning Source UK Ltd.
Milton Keynes UK
UKHW012135290119
336431UK00008B/305/P